Handbook of

Psychotropic
Drugs

Handbook of

Psychotropic Drugs

Springhouse Corporation
Springhouse, Pennsylvania

Staff

Executive Director, Editorial
Stanley Loeb

Editorial Director
Helen Klusek Hamilton

Clinical Director
Barbara McVan, RN

Art Director
John Hubbard

Drug Information Editor
George J. Blake, RPh, MS

Copy Editors
Jane V. Cray (supervisor), Traci A. Ginnona

Designers
Stephanie Peters (associate art director), Maryanne
Buschini, Mary Stangl

Art Production
Robert Perry (manager), Heather Bernhardt, Donald
Knauss, Robert Wieder

Typography
David Kosten (director), Diane Paluba (manager),
Liz Bergman, Joyce Rossi Biletz, Phyllis Marron, Robin
Rantz, Valerie Rosenberger

Manufacturing
Deborah Meiris (manager), T.A. Landis, Jennifer Suter

Production Coordination
Colleen Hayman

Editorial Assistants
Maree DeRosa, Beverly Lane, Mary Madden

PSYCHO-021293

Library of Congress Cataloging-in-Publication Data
Handbook of psychotropic drugs.
     p.   cm.
  Includes bibliographical references and index.
  1. Psychotropic drugs – Handbooks, manuals, etc.
I. Springhouse Corporation.
[DNLM: 1. Psychotropic Drugs – handbooks.
QV 39 H23642]
RM315.H347   1992
615′.78 – dc20
DNLM/DLC   91-5206
ISBN 0-87434-391-7   CIP

Contents

Therapeutic classes and generic drugs

Pharmacologic classes

Contributors and consultants

William R. Dubin, MD, FAPA
Deputy Medical Director, Philadelphia
Psychiatric Center; Professor of Psychiatry,
Temple University School of Medicine,
Philadelphia

Susan Gatzert-Snyder, RN, MS, CS
Staff Nurse, Northwestern Institute, Fort
Washington, Pa.

Cathleen M. Jaeger, RN, MSHA, CNA
Director of Nursing, Philadelphia Psychiatric
Center

Richard Jaffee, MD
Assistant Director of Residency Training,
Philadelphia Psychiatric Center

Arthur Lazarus, MD
Director, Diagnostic and Evaluation Unit,
Philadelphia Psychiatric Center

Roberta Schweitzer, RN, MSN, CS
Private Consultant, Phoenix

Joanne M. Sica, RPh, MHA
Administrator, Pharmacy Program, Greater
Atlantic Health Service, Philadelphia

Michelle Spurlock, RN, BSN
Head Nurse, Adult Psychiatry, Norton Hospital –
Norton Psychiatric Clinic, Louisville, Ky.

How to use this book

The Handbook of Psychotropic Drugs provides exhaustively reviewed, completely updated drug information on virtually every drug in current use for management of mental and emotional disorders. Organized by therapeutic use, individual chapters describe and list anticonvulsants, antidepressants, antimanic agents, antiparkinsonian agents, antipsychotic agents, anxiolytics, CNS stimulants, and sedative-hypnotics. Each chapter provides an overview of all aspects of drug information from fundamental pharmacology to specific management of toxicity and overdose.

Each chapter begins with a list of all relevant generic drugs. The primary drug entry for those drugs that have multiple uses appears in the chapter that reflects its most common use. However, the drug is also listed (with a cross-reference to the primary listing) in drug groups that share its secondary applications. For example, diazepam is listed among the anticonvulsants with a cross-reference to the primary entry in the chapter on sedative-hypnotics.

Generic drug entries

In each drug entry, the generic name (with alternate generic names following in parentheses) precedes an alphabetically arranged list of current trade names. (An asterisk signals products available only in Canada.)

Next, the pharmacologic and therapeutic classifications identify the drug's pharmacologic or chemical category and its major clinical uses. Listing both classifications helps the reader grasp the multiple, varying, and sometimes overlapping uses of drugs within a single pharmacologic class and among different classes. If appropriate, the next line identifies any drug that the Drug Enforcement Administration (DEA) lists as a controlled substance and specifies the schedule of control as II, III, IV, or V.

The pregnancy risk category identifies the potential risk to the fetus. Categories listed were determined by application of the Food and Drug Administration (FDA) definitions to available clinical data to define a drug's potential to cause birth defects or fetal death. These categories, labeled A, B, C, D, and X, are listed below with an explanation of each. Drugs in category A usually are considered safe to use in pregnancy; drugs in category X usually are contraindicated.

A: Adequate studies in pregnant women have failed to show a risk to the fetus in the first trimester of pregnancy—and there is no evidence of risk in later trimesters.

B: Animal studies have not shown an adverse effect on the fetus, but there are no adequate clinical studies in pregnant women.

C: Animal studies have shown an adverse effect on the fetus, but there are no adequate studies in humans. The drug may be useful in pregnant women despite its potential risks.

D: There is evidence of risk to the human fetus, but the potential benefits of use in pregnant women may be acceptable despite potential risks.

X: Studies in animals or humans show fetal abnormalities, or adverse reaction reports indicate evidence of fetal risk. The risks involved clearly outweigh potential benefits.

Pregnancy risk classifications were assigned for all appropriate generic drugs according to the above criteria.

How supplied lists the preparations available for each drug (for example, tablets, capsules, solution, injection), specifying available dosage forms and strengths.

Indications, route, and dosage presents all clinically accepted psychiatric or neurologic indications with general dosage recommendations for adults and children; specific recommendations for infants, elderly patients, or other special patient groups are included when appropriate. A preceding dagger signals clinically accepted but unlabeled uses. Dosage instructions reflect current clinical trends in therapeutics and should not be considered an absolute and universal recommendations. For individual application, dosage must be considered according to the patient's condition.

Pharmacodynamics explains the mechanism and effects of the drug's physiologic action.

Pharmacokinetics describes absorption, distribution, metabolism, and excretion of the drug; it specifies onset and duration of action and half-life as appropriate.

Contraindications and precautions lists conditions that are associated with special risks in patients who receive the drug and includes the rationale for each warning.

Interactions specifies the clinically significant additive, synergistic, or antagonistic effects that result from combined use of the drug with other drugs.

Effects on diagnostic tests lists significant interference with a diagnostic test or its result by direct effects on the test itself or by systemic drug effects that lead to misleading test results.

Adverse reactions lists the undesirable effects that may follow use of the drug; these effects are arranged by body systems (CNS, CV, DERM, EENT, GI, GU, HEMA, Hepatic, Metabolic, Respiratory, Local, and Other). Local effects occur at the site of drug administration (by application, infusion, or injection); adverse reactions not specific to a single body system (for example, the effects of hypersensitivity) are listed under *Other*. Throughout, life-threatening reactions are italicized. At the end of this section, *Note* signals a list of severe and hazardous reactions that mandate discontinuation of the drug.

Overdose and treatment summarizes the clinical manifestations of drug overdose and recommends specific treatment as appropriate. Usually, this segment recommends emesis or gastric lavage, followed by activated charcoal to reduce the amount of drug absorbed and possibly a cathartic to eliminate the toxin. This section specifies antidotes, drug therapy, and other special care, if known. It also specifies the effects of hemodialysis or peritoneal dialysis for dialyzable drugs.

Special considerations offers detailed recommendations specific to the drug for preparation and administration, care and teaching of the patient during therapy, and use in elderly patients, children, and breast-feeding women. This section includes recommendations for monitoring the effects of drug therapy, preventing and treating adverse reactions, promoting patient comfort, and storing the drug.

Pharmacologic class entries
Clustered in a separate section, pharmacologic class entries describe the pharmacology, clinical indications and actions, adverse reactions, and special implications of drugs that fall into a major pharmacologic group (for example, benzodiazepines or phenothiazines). This allows the reader to compare the effects and uses of drugs within each class. Pharmacologic class entries list special considerations that are common to all generic members of the class and include geriatric, pediatric, and breast-feeding use. If specific considerations are unknown, these headings are omitted.

Graphic enhancement
Selected charts and tables compare uses, effects, or dosages of drugs within a therapeutic class.

Selected references
This section provides a list of supplementary readings related to psychotropic drugs.

Appendices
The appendices include a charted summary of laboratory tests recommended during chronic drug therapy; psychotropic drugs listed by trade name, with manufacturers; psychiatric adverse reactions to specific drugs; a complete list of *DSM-III-R* and *ICD-9-CM* codes, listed numerically and by diagnoses; the schedule of controlled substances and a charted summary of the management of acute substance abuse.

ABBREVIATIONS			
Abbreviation	**Meaning**	**Abbreviation**	**Meaning**
ALT	serum alanine aminotransferase, formerly SGPT	I.V.	intravenous
		kg	kilogram
AST	serum aspartate aminotransferase, formerly SGOT	L	liter
		m^2	square meter
ATP	adenosine triphosphate	mm^3	cubic millimeter
AV	atrioventricular	MAO	monoamine oxidase
b.i.d.	twice a day	mcg or μg	microgram
BUN	blood urea nitrogen	mEq	milliequivalent
cAMP	adenosine 3':5'-cyclic phosphate	mg	milligram
CBC	complete blood count	MI	myocardial infarction
CHF	congestive heart failure	ml	milliliter
CNS	central nervous system	ng	nanogram (millimicrogram)
CPK	creatine phosphokinase	OTC	over-the-counter
CPR	cardiopulmonary resuscitation	P.O.	by mouth
CSF	cerebrospinal fluid	p.r.n.	as needed
CV	cardiovascular	q	every
CVP	central venous pressure	q.i.d.	four times a day
DNA	deoxyribonucleic acid	RBC	red blood cell
ECG	electrocardiogram	RNA	ribonucleic acid
EEG	electroencephalogram	SA	sinoatrial
FDA	Food and Drug Administration	S.C.	subcutaneous
g	gram	SGOT	serum glutamic-oxaloacetic transaminase
G	gauge		
GI	gastrointestinal	SGPT	serum glutamic-pyruvic transaminase
GU	genitourinary		
h.s.	at bedtime	TCA	tricyclic antidepressant
I.M.	intramuscular	t.i.d.	three times a day
IU	International Unit	WBC	white blood cell

Foreword

Dramatic advances in psychopharmacology offer new treatment options to psychiatric patients who previously resisted or could not tolerate existing drugs. For example, several recently developed antidepressant agents offer the benefits of milder, more tolerable adverse reactions; fluoxetine (Prozac) and clomipramine (Anafranil) offer treatment of obsessive-compulsive disorder; and clozapine (Clozaril) now offers hope for schizophrenic patients who previously had no hope of recovery or improvement.

These expanding therapeutic options offer psychiatric patients real benefits, but not without some associated clinical problems. These problems fall into three categories: the associated risk of adverse reactions, the potential for adverse interactions, and the need to keep up with new uses and indications for known drugs.

Most important is these drugs' potential to provoke severe and sometimes life-threatening adverse reactions. For example, physicians and nurses who manage the care of psychiatric patients are well aware of the risk of neuroleptic malignant syndrome, a potentially fatal reaction to certain antipsychotic drugs. Such clinicians also express growing concern about the risk of agranulocytosis with certain anticonvulsants (carbamazepine) and antipsychotics (haloperidol, clozapine) and about the risk of akathisia and akinesia with their implications for diagnosis, recovery, and compliance. The widespread prevalence of depressive illness and the corresponding increase in the use of antidepressants also require health care professionals to consider these drugs' cardiac effects and their impact on sexual function. Most adverse reactions to psychotropic drugs do not usually contraindicate their use, but they always require a well-informed and cautious approach to drug treatment.

Another major concern is the potential for drug interactions, which can adversely affect treatment and prolong morbidity. For example, lithium interacts with thiazide diuretics to increase lithium toxicity, with haloperidol to cause severe encephalopathy, and with chlorpromazine to decrease its therapeutic effect. Tricyclic antidepressants interact with quinidine to cause additive cardiac effects and with clonidine to cause dangerous hypertension. Clearly, reviewing potential interactions is absolutely essential for safe treatment.

A significant area of expanding information is the application to psychiatric illness of drugs formerly used solely for medical indications; for example, anticonvulsants have recently been found to aid treatment of affective disorders; antidepressants have been found to aid treatment of obsessive-compulsive disorders.

These rapid developments challenge clinicians' ability to keep up with new information and clearly require a reliable and current drug reference. The new *Handbook of Psychotropic Drugs* meets this need in an easily accessible format. It provides reliable, comprehensive, and current information about all drugs currently in use for psychiatric indications. Each of these drugs is described in detail in a complete and independent entry that has been reviewed by a practicing psychiatrist for relevance and accuracy.

To allow easy comparison of drugs that share similar uses, the book is organized by therapeutic classes: anticonvulsants, antidepressants, antimanic agents, antiparkinsonian agents, antipsychotic agents, anxiolytics, CNS stimulants, and sedative-hypnotics.

Each chapter begins with a list of all relevant generic drugs. Drugs that have multiple uses are classified according to their most common use; they are also listed (with a cross-reference to the major drug entry) in drug groups that share their secondary applications. For example, diazepam is listed among the anticonvulsants with a cross-reference to the chapter on sedative-hypnotics.

The chapter continues with a summary of these drugs' pharmacologic effects, comparative clinical considerations, and recommendations for administering, monitoring, and patient teaching. The chapter further includes a separate and detailed entry for each generic drug listed in the chapter.

Each generic drug entry lists all trade names, pharmacologic and therapeutic classifications, available dosage forms and strengths, the Drug Enforcement Administration category for controlled substances, and the pregnancy risk category. It also includes all clinically accepted psychiatric indications (unlabeled indications are identified with a graphic symbol), mechanism of action, pharmacokinetics, contraindications and precautions, interactions, adverse reactions, treatment of overdose, and an especially helpful summary of the drug's effects on diagnostic tests.

The final section, Special Considerations, lists recommendations for administration, monitoring and prevention of complications, patient safety, and for use in children, elderly patients, and breast-feeding women. A uniquely useful feature, Information for the Patient, summarizes drug information that clinicians should include in all discussions with patients who receive psychotropic medications. One of the most important clinical changes in recent years has been the growing emphasis on teaching patients and their families about the medications they are taking. The *Handbook of Psychotropic Drugs* is a valuable resource for all health care professionals who need reliable information about drugs that are prescribed for psychiatric patients.

William R. Dubin, MD, FAPA
Deputy Medical Director;
Philadelphia Psychiatric Center;
Professor of Psychiatry,
Temple University School of Medicine

Cathleen M. Jaeger, RN, MSHA, CNA
Director of Nursing,
Philadelphia Psychiatric Center

Anticonvulsants

acetazolamide
acetazolamide sodium
carbamazepine
clonazepam
clorazepate dipotassium
diazepam (See *ANXIOLYTICS.*)
divalproex sodium
ethosuximide
ethotoin
lorazepam (See *ANXIOLYTICS.*)
magnesium sulfate
mephenytoin
mephobarbital
methsuximide
paraldehyde
paramethadione
phenacemide
phenobarbital (See *SEDATIVE-*
  HYPNOTICS.)
phensuximide
phenytoin
phenytoin sodium
phenytoin sodium (extended)
phenytoin sodium (prompt)
primidone
trimethadione
valproate sodium
valproic acid

Anticonvulsant drugs elevate the seizure threshold of the motor cortex to chemical or electrical stimuli or limit the propagation of seizure-evoking stimuli from seizure foci to effector organs. Anticonvulsant therapy achieves complete control of seizure activity in about 50% of patients; it improves symptoms in about 25%. Seizure type and associated neurologic abnormalities determine the degree of benefit achieved. All anticonvulsants produce some CNS depression, which varies according to the specific drug. Therapy must be individualized by selecting the drug or combination of drugs that controls seizures without producing an unacceptable level of adverse reactions.

The principal anticonvulsants include derivatives of barbiturates, benzodiazepines, hydantoins, oxazolidinediones, succinimides, and a miscellaneous group that is structurally unrelated to all other agents.

Pharmacologic effects

• *Barbiturates* (mephobarbital, phenobarbital, primidone) are used for prophylaxis of various seizure types, principally generalized tonic-clonic and partial seizures.

• *Benzodiazepines* (clonazepam, clorazepate, diazepam, lorazepam) are used mainly for absence seizures. Clonazepam is the most commonly used benzodiazepine; it is frequently combined with other anticonvulsants. I.V. diazepam is the drug of choice for terminating status epilepticus. The usefulness of benzodiazepines has yet to be established because tolerance to their anticonvulsant effects develops quickly.

• *Hydantoins* (ethotoin, mephenytoin, phenacemide, phenytoin) are used primarily to control generalized tonic-clonic and complex partial seizures. Hydantoins should not be used for absence seizures because they may increase their frequency. Because of its extreme toxicity, phenacemide should be reserved for patients whose seizures resist treatment to all other anticonvulsants.

• *Oxazolidinediones* (paramethadione, trimethadione) were once the drugs of choice for absence seizures but are now used only for refractory seizures. They are not effective for generalized tonic-clonic seizures and may precipitate new generalized tonic-clonic seizures or increase their frequency.

• *Succinimides* (ethosuximide, methsuximide, phensuximide) are used mainly for absence seizures. Ethosuximide is the drug of choice; phensuximide is least effective and least toxic.

• *Miscellaneous agents* (acetazolamide, carbamazepine, divalproex sodium, paraldehyde, valproic acid, valproate sodium) may have limited usefulness.

Mechanism of action

The exact mechanism of anticonvulsant action has not been confirmed and is poorly understood. It is probably related to stabilization of the cell membrane secondary to modification of cation transport via the sodium reflux sys-

---

CLASSIFICATION OF SEIZURES

SEIZURE TYPE	CLINICAL CHARACTERISTICS	USEFUL DRUGS
Partial seizures		
Simple partial	Various manifestations, without impairment of consciousness, including seizures confined to a single limb or muscle group *(Jacksonian motor seizures)*, specific and localized sensory disturbances *(Jacksonian sensory seizures)*, and other limited signs and symptoms depending on the particular cortical area producing the abnormal discharge	carbamazepine (1), divalproex sodium (15), mephenytoin (5), phenobarbital (10), phenytoin (12), valproate sodium (15), valproic acid (15)
Complex partial	Attacks of confused behavior, impaired consciousness, various clinical manifestations, bizarre generalized EEG activity during the seizure, commonly associated with evidence of anterior temporal lobe focal abnormalities in the interseizure period	carbamazepine (1), clonazepam (2), divalproex sodium (15), ethotoin (4), mephenytoin (5), methsuximide (7), phenacemide (9), phenobarbital (10), phenytoin (12), primidone (13), valproate sodium (15), valproic acid (15)
Partial seizures secondarily generalized	Loss of consciousness with convulsive motor activity which may occur immediately or within 2 minutes.	carbamazepine (1), divalproex sodium (15), phenobarbital (10), phenytoin (12), valproate sodium (15), valproic acid (15)
Generalized seizures (convulsive or nonconvulsive)		
Absence seizures	Brief and abrupt loss of consciousness associated with high-voltage, bilaterally synchronous, 3-per-second spike-and-wave pattern in the EEG, usually with some symmetrical clonic motor activity varying from eyelid blinking to jerking of the entire body; sometimes without motor activity	carbamazepine (1), divalproex sodium (15), ethosuximide (3), mephobarbital (6), methsuximide (7), paramethadione (8), phenacemide (9), phensuximide (11), trimethadione (14), valproate sodium (15), valproic acid (15)
Atypical absence seizures	Attacks with slower onset and cessation than is usual for absence seizures, associated with a more heterogeneous EEG	carbamazepine (1), divalproex sodium (15), valproate sodium (15), valproic acid (15)

(1) Carbamazepine: Response may be variable in mixed seizures. May be given with other anticonvulsants; however, use cautiously with phenacemide, mephenytoin, trimethadione, or paramethadione because toxicity may be additive.
(2) Clonazepam: Particularly useful in Lennox-Gastaut syndrome.
(3) Ethosuximide: Generally considered drug of choice in absence seizures, although some clinicians prefer valproic acid. May precipitate generalized tonic-clonic seizures; should be used with phenytoin or phenobarbital.
(4) Ethotoin: Less toxic and less effective than phenytoin.
(5) Mephenytoin: Generally not used unless less toxic alternatives are ineffective.
(6) Mephobarbital: Used to replace phenobarbital when patients cannot tolerate the latter drug.
(7) Methsuximide: Usually used when other drugs have failed. Does not usually precipitate tonic-clonic seizures in mixed seizures.
(8) Paramethadione: Used when other drugs are ineffective. Less toxic but generally less effective than trimethadione. May

precipitate or worsen generalized tonic-clonic seizures.
(9) Phenacemide: Extremely toxic – do not use unless other drugs are ineffective.
(10) Phenobarbital: May be used as the initial drug, particularly in infants and children. Often administered with phenytoin.
(11) Phensuximide: Least toxic yet least effective; beneficial effects of the drug may decrease with prolonged use.
(12) Phenyton: Not recommended for absence seizures because it may increase their frequency.
(13) Primidone: Some clinicians consider the drug of choice for this indication; particularly useful for refracting seizures.
(14) Trimethadione: Usually used in patients refractory to other drugs; may precipitate or worsen generalized tonic-clonic seizures.
(15) Valproate sodium, valproic acid, divalproex sodium: Some clinicians use these drugs only as an adjunct to other drugs; some consider them the primary agents for most generalized seizures.

CLASSIFICATION OF SEIZURES *(continued)*

SEIZURE TYPE	CLINICAL CHARACTERISTICS	USEFUL DRUGS
Generalized seizures (convulsive or nonconvulsive)		
Myoclonic seizures	Isolated clonic jerks associated with brief bursts of multiple spikes in the EEG	carbamazepine (1), divalproex sodium (15), phenytoin (12), valproate sodium (15), valproic acid (15)
Clonic seizures	Rhythmic clonic contractions of all muscles, with loss of consciousness and marked autonomic manifestations	carbamazepine (1), divalproex sodium (15), phenytoin (12), valproate sodium (15), valproic acid (15)
Tonic seizures	Opisthotonus, loss of consciousness, and marked autonomic manifestations	carbamazepine (1), divalproex sodium (15), phenytoin (12), valproate sodium (15), valproic acid (15)
Tonic-clonic seizures	Major seizures, usually a sequence of maximal tonic spasm of all body musculature followed by synchronous clonic jerking and a prolonged depression of all central functions	carbamazepine (1), divalproex sodium (15), ethotoin (4), mephenytoin (5), mephobarbital (6), phenacemide (9), phenobarbital (10), phenytoin (12), primidone (13), valproate sodium (15), valproic acid (15)
Atonic seizures	Loss of postural tone, with sagging of the head or falling	carbamazepine (1), divalproex sodium (15), phenytoin (12), valproate sodium (15), valproic acid (15)

(1) Carbamazepine: Response may be variable in mixed seizures. May be given with other anticonvulsants; however, use cautiously with phenacemide, mephenytoin, trimethadione, or paramethadione because toxicity may be additive.

(2) Clonazepam: Particularly useful in Lennox-Gastaut syndrome.

(3) Ethosuximide: Generally considered drug of choice in absence seizures, although some clinicians prefer valproic acid. May precipitate generalized tonic-clonic seizures; should be used with phenytoin or phenobarbital.

(4) Ethotoin: Less toxic and less effective than phenytoin.

(5) Mephenytoin: Generally not used unless less toxic alternatives are ineffective.

(6) Mephobarbital: Used to replace phenobarbital when patients cannot tolerate the latter drug.

(7) Methsuximide: Usually used when other drugs have failed. Does not usually precipitate tonic-clonic seizures in mixed seizures.

(8) Paramethadione: Used when other drugs are ineffective. Less toxic but generally less effective than trimethadione. May

precipitate or worsen generalized tonic-clonic seizures.

(9) Phenacemide: Extremely toxic – do not use unless other drugs are ineffective.

(10) Phenobarbital: May be used as the initial drug, particularly in infants and children. Often administered with phenytoin.

(11) Phensuximide: Least toxic yet least effective; beneficial effects of the drug may decrease with prolonged use.

(12) Phenyton: Not recommended for absence seizures because it may increase their frequency.

(13) Primidone: Some clinicians consider the drug of choice for this indication; particularly useful for refracting seizures.

(14) Trimethadione: Usually used in patients refractory to other drugs; may precipitate or worsen generalized tonic-clonic seizures.

(15) Valproate sodium, valproic acid, divalproex sodium: Some clinicians use these drugs only as an adjunct to other drugs; some consider them the primary agents for most generalized seizures.

tem. Anticonvulsants may also cause some mutually reinforcing actions that produce therapeutic responses without disrupting normal function.

Pharmacokinetics

• *Absorption and distribution:* The rate and degree of absorption of anticonvulsants is unknown. Onset and duration of action vary with the drug as well as among patients using the same drug. Most anticonvulsants have relatively long half-lives and may require from several days to several weeks to achieve steady-state plasma levels. They are widely distributed in the body with high concentrations in the brain and liver; many cross the placental barrier. The hydantoins also accumulate in salivary glands; the oxazolidinediones and succinimides, in body fluid. Barbiturates, phenytoin, and primidone are distributed in breast milk.

• *Metabolism and excretion:* Most anticonvulsants are metabolized in the liver by the microsomal enzyme process. Metabolites are excreted in bile and in urine. Note that phenytoin and phenobarbital (and probably other barbiturates) induce the microsomal enzyme process and thus accelerate the metabolism of other concomitantly used anticonvulsants. There is no evidence that they accelerate their own metabolism.

Adverse reactions and toxicity

Consider the slow rate of elimination when treating acute toxicity of anticonvulsants. Barbiturate overdosage can produce profound CNS depression and shock and can result in death. Treatment is mainly supportive. Hydantoin overdosage produces various CNS effects that may include hydantoin-like deep coma and nausea and vomiting. Treatment includes induced emesis, gastric lavage, and supportive measures. Oxazolidinedione overdosage produces similar effects and requires similar treatment. Succinimide overdosage is rare but produces profound CNS depression; treatment is the same as for hydantoin toxicity but may also include hemodialysis. Benzodiazepine overdosage can lead to apnea and death.

Many different types of adverse reactions to anticonvulsants can be expected. Drug selection may sometimes be based on the adverse reaction profile.

Acute adverse reactions may differ from those seen with continued therapy because tolerance can develop (for example, most anticonvulsants produce sedation early in therapy). Skin reactions ranging from erythematous rashes to exfoliative dermatitis (rarely) can occur with carbamazepine, phenytoin, primidone, and phenobarbital and may reflect some form of acute hypersensitivity reaction. Most of these drugs can produce some idiosyncratic reactions (such as a lupuslike syndrome, hepatitis, or vasculitis). Valproic acid and its derivatives are associated with the development of acute hepatic failure, especially when given to young children in high doses.

With long-term use, cosmetic changes have been reported with these drugs. Phenytoin can cause a coarsening of facial features, increased body hair, and hypertrophy of the gums (especially in patients with poor dental hygiene). High-dose valproate therapy can cause alopecia. Phenobarbital and primidone may be associated with some connective tissue disorders. Lymphoproliferative disorders have been reported with phenytoin. Several of these drugs have been associated with the development of blood dyscrasias, including leukopenia, granulocytopenia, and agranulocytosis.

Clinical considerations

● Selection depends on the type of seizure(s) and may require multiple drug therapy.

● Anticonvulsant therapy is highly individualized. Proceed slowly when increasing or decreasing dosage or when adding a new drug to an existing regimen.

● Some patients require more than one drug to control their seizures adequately. Most clinicians limit such therapy to no more than three agents, if possible. Commercially available fixed-combination preparations should not be used initially. Instead, titrate the dosage of each individual component until the patient exhibits adequate seizure control.

● Status epilepticus must be treated immediately or it may be fatal. I.V. diazepam remains the drug of choice. Phenytoin is preferred by some clinicians but it must be given slowly; therefore, its onset of action may be delayed. Phenobarbital may be used, but it also has a relatively slow onset. Some investigators advocate simultaneous treatment with phenytoin and diazepam. Supportive care should include continuous monitoring of blood pressure and ECG, maintenance of a patent airway, and monitoring of blood glucose levels, serum electrolyte levels, and fluid and acid-base status. If drug treatment doesn't adequately control status epilepticus, general anesthesia may be considered.

● If maximal doses of a single drug fail to produce adequate control of seizures, another drug should be substituted. In the absence of serious adverse reactions, the initial drug should be gradually withdrawn while the new drug is initiated. If the new drug fails to control seizure activity, many clinicians will substitute a third agent before using a multiple drug regimen.

● All anticonvulsants cause some degree of CNS depression, which commonly subsides or disappears with continued use. Starting with a low dosage that increases gradually may minimize adverse CNS effects.

● Some clinicians recommend that pregnant women who must receive treatment with phenytoin, barbiturates, primidone, phenacemide, paramethadione, or trimethadione should receive prophylactic vitamin K 1 month before and during delivery to reduce the risk of drug-induced hemorrhagic disease in the neonate. Neonates should also receive vitamin K immediately after birth.

● Withdraw anticonvulsants gradually because rapid discontinuation of these drugs can precipitate status epilepticus. Most clinicians consider the decision to withdraw the drug at least as important as the drug selection at the be-

---

ginning of therapy.

- Although a causal relationship has not been established, a two to three times greater incidence of birth defects has been reported in women with seizure disorders who take these drugs in early stages of pregnancy. Extensive data exists about such effects after use of paramethadione, trimethadione, phenobarbital, and hydantoins.

- Growing evidence suggests that anticonvulsant therapy in children may adversely influence behavioral and cognitive function. Children receiving an anticonvulsant medication should be under the care of a clinician experienced in pediatric anticonvulsant therapy. Follow-up examinations should assess mood, behavior, and cognitive function, and clinicians should consider the observations of parents and teachers.

- Blood counts, hepatic function, and renal function should be tested to establish a baseline before therapy and repeated regularly throughout long-term therapy. Drug levels should also be monitored regularly.

- Bone marrow depression progressing to fatal aplastic anemia has been reported with nearly all of the anticonvulsants.

- Observe carefully for the signs that precede the onset of drug-induced cutaneous lesions and reactions: high fever, severe headache, stomatitis, rhinitis, urethritis, conjunctivitis.

- Phenytoin produces gingival hyperplasia, particularly in children, and may require surgical removal. Good oral hygiene and gum massage can minimize the inflammatory changes that cause it. This effect has not been reported with the other hydantoins.

- Warn patients to avoid hazardous activities that require mental alertness or physical coordination until drug's effects are known.

**acetazolamide,
acetazolamide sodium**
Ak-Zol, Diamox, Diamox Sequels

- Pharmacologic classification: carbonic anhydrase inhibitor
- Therapeutic classification: anticonvulsant, management of edema
- Pregnancy risk category C

How supplied
Available by prescription only
Tablets: 125 mg, 250 mg

Capsules (extended-release): 500 mg
Powder for injection: 500 mg

Indications, route, and dosage
Myoclonic seizures, refractory generalized tonic-clonic or absence seizures, mixed seizures
Adults: 375 mg P.O., I.M., or I.V. daily up to 250 mg q.i.d. Or Diamox Sequels 250 to 500 mg daily or b.i.d. Initial dosage when used with other anticonvulsants usually is 250 mg daily.
Children: 8 to 30 mg/kg P.O., I.M., or I.V. daily divided t.i.d. or q.i.d. Maximum dosage is 1.5 g daily or 300 to 900 mg/m² daily.
†*Treatment of pseudotumor cerebri*
Adults: 250 to 375 mg P.O., I.M., or I.V. daily in a.m.
Children: 5 mg/kg P.O., I.M., or I.V. daily in a.m.
†*Treatment of periodic paralysis*
Adults: 250 mg P.O. b.i.d. or t.i.d. Effective dosage range 250 mg to 1.5 g daily.

Pharmacodynamics
Anticonvulsant action: The mechanism is unknown. Acetazolamide is used with other anticonvulsants in various types of seizure disorders, particularly absence seizures.

Pharmacokinetics
- *Absorption:* Acetazolamide is well absorbed from the GI tract after oral administration.
- *Distribution:* Acetazolamide is distributed throughout body tissues.
- *Metabolism:* None.
- *Excretion:* Acetazolamide is excreted primarily in urine via tubular secretion and passive reabsorption.

Contraindications and precautions
Acetazolamide is contraindicated in patients with hepatic insufficiency because the drug may precipitate hepatic coma; in patients with low potassium or sodium concentration level or hyperchloremic acidosis because it may worsen electrolyte imbalance; and in patients with severe renal impairment because nephrotoxicity has been reported.

Acetazolamide should be used cautiously in patients with respiratory acidosis or other severe respiratory problems because the drug may produce acidosis; in patients with diabetes because it may cause hyperglycemia and glycosuria; in patients taking cardiac glycosides because they are more susceptible to digitalis toxicity from acetazolamide-induced hypokalemia; and in patients taking diuretics.

Interactions
Acetazolamide alkalinizes urine and thus may decrease excretion of amphetamines, procainamide, quinidine, and flecainide. Acetazolamide may increase excretion of salicylates, phenobarbital, and lithium, lowering plasma levels of these drugs and possibly necessitating dosage adjustments.

Effects on diagnostic tests
Because it alkalinizes urine, acetazolamide may cause false-positive proteinuria in Albustix or Albutest. Acetazolamide may also decrease thyroid iodine uptake.

Adverse reactions
● CNS: drowsiness, paresthesia, confusion.
● DERM: rash.
● EENT: transient myopia.
● GI: nausea, vomiting, anorexia.
● GU: crystalluria, renal calculi, hematuria.
● HEMA: *aplastic anemia,* hemolytic anemia, leukopenia.
● Metabolic: *hyperchloremic acidosis,* hypokalemia, asymptomatic hyperuricemia.
● Local: pain at injection site, sterile abscesses.
   Note: Drug should be discontinued if blood pH is below 7.2.

Overdose and treatment
Specific recommendations are unavailable. Treatment is supportive and symptomatic. Acetazolamide increases bicarbonate excretion and may cause hypokalemia and hyperchloremic acidosis. Induce emesis or perform gastric lavage. Do not induce catharsis because this may exacerbate electrolyte disturbances. Monitor fluid and electrolyte levels.

▶ Special considerations
● For patients who have difficulty swallowing tablets, a single dose may be prepared by softening 1 tablet in 2 teaspoons of warm water and adding 2 teaspoonfuls of honey or syrup (chocolate, cherry) and then taken immediately.
● Suspensions containing 250 mg/5 ml of syrup are the most palatable and can be made by a pharmacist. These will remain stable for about 1 week. Tablets will not dissolve in fruit juice.
● Reconstitute powder by adding at least 5 ml sterile water for injection.
● I.M. injection is painful because of alkalinity of solution. Direct I.V. administration is preferred if drug must be given parenterally.
● Acetazolamide has been used for periodic paralysis in dosages up to 1.5 g daily in divided doses b.i.d. or t.i.d.

● May be useful in treating idiopathic pseudotumor cerebri or pseudotumor cerebri as a complication of lithium therapy. However, the drug may not be consistently effective in lowering intracranial pressure.

Geriatric use
Elderly and debilitated patients require close observation, as they are more susceptible to drug-induced diuresis. Excessive diuresis promotes rapid dehydration, leading to hypovolemia, hypokalemia, and hyponatremia, and may cause circulatory collapse. Reduced dosages may be indicated.

Breast-feeding
Safety of acetazolamide in breast-feeding women has not been established.

---

carbamazepine
Epitol, Mazepine, Tegretol

● Pharmacologic classification: iminostilbene derivative; chemically related to tricyclic antidepressants (TCAs)
● Therapeutic classification: anticonvulsant
● Pregnancy risk category C

How supplied
Available by prescription only
Tablets: 200 mg
Tablets (chewable): 100 mg
Oral suspension: 100 mg/5 ml

Indications, route, and dosage
Generalized tonic-clonic, complex-partial, mixed seizure patterns
Adults and children over age 12: 200 mg P.O. b.i.d. on day 1. May increase by 200 mg/day P.O. in divided doses at 6- to 8-hour intervals. Adjust to minimum effective level when control is achieved; do not exceed 1,000 mg/day in children ages 12 to 15 or 1,200 mg/day in those over age 15. In rare instances, dosages up to 1,600 mg/day have been used in adults.
Children ages 6 to 12: Initially, 100 mg P.O. b.i.d. Increase at weekly intervals by adding 100 mg P.O. daily, using first a t.i.d. schedule, then q.i.d. if necessary. Adjust dosage based on the response. Generally, dosage should not exceed 1,000 mg/day.

†*Bipolar affective disorder,* †*intermittent explosive disorder*

Adults: Initially, 200 mg P.O. b.i.d., increased as needed q 3 to 4 days. Maintenance dosage may range from 600 to 1,600 mg/day.

†*Alcohol withdrawal*

Adults: Initially, 200 mg P.O. q.i.d. Maintenance dosage is 800 to 1,000 mg/day.

†*Nonneuritic pain syndromes (such as phantom limb pain)*

Adults: Initially, 100 mg P.O. b.i.d. Maintenance dosage is 600 to 1,400 mg/day usually combined with a TCA.

†*Benzodiazepine withdrawal*

Adults: Initially, 200 mg P.O. b.i.d. Maintenance dosage is 400 to 800 mg/day.

Pharmacodynamics

Anticonvulsant action: Carbamazepine is chemically unrelated to other anticonvulsants and its mechanism of action is unknown. It appears to limit seizure propagation by reducing polysynaptic responses.

Pharmacokinetics

● *Absorption:* Carbamazepine is absorbed slowly from the GI tract; peak plasma concentrations occur at 2 to 8 hours.

● *Distribution:* Carbamazepine is distributed widely throughout the body; it crosses the placenta and accumulates in fetal tissue. The drug is approximately 75% protein-bound. Therapeutic serum levels are 3 to 14 mcg/ml; nystagmus can occur above 4 mcg/ml and ataxia, dizziness, and anorexia at or above 10 mcg/ml. Serum levels may be misleading because an unmeasured active metabolite also can cause toxicity.

● *Metabolism:* Carbamazepine is metabolized by the liver to an active metabolite. It may also induce its own metabolism; over time, higher doses are needed to maintain plasma levels.

● *Excretion:* Carbamazepine is excreted in urine (70%) and feces (30%); carbamazepine levels in breast milk approach 60% of serum levels.

Contraindications and precautions

Carbamazepine is contraindicated in patients with known hypersensitivity to carbamazepine and TCAs and in patients with past or present bone marrow depression; it also is contraindicated for use with monoamine oxidase (MAO) inhibitors or within 14 days of such use.

Use carbamazepine with caution in patients with cardiovascular, renal, or hepatic damage; increased intraocular pressure; or atypical absence seizures. It also may activate latent psychosis, agitation, or confusion in elderly patients.

Interactions

Concomitant use of carbamazepine with MAO inhibitors may cause hypertensive crisis; use with calcium channel blockers (verapamil and possibly diltiazem) may increase serum levels of carbamazepine significantly (therefore, carbamazepine dosage should be decreased by 40% to 50% when given with verapamil); concomitant use with erythromycin, cimetidine, isoniazid, or propoxyphene also may increase serum carbamazepine levels.

Concomitant use with phenobarbital, phenytoin, or primidone lowers serum carbamazepine levels. When used with warfarin, phenytoin, haloperidol, ethosuximide, or valproic acid, carbamazepine may increase the metabolism of these drugs; it may decrease the effectiveness of theophylline and oral contraceptives.

Effects on diagnostic tests

Carbamazepine may elevate liver enzyme levels; it also may decrease values of thyroid function tests.

Adverse reactions

● CNS: dizziness, vertigo, drowsiness, fatigue, ataxia, worsening of seizures, hallucinations, speech disturbances, paralysis, abnormal movements.

● CV: *CHF,* hypertension, hypotension, aggravation of coronary artery disease, thrombophlebitis, *arrhythmias* (deaths have occurred).

● DERM: rash, urticaria, erythema multiforme, *Stevens-Johnson syndrome.*

● EENT: conjunctivitis, dry mouth and pharynx, blurred vision, diplopia, nystagmus.

● GI: nausea, vomiting, abdominal pain, diarrhea, anorexia, stomatitis, glossitis, dry mouth.

● GU: urinary frequency, urine retention, impotence, albuminuria, glycosuria, elevated blood urea nitrogen levels.

● HEMA: *aplastic anemia, agranulocytosis,* eosinophilia, leukocytosis, *thrombocytopenia.*

● Hepatic: abnormal liver function tests, hepatitis.

● Metabolic: water intoxication, hypocalcemia.

● Other: diaphoresis, fever, chills, pulmonary hypersensitivity, leg cramps, joint pain.

Note: Drug should be discontinued if signs of hypersensitivity, significant elevation of liver function tests, or hematologic abnormalities occur; or if any of the following signs of bone marrow depression appear: fever, sore throat, mouth ulcers, easy bruising, or petechial or purpuric hemorrhage.

Overdose and treatment
Symptoms of overdose may include irregular breathing, respiratory depression, tachycardia, blood pressure changes, shock, arrhythmias, impaired consciousness (ranging to deep coma), seizures, restlessness, drowsiness, psychomotor disturbances, nausea, vomiting, anuria, or oliguria.

Treat overdose with repeated gastric lavage, especially if the patient ingested alcohol concurrently. Oral charcoal and laxatives may hasten excretion. Carefully monitor vital signs, ECG, and fluid and electrolyte balance. Diazepam may control seizures but can exacerbate respiratory depression.

▶ Special considerations
● Many clinicians consider carbamazepine the drug of choice for initial anticonvulsant therapy, especially in women and children; it is increasingly preferred to phenobarbital in children because it has less effect on alertness and behavior. In seizure disorders, carbamazepine can be used alone or with other anticonvulsants.
● Carbamazepine dosage should be adjusted according to individual response as well as therapeutic serum levels (3 to 14 mcg/ml).
● Hematologic toxicity is rare but serious. Perform baseline hematologic testing before treatment.
● Chewable tablets are available for children.
● Reduced bioavailability has been reported with use of improperly stored carbamazepine tablets.

Information for the patient
● Tell patient that carbamazepine may cause GI distress. Patient should take drug with food at equally spaced intervals.
● Advise patient to wear medical identification indicating medication and seizure disorder.
● Warn patient not to stop drug abruptly.
● Encourage patient to promptly report unusual bleeding, bruising, jaundice, dark urine, pale stools, abdominal pain, impotence, fever, chills, sore throat, mouth ulcers, edema, or disturbances in mood, alertness, or coordination.
● Emphasize importance of follow-up laboratory tests and continued medical supervision. Periodic eye examinations are recommended.
● Warn patient that drug may cause drowsiness, dizziness, and blurred vision. Patient should avoid hazardous activities that require alertness, especially during first week of therapy and when dosage is increased.
● Remind patient to shake suspension well before using and to store drug in a cool, dry place, not in the medicine cabinet.

Geriatric use
Carbamazepine may activate latent psychosis, confusion, or agitation in elderly patients and should be used with caution.

Pediatric use
Safety and efficacy have not been established for children under age 6.

Breast-feeding
Significant amounts of carbamazepine appear in breast milk; alternate feeding method is recommended during therapy.

---

clonazepam
Klonopin, Rivotril

● Pharmacologic classification: benzodiazepine
● Therapeutic classification: anticonvulsant
● Controlled substance schedule IV
● Pregnancy risk category C

How supplied
Available by prescription only
Tablets: 0.5 mg, 1 mg, 2 mg

Indications, route, and dosage
Absence and atypical absence seizures; akinetic and myoclonic seizures
Adults: Initial dosage should not exceed 1.5 mg P.O. daily, divided into three doses. May be increased by 0.5 to 1 mg q 3 days until seizures are controlled. Maximum recommended daily dosage is 20 mg.
Children up to age 10 or weighing 30 kg or less: 0.01 to 0.03 mg/kg P.O. daily (not to exceed 0.05 mg/kg daily), divided q 8 hours. Increase dosage by 0.25 to 0.5 mg q third day to a maximum maintenance dosage of 0.1 to 0.2 mg/kg daily.
Nocturnal myoclonus
Adults: 0.5 mg t.i.d. or 1.5 mg h.s.
†Bipolar disorder
Adults: 0.5 mg t.i.d. or 1.5 mg h.s.

Pharmacodynamics
Anticonvulsant action: Mechanism of anticonvulsant activity is unknown; clonazepam ap-

---

pears to act in the limbic system, thalamus, and hypothalamus.

Pharmacokinetics
• *Absorption:* Clonazepam is well absorbed from the GI tract; action begins in 20 to 60 minutes and persists for 6 to 8 hours in infants and children and up to 12 hours in adults.
• *Distribution:* Clonazepam is distributed widely throughout the body; it is approximately 47% protein-bound.
• *Metabolism:* Clonazepam is metabolized by the liver to several metabolites.
• *Excretion:* Clonazepam is excreted in urine.

Contraindications and precautions
Clonazepam is contraindicated in patients with known hypersensitivity to clonazepam and other benzodiazepines and in patients with significant hepatic disease, chronic respiratory disease, and untreated open-angle glaucoma or narrow-angle glaucoma. It should be used with caution (and at lower doses) in patients with decreased renal function.

Interactions
Concomitant use of clonazepam with other CNS depressants (alcohol, narcotics, tranquilizers, anxiolytics, barbiturates) and other anticonvulsants will produce additive CNS depressant effects. Concomitant use with valproic acid may induce absence seizures.

Effects on diagnostic tests
Clonazepam may elevate liver function test values.

Adverse reactions
• CNS: drowsiness, ataxia, behavioral disturbances (especially in children), slurred speech, tremor, confusion, headache.
• CV: thrombophlebitis, *arrhythmias* (deaths have occurred).
• DERM: rash.
• EENT: increased salivation, diplopia, nystagmus, abnormal eye movements, rhinorrhea.
• GI: constipation, gastritis, change in appetite, nausea, abnormal thirst, sore gums.
• GU: dysuria, enuresis, nocturia, urine retention.
• HEMA: leukopenia, thrombocytopenia, eosinophilia.
• Metabolic: hypocalcemia.
• Respiratory: *respiratory depression,* chest congestion, shortness of breath.
  Note: Drug should be discontinued if signs of hypersensitivity occur or if liver function or

hematologic tests show significant abnormalities.

Overdose and treatment
Symptoms of overdose may include ataxia, confusion, coma, decreased reflexes, and hypotension. Treat overdose with gastric lavage and supportive therapy. Vasopressors should be used to treat hypotension. Carefully monitor vital signs, ECG, and fluid and electrolyte balance. Clonazepam is not dialyzable.

▶ Special considerations
Besides those relevant to all *benzodiazepines,* consider the following recommendations.
• Clonazepam is used to treat myoclonic, atonic, and absence seizures resistant to other anticonvulsants and to suppress or eliminate attacks of sleep-related nocturnal myoclonus (restless legs syndrome).
• Abrupt withdrawal may precipitate status epilepticus; after long-term use, lower dosage gradually.
• Concomitant use with barbiturates or other CNS depressants may impair ability to perform tasks requiring mental alertness, such as driving a car. Warn patient to avoid such combined use.
• Monitor complete blood counts and liver function tests periodically.
• Monitor for oversedation, especially in elderly patients.

Information for the patient
• Explain rationale for therapy and for risks and benefits that may be anticipated.
• Teach patient signs and symptoms of adverse reactions and emphasize need to report them promptly.
• Tell patient to avoid alcohol and other sedatives to prevent added CNS depression.
• Warn patient not to discontinue drug or change dosage unless prescribed.
• Advise patient to avoid tasks that require mental alertness until degree of sedative effect is determined.

Geriatric use
Elderly patients may require lower doses because of diminished renal function; such patients also are at greater risk for oversedation from CNS depressants.

Pediatric use
Long-term safety in children has not been established.

Breast-feeding
Alternate feeding method is recommended during clonazepam therapy.

---

clorazepate dipotassium
Novoclopate∗, Tranxene-SD, Tranxene-SD Half Strength, Tranxene T-Tab

- Pharmacologic classification: benzodiazepine
- Therapeutic classification: anticonvulsant, anxiolytic, sedative-hypnotic
- Controlled substance schedule IV
- Pregnancy risk category D

How supplied
Available by prescription only
Capsules: 3.75 mg, 7.5 mg, 15 mg
Tablets: 3.75 mg, 7.5 mg, 11.25 mg, 15 mg, 22.5 mg

Indications, route, and dosage
Acute alcohol withdrawal
Adults: Day 1 – initially, 30 mg P.O., followed by 30 to 60 mg P.O. in divided doses; Day 2 – 45 to 90 mg P.O. in divided doses; Day 3 – 22.5 to 45 mg P.O. in divided doses; Day 4 – 15 to 30 mg P.O. in divided doses; gradually reduce daily dose to 7.5 to 15 mg.
Anxiety
Adults: 15 to 60 mg P.O. daily; usual dosage is 30 mg daily.
Elderly or debilitated adults: Begin treatment at 7.5 to 15 mg daily; adjust dosage according to patient tolerance and response.
Adjunct in seizure management
Adults and children over age 12: Maximum recommended initial dosage is 7.5 mg P.O. t.i.d. Dosage increases should be no greater than 7.5 mg/week. Maximum daily dosage should not exceed 90 mg.
Children between ages 9 and 12: Maximum recommended initial dosage is 7.5 mg P.O. b.i.d. Dosage increases should be no greater than 7.5 mg/week. Maximum daily dosage should not exceed 60 mg/day.

Pharmacodynamics
- *Anxiolytic and sedative actions:* Clorazepate depresses the CNS at the limbic and subcortical levels of the brain. It produces an anxiolytic effect by enhancing the effect of the neurotransmitter gamma-aminobutyric acid on its receptor in the ascending reticular activating system, which increases inhibition and blocks both cortical and limbic arousal.
- *Anticonvulsant action:* Clorazepate suppresses the spread of seizure activity produced by epileptogenic foci in the cortex, thalamus, and limbic structures by enhancing presynaptic inhibition.

Pharmacokinetics
- *Absorption:* After oral administration, clorazepate is hydrolyzed in the stomach to desmethyldiazepam, which is absorbed completely and rapidly. Peak serum levels occur at 1 to 2 hours.
- *Distribution:* Clorazepate is distributed widely throughout the body. Approximately 80% to 95% of an administered dose is bound to plasma protein.
- *Metabolism:* Desmethyldiazepam is metabolized in the liver to oxazepam.
- *Excretion:* Inactive glucuronide metabolites are excreted in urine. The half-life of desmethyldiazepam ranges from 30 to 200 hours.

Contraindications and precautions
Clorazepate is contraindicated in patients with known hypersensitivity to the drug; in patients with acute narrow-angle glaucoma or untreated open-angle glaucoma, because of the drug's possible anticholinergic effect; in patients in shock or coma, because the drug's hypnotic or hypotensive effect may be prolonged or intensified; in patients with acute alcohol intoxication who have depressed vital signs, because the drug will worsen CNS depression; and in neonates, in whom slow metabolism of the drug causes it to accumulate. Patients with depression and anxiety who exhibit suicidal ideation should not be given benzodiazepines.

Clorazepate should be used cautiously in patients with psychoses, because the drug is rarely beneficial in such patients and may induce paradoxical reactions; in patients with myasthenia gravis or Parkinson's disease, because it may exacerbate the disorder; in patients with impaired renal or hepatic function, which prolongs elimination of the drug; in elderly or debilitated patients, who are usually more sensitive to the drug's CNS effects; and in individuals prone to addiction or drug abuse.

Patients on long-term therapy may experience withdrawal symptoms (including nervousness, anxiety, irritability, diarrhea, muscle aches) after abrupt discontinuation of the drug.

Interactions

Clorazepate potentiates the CNS depressant effects of phenothiazines, narcotics, barbiturates, alcohol, antihistamines, monoamine oxidase inhibitors, general anesthetics, and antidepressants. Concomitant use with cimetidine and possibly disulfiram causes diminished hepatic metabolism of clorazepate, which increases its plasma concentration.

Heavy smoking accelerates clorazepate's metabolism, thus lowering clinical effectiveness. Antacids delay the drug's absorption and reduce the total amount absorbed.

Benzodiazepines may reduce serum levels of haloperidol. Clorazepate may decrease the therapeutic effectiveness of levodopa.

Effects on diagnostic tests

Clorazepate therapy may elevate liver function test results. Minor changes in EEG patterns, usually low-voltage, fast activity, may occur during and after clorazepate therapy.

Adverse reactions

- CNS: confusion, depression, drowsiness, lethargy, hangover effect, ataxia, dizziness, syncope, nightmares, fatigue, slurred speech, tremors, vertigo, headache, paradoxical reactions.
- CV: bradycardia, palpitations, *CV collapse,* transient hypotension.
- DERM: rash, urticaria.
- EENT: diplopia, blurred vision, nystagmus.
- GI: constipation, dry mouth, nausea, vomiting, anorexia, dysphagia, abdominal discomfort.
- GU: urinary incontinence, urine retention.
- Other: *respiratory depression,* dysarthria, behavior problems, hepatic dysfunction, changes in libido.

Note: Drug should be discontinued if hypersensitivity or the following paradoxical reactions occur: acute hyperexcited state, anxiety, hallucinations, increased muscle spasticity, insomnia, or rage.

Overdose and treatment

Clinical manifestations of overdose include somnolence, confusion, coma, hypoactive reflexes, dyspnea, labored breathing, hypotension, bradycardia, slurred speech, and unsteady gait or impaired coordination.

Support blood pressure and respiration until drug effects subside; monitor vital signs. Mechanical ventilatory assistance via endotracheal tube may be required to maintain a patent airway and support adequate oxygenation. Treat hypotension with I.V. fluids and vasopressors such as dopamine and phenylephrine as needed.

Induce emesis if patient is conscious. Use gastric lavage if ingestion was recent, but only if an endotracheal tube is present to prevent aspiration. After emesis or lavage, administer activated charcoal with a cathartic as a single dose. Dialysis is of limited value. Do not use barbiturates if excitation occurs, because of possible exacerbation of excitation or CNS depression.

▶ Special considerations

Besides those relevant to all *benzodiazepines,* consider the following recommendations.
- Use cautiously in patients who may have the potential to develop drug dependence.
- Lower doses are effective in elderly patients and patients with renal or hepatic dysfunction.
- Store in a cool, dry place away from direct light.

Information for the patient

- Advise patient to avoid driving and other hazardous activities that require alertnesss until the adverse CNS effects of the drug are known.
- Advise patient of potential for physical and psychological dependence with chronic use of clorazepate.
- Instruct patient not to alter drug regimen in any way without medical approval.
- Warn patient that sudden position changes may cause dizziness. Advise patient to dangle legs for a few minutes before getting out of bed to prevent falls and injury.
- Advise patient to take antacids 1 hour before or after clorazepate.

Geriatric use

- Lower doses are usually effective in elderly patients because of decreased elimination. Use with caution.
- Elderly patients who receive this drug require supervision with ambulation and activities of daily living during initiation of therapy or after an increase in dosage.

Pediatric use

Safety has not been established in children under age 9.

Breast-feeding

The breast-fed infant of a woman who uses clorazepate may become sedated, have feeding difficulties, or lose weight. Avoid use in breast-feeding women.

---

ethosuximide
Zarontin

- Pharmacologic classification: succinimide derivative
- Therapeutic classification: anticonvulsant
- Pregnancy risk category C

How supplied
Available by prescription only
Capsules: 250 mg
Syrup: 250 mg/5 ml

Indications, route, and dosage
Absence seizures
Adults and children over age 6: Initially, 250 mg P.O. b.i.d. May increase by 250 mg q 4 to 7 days up to 1.5 g daily.
Children ages 3 to 6: 20 mg/kg or 1.2 g/m² P.O. daily in a single dose or divided b.i.d. up to 1.5 g daily.

Pharmacodynamics
Anticonvulsant action: Ethosuximide raises the seizure threshold; it suppresses characteristic spike-and-wave pattern by depressing neuronal transmission in the motor cortex and basal ganglia.

Pharmacokinetics
- *Absorption:* Ethosuximide is absorbed from the GI tract; steady-state plasma levels occur in 4 to 7 days.
- *Distribution:* Ethosuximide is distributed widely throughout the body; protein binding is minimal.
- *Metabolism:* Ethosuximide is metabolized extensively in the liver to several inactive metabolites.
- *Excretion:* Ethosuximide is excreted in urine, with small amounts excreted in bile and feces.

Contraindications and precautions
Ethosuximide is contraindicated in patients with known hypersensitivity to succinimides. It should be used with extreme caution in patients with hepatic or renal disease and in those taking other CNS depressants or anticonvulsants. Ethosuximide may increase the incidence of generalized tonic-clonic seizures if used alone to treat patient with mixed seizures; abrupt withdrawal may precipitate absence seizures. Anticonvulsants have been associated with an increased incidence of birth defects.

Interactions
Concomitant use of ethosuximide and other CNS depressants (alcohol, narcotics, anxiolytics, antidepressants, antipsychotics, and other anticonvulsants) causes additive CNS depression and sedation.

Effects on diagnostic tests
Ethosuximide may elevate liver enzyme levels and may cause false-positive Coombs' test results. It may also cause abnormal results of renal function tests.

Adverse reactions
- CNS: drowsiness, headache, fatigue, dizziness, ataxia, irritability, hiccups, euphoria, lethargy, paranoid or psychotic behavior.
- DERM: urticaria, pruritic and erythematous rashes, hirsutism, *Stevens-Johnson syndrome,* lupuslike syndrome.
- EENT: myopia.
- GI: nausea, vomiting, diarrhea, gum hypertrophy, weight loss, cramps, tongue swelling, anorexia, epigastric and abdominal pain.
- GU: vaginal bleeding.
- HEMA: leukopenia, eosinophilia, *agranulocytosis, pancytopenia, aplastic anemia.*
  Note: Drug should be discontinued if signs of hypersensitivity, rash, or unusual skin lesions or any of the following signs of blood dyscrasia occur: joint pain, fever, sore throat, or unusual bleeding or bruising.

Overdose and treatment
Symptoms of ethosuximide overdose, when used alone or with other anticonvulsants, include CNS depression, ataxia, stupor, and coma. Treatment is symptomatic and supportive. Carefully monitor vital signs and fluid and electrolyte balance.

▶ Special considerations
Besides those relevant to all *succinimide derivatives,* consider the following recommendations.
- Ethosuximide is indicated for absence seizures refractory to other drugs.
- Perform baseline hematologic testing before therapy, and repeat blood studies regularly during long-term treatment.
- Administer ethosuximide with food to minimize GI distress.
- Avoid abrupt discontinuation of drug. This may precipitate absence seizures.
- Observe patient for dermatologic reactions,

joint pain, unexplained fever, or unusual bruising or bleeding (which may signal hematologic or other severe adverse reactions).

Information for the patient
● Tell patient to take drug with food or milk to prevent GI distress, to avoid use with alcoholic beverages, and to avoid hazardous tasks that require alertness if drug causes drowsiness, dizziness, or blurred vision.
● Warn patient not to discontinue drug abruptly; this may cause seizures.
● Encourage patient to wear medical identification.
● Tell patient to report the following effects: skin rash, joint pain, fever, sore throat, or unusual bleeding or bruising.
● If pregnancy occurs, patient should notify physician promptly.
● Tell patient to protect pediatric syrup from freezing.

Geriatric use
Use with caution in elderly patients.

Pediatric use
Ethosuximide is not recommended for children under age 3.

Breast-feeding
Safe use has not been established. Alternate feeding method is recommended during therapy with ethosuximide.

---

ethotoin
Peganone

● Pharmacologic classification: hydantoin derivative
● Therapeutic classification: anticonvulsant
● Pregnancy risk category D

How supplied
Available by prescription only
Tablets: 250 mg, 500 mg

Indications, route, and dosage
Generalized tonic-clonic or complex-partial seizures
Adults: Initially, 250 mg P.O. q.i.d. after meals; may increase slowly over several days to 3 g/day divided q.i.d.
Children: 80 mg/kg or 2.5 mg/m^2 P.O. daily or divided b.i.d.

Pharmacodynamics
Anticonvulsant action: Like other hydantoin derivatives, ethotoin stabilizes neuronal membranes and limits seizure activity by increasing efflux of sodium ions across cell membranes in the motor cortex during generation of nerve impulses. However, ethotoin lacks the antiarrhythmic effects of phenytoin.

Pharmacokinetics
● *Absorption:* Ethotoin is absorbed rapidly from the GI tract.
● *Distribution:* Ethotoin is distributed widely throughout the body; its therapeutic range is believed to be 15 to 50 mcg/ml.
● *Metabolism:* Ethotoin is metabolized by the liver, probably by a saturable mechanism (at high doses, a small increase in dosage may produce a large increase in plasma levels).
● *Excretion:* Ethotoin is excreted in urine and feces; small amounts appear in saliva and breast milk.

Contraindications and precautions
Ethotoin is contraindicated in patients with hepatic dysfunction or hematologic disorders. It should be used with caution in patients taking other hydantoin derivatives; concomitant use with phenacemide has caused extreme paranoid symptoms.

Interactions
Concomitant use of ethotoin with phenacemide may cause extreme paranoia. Use of ethotoin with oral contraceptives may decrease the efficacy of oral contraceptives.
The use of anticonvulsants during pregnancy has been associated with an increased incidence of birth defects.

Effects on diagnostic tests
Ethotoin may raise liver enzyme levels.

Adverse reactions
● CNS: fatigue, insomnia, dizziness, headache, numbness.
● CV: chest pain.
● DERM: rash.
● EENT: diplopia, nystagmus.
● GI: nausea, vomiting, diarrhea, gingival hyperplasia (rare).
● HEMA: thrombocytopenia, leukopenia, *agranulocytosis,* pancytopenia, megaloblastic anemia.
● Other: fever, lymphadenopathy.
  Note: Drug should be discontinued if signs of hypersensitivity occur, if a lymphoma-like

---

syndrome develops, or if laboratory tests show hepatic or hematologic changes.

Overdose and treatment

Symptoms of overdose may include drowsiness, nausea, nystagmus, ataxia, and dysarthria; hypotension, respiratory depression, and coma may follow.

Treat overdose with gastric lavage or emesis and follow with supportive treatment. Carefully monitor vital signs and fluid and electrolyte balance. Hemodialysis or total exchange transfusion has been used for managing severe overdose, especially in children.

▶ Special considerations

Besides those relevant to all *hydantoin derivatives,* consider the following recommendations.
● Ethotoin is indicated for generalized tonic-clonic and partial seizures. It is less toxic and less effective than phenytoin and usually is given with other anticonvulsants.
● Use with extreme caution in patients receiving phenacemide.
● Obtain CBC and urinalysis at start of therapy and monthly thereafter.
● Administer ethotoin after meals. Schedule doses as evenly as possible over 24 hours.
● Ethotoin generally produces milder adverse reactions than phenytoin; however, larger doses needed to maintain therapeutic effect frequently cause GI distress.
● In patients with generalized tonic-clonic seizures, ethotoin may be combined with methobarbital or phenobarbital. In patients with mixed absence and generalized tonic-clonic seizures, combined therapy with trimethadione or paramethadione may be useful.
● Ethotoin may be removed by hemodialysis. Dosage adjustments may be necessary in patients undergoing dialysis.

Information for the patient

● Warn patient to avoid hazardous activities that require alertness until CNS response to drug has been determined.
● Tell patient to avoid alcohol while taking this drug, to take drug with food or milk to prevent GI distress, and never to discontinue drug abruptly.
● Patient should call physician at once if adverse reactions, especially rash, swollen glands, bleeding or bruising, yellow skin or eyes, fever, sore throat, or infection, occur.
● Warn patient that pregnancy should be avoided during therapy. Patient should call physician promptly if pregnancy is suspected.

Geriatric use

Use with caution in elderly patients.

Pediatric use

Pediatric dosage form unavailable.

Breast-feeding

Ethotoin appears in breast milk. Alternate feeding method is recommended during therapy with ethotoin.

---

magnesium sulfate

● Pharmacologic classification: mineral/electrolyte
● Therapeutic classification: anticonvulsant
● Pregnancy risk category B

How supplied

Injectable solutions: 10%, 12.5%, 25%, 50% in 2-ml, 5-ml, 10-ml, 20-ml, and 30-ml ampules, vials, and prefilled syringes

Indications, route, and dosage
Hypomagnesemic seizures

Adults: 1 to 2 g (as 10% solution) I.V. over 15 minutes, then 1 g I.M. q 4 to 6 hours, based on patient's response and magnesium blood levels.
Children: 0.2 ml/kg of 50% solution I.M. q 4 to 6 hours p.r.n., or 100 mg/kg of 10% solution I.V. given slowly. Titrate dosage according to magnesium blood levels and seizure response.
Prevention or control of seizures in preeclampsia or eclampsia

Adults: Initially, 4 g I.V. in 250 ml dextrose 5% in water and 4 g deep I.M. each buttock; then 4 g deep I.M. into alternate buttock q 4 hours p.r.n. Alternatively, 4 g I.V. as a loading dose followed by 1 to 4 g hourly as an I.V. infusion.

Pharmacodynamics

Anticonvulsant action: Magnesium sulfate has CNS and respiratory depressant effects. It acts peripherally, causing vasodilation; moderate doses cause flushing and sweating, whereas high doses cause hypotension. It prevents or controls seizures by blocking neuromuscular transmission.

Pharmacokinetics

● *Absorption:* I.V. magnesium sulfate acts immediately; effects last about 30 minutes. After I.M. injection, it acts within 60 minutes and lasts

---

for 3 to 4 hours. Effective anticonvulsant serum levels are 2.5 to 7.5 mEq/liter.
● *Distribution:* Magnesium sulfate is distributed widely throughout the body.
● *Metabolism:* None.
● *Excretion:* Magnesium sulfate is excreted unchanged in urine; some is excreted in breast milk.

Contraindications and precautions
Magnesium sulfate is contraindicated in patients with known heart block, myocardial damage, respiratory depression, or renal failure and in patients with eclampsia, for 2 hours preceding induced delivery, to prevent toxicity and respiratory and CNS depression in the newborn.

Patient's urine output should be maintained at 100 ml/4 hours; magnesium sulfate should be used with caution in patients with decreased renal function.

Interactions
Concomitant use with alcohol, narcotics, anxiolytics, barbiturates, antidepressants, hypnotics, antipsychotics, or general anesthetics may increase CNS depressant effects; reduced dosages may be required. Concomitant use of magnesium sulfate with succinylcholine or tubocurarine potentiates and prolongs neuromuscular blocking action of these drugs; use with caution.

Extreme caution should be used when magnesium sulfate is used concomitantly with cardiac glycosides; changes in cardiac conduction in digitalized patients may lead to heart block if I.V. calcium is administered.

Effects on diagnostic tests
None reported.

Adverse reactions
● CNS: sweating, drowsiness, depressed reflexes, flaccid paralysis, hypothermia.
● CV: hypotension, flushing, *circulatory collapse, depressed cardiac function, heart block.*
● Other: *respiratory paralysis,* hypocalcemia, pain at infusion site.
Note: Drug should be discontinued if signs of hypersensitivity, anuria, toxic symptoms, or toxic serum levels occur.

Overdose and treatment
Clinical manifestations of overdose with magnesium sulfate include a sharp drop in blood pressure and respiratory paralysis, ECG changes (increased PR, QRS, and QT intervals), heart block, and asystole.

Treatment requires artificial ventilation and I.V. calcium salts to reverse respiratory depression and heart block. Usual dosage is 5 to 10 mEq of calcium (10 to 20 ml of a 10% calcium gluconate solution).

▶ **Special considerations**
● Magnesium sulfate is sometimes used in pregnant women to prevent or control preeclamptic or eclamptic seizures; it also is used to treat hypomagnesemic seizures in adults and in children with acute nephritis.
● I.V. bolus *must* be injected slowly (to avoid respiratory or cardiac arrest).
● If available, administer by infusion pump; maximum infusion rate is 150 mg/minute. Rapid drip causes feeling of heat.
● Discontinue drug as soon as needed effect is achieved.
● When giving repeated doses, test knee jerk reflex before each dose; if absent, discontinue magnesium because continued use risks respiratory center failure.
● Respiratory rate must be 16 breaths per minute or more before each dose. Keep I.V. calcium salts on hand.
● To calculate grams of magnesium in a percentage of solution: X% = X g/100 ml (for example, 25% = 25 g/100 ml = 250 mg/ml).
● Monitor serum magnesium load and clinical status to avoid overdose.
● After use in toxemic women within 24 hours before delivery, watch neonate for signs of magnesium toxicity, including neuromuscular and respiratory depression.

Pediatric use
Magnesium sulfate is not indicated for pediatric use.

Breast-feeding
Magnesium sulfate is excreted in breast milk; in patients with normal renal function, all magnesium sulfate is excreted within 24 hours of discontinuing drug. Alternate feeding method is recommended during therapy.

---

mephenytoin
Mesantoin

- Pharmacologic classification: hydantoin derivative
- Therapeutic classification: anticonvulsant
- Pregnancy risk category C

How supplied
Available by prescription only
Tablets: 100 mg

Indications, route, and dosage
Generalized tonic-clonic or complex-partial seizures
Adults: 50 to 100 mg P.O. daily; may increase by 50 to 100 mg at weekly intervals, up to 200 mg P.O. q 8 hours. Dosages up to 800 mg/day may be required.
Children: Initial dosage is 50 to 100 mg P.O. daily (3 to 15 mg/kg/day or 100 to 450 mg/m²/day) in three divided doses. May increase slowly by 50 to 100 mg at weekly intervals up to 200 mg P.O. t.i.d. divided q 8 hours. Dosage must be adjusted individually. Usual maintenance dosage in children is 100 to 400 mg/day divided q 8 hours.

Pharmacodynamics
Anticonvulsant action: Like other hydantoin derivatives, mephenytoin stabilizes the neuronal membranes and limits seizure activity either by increasing efflux or by decreasing influx of sodium ions across cell membranes in the motor cortex during generation of nerve impulses. Like phenytoin, mephenytoin appears to have antiarrhythmic effects.

Pharmacokinetics
- *Absorption:* Mephenytoin is absorbed from the GI tract. Onset of action occurs in 30 minutes and persists for 24 to 48 hours.
- *Distribution:* Mephenytoin is distributed widely throughout the body; good seizure control without toxicity occurs when serum concentrations of drug and major metabolite reach 25 to 40 mcg/ml.
- *Metabolism:* Mephenytoin is metabolized by the liver.
- *Excretion:* Mephenytoin is excreted in urine.

Contraindications and precautions
Mephenytoin is contraindicated in patients with hypersensitivity to hydantoins. Generally, it is used only when other anticonvulsants have failed. It should be used with caution. Patients should be monitored carefully for toxic reactions, including potentially fatal blood dyscrasias and mucocutaneous syndromes. Such have occurred within 2 weeks to 2 years after initiation of therapy.

Interactions
Mephenytoin's therapeutic effects and toxicity may be increased by concomitant use with oral anticoagulants, antihistamines, chloramphenicol, cimetidine, diazepam, diazoxide, disulfiram, isoniazid, phenylbutazone, salicylates, sulfamethizole, or valproate. Mephenytoin's therapeutic effects may be decreased by concomitant use of alcohol or folic acid. Mephenytoin may decrease the effects of oral contraceptives.

Effects on diagnostic tests
Mephenytoin may elevate liver function test results.

Adverse reactions
- CNS: ataxia, drowsiness, fatigue, irritability, choreiform movements, depression, tremor, sleeplessness, dizziness (usually transient).
- DERM: rashes, *exfoliative dermatitis.*
- EENT: photophobia, conjunctivitis, diplopia, nystagmus.
- GI: gingival hyperplasia, nausea and vomiting (with prolonged use).
- HEMA: *leukopenia,* neutropenia, *agranulocytosis,* thrombocytopenia, pancytopenia, eosinophilia.
- Other: alopecia, weight gain.
  Note: Drug should be discontinued if signs of hypersensitivity or hepatotoxicity occur; if neutrophil count decreases by 1,600 to 2,500/mm³ or other signs of hematologic abnormalities occur; or if lymphadenopathy or rash occurs.

Overdose and treatment
Signs of acute mephenytoin toxicity may include restlessness, dizziness, drowsiness, nausea, vomiting, nystagmus, ataxia, dysarthria, tremor, and slurred speech; hypotension, respiratory depression, and coma may follow. Death may result from respiratory and circulatory depression.

Treat overdose with gastric lavage or emesis and follow with supportive treatment. Carefully monitor vital signs and fluid and electrolyte balance. Forced diuresis is of little or no value. Hemodialysis or peritoneal dialysis may be helpful.

▶ **Special considerations**

Besides those relevant to all *hydantoin derivatives,* consider the following recommendations.

● Mephenytoin is used for prophylaxis of generalized tonic-clonic, psychomotor, focal, and jacksonian-type partial seizures in patients refractory to less toxic agents. It usually is combined with phenytoin, phenobarbital, or primidone; phenytoin is preferred because it causes less sedation than barbiturates. Mephenytoin also is used with succinimides to control combined absence and generalized tonic-clonic disorders; combined use with oxazolidinediones is not recommended because of the increased hazard of blood dyscrasias.

● Decreased alertness and coordination are most pronounced at start of treatment. Patient may need help with walking and other activities for first few days.

● Drug should not be discontinued abruptly. Transition from mephenytoin to other anticonvulsant drug should progress over 6 weeks.

Information for the patient

● Tell patient never to discontinue drug or change dosage except as prescribed and to avoid alcohol, which decreases effectiveness of drug and increases sedative effects.

● Explain to patient that follow-up laboratory tests are essential for safe use.

● Instruct patient to report any unusual changes immediately (cutaneous reaction, sore throat, glandular swelling, fever, mucous membrane swelling).

Pediatric use

Children usually require from 100 to 400 mg/day.

Breast-feeding

Safe use in breast-feeding has not been established. Alternate feeding method is recommended during therapy with mephenytoin.

mephobarbital
Mebaral

● Pharmacologic classification: barbiturate
● Therapeutic classification: anticonvulsant, nonspecific CNS depressant
● Controlled substance schedule IV
● Pregnancy risk category D

How supplied

Available by prescription only
Tablets: 32 mg, 50 mg, 100 mg

Indications, route, and dosage
Generalized tonic-clonic or absence seizures

Adults: 400 to 600 mg P.O. daily or in divided doses.

Children: 6 to 12 mg/kg P.O. daily divided q 6 to 8 hours (smaller doses are given initially and increased over 4 to 5 days as needed).

Sedation

Adults: 32 to 100 mg P.O. t.i.d. or q.i.d. Usual dose is 50 mg P.O. t.i.d. or q.i.d.

Children: 16 to 32 mg P.O. t.i.d. or q.i.d.

Pharmacodynamics

Anticonvulsant and sedative actions: Mephobarbital raises seizure threshold in the motor cortex. It is indicated to treat generalized tonic-clonic, absence, myoclonic, and mixed seizures and, as a sedative, to relieve anxiety and tension. It is used chiefly to replace phenobarbital when less sedation is needed (no data support this rationale) and in children with hyperexcitability states or other mood disturbances.

Pharmacokinetics

● *Absorption:* About 50% of an oral dose of mephobarbital is absorbed from the GI tract; action begins within 30 to 60 minutes and lasts 10 to 16 hours.

● *Distribution:* Mephobarbital is distributed widely throughout the body.

● *Metabolism:* Mephobarbital is metabolized by the liver to phenobarbital; about 75% of a given dose is converted in 24 hours. Therapeutic blood levels of phenobarbital are 15 to 40 mcg/ml.

● *Excretion:* Mephobarbital is excreted primarily in urine; small amounts are excreted in breast milk.

Contraindications and precautions

Mephobarbital is contraindicated in patients with known hypersensitivity to barbiturates; in suspected pregnancy and pregnancy near term because of the hazard of respiratory depression and neonatal coagulation defects; in patients with severe respiratory disease or status asthmaticus because it may cause respiratory depression; or in patients with a history of porphyria or marked hepatic impairment because it may exacerbate porphyria. Drug should be used with caution in patients taking alcohol, CNS depressants, monoamine oxidase (MAO) inhibitors, narcotic analgesics, or anticoagulants.

Interactions

Alcohol and other CNS depressants, including narcotic analgesics, cause excessive depression in patients taking mephobarbital. Although concrete data are lacking, mephobarbital is assumed to be an enzyme inducer (like phenobarbital); therefore, all cautions for phenobarbital drug interactions apply. Barbiturates can induce hepatic metabolism of oral anticoagulants, combination oral contraceptives, and doxycycline. Concomitant use with MAO inhibitors potentiates the CNS depressant effects of barbiturates; rifampin may decrease barbiturate levels and thereby decrease efficacy.

Effects on diagnostic tests

Mephobarbital may elevate liver function test results.

Adverse reactions

● CNS: dizziness, headache, hangover, confusion, paradoxical excitation, exacerbation of existing pain, drowsiness, nightmares, hallucinations.
● CV: hypotension.
● DERM: urticaria, morbilliform rash, blisters, purpura, *erythema multiforme, Stevens-Johnson syndrome.*
● GI: nausea, vomiting, epigastric pain, constipation.
● HEMA: megaloblastic anemia, *agranulocytosis,* thrombocytopenia.
● Other: allergic reactions (facial edema).
Note: Drug should be discontinued if signs of hypersensitivity or hepatic dysfunction occur.

Overdose and treatment

Symptoms of acute overdose include CNS and respiratory depression, areflexia, oliguria, tachycardia, hypotension, hypothermia, and coma. Shock may occur. In massive overdose, ECG may be flat, even if patient is not clinically dead.

Treat overdose symptomatically and supportively: in conscious patient with intact gag reflex, induce emesis with ipecac syrup; follow in 30 minutes with repeated doses of activated charcoal. Forced diuresis and alkalinization of urine may hasten excretion. Hemodialysis may be necessary. Monitor vital signs and fluid and electrolyte balance.

▶ Special considerations

Besides those relevant to all *barbiturates,* consider the following recommendations.
● Monitor for signs of bleeding if patient is on stable anticoagulant regimen.
● Do not withdraw drug abruptly; after long-term use, lower dosage gradually.
● Mephobarbital impairs ability to perform tasks requiring mental alertness, such as driving a car.
● Use caution in patients who may have the potential to develop drug dependence.

Information for the patient

● Explain rationale for therapy and the potential risks and benefits.
● Teach patient how to recognize signs and symptoms of adverse reactions and what to do if they occur.
● Tell patient to avoid alcohol and other sedatives to prevent added CNS depression.
● Barbiturates carry a risk of physical and psychological dependence; warn patient not to discontinue drug abruptly or to alter dosage.
● Explain that barbiturates may render oral contraceptives ineffective; advise consideration of different birth control method.
● Advise patient to avoid hazardous tasks that require mental alertness until degree of sedative effect is determined.

Geriatric use

Some clinicians avoid using mephobarbital in elderly patients because it can cause excessive CNS depression or paradoxical excitement.

Pediatric use

Mephobarbital is not recommended for children under age 6.

Breast-feeding

Some mephobarbital is excreted in breast milk. Alternate feeding method is recommended during therapy with mephobarbital.

methsuximide
Celontin Half Strength Kapseals, Celontin
Kapseals

- Pharmacologic classification: succinimide derivative
- Therapeutic classification: anticonvulsant
- Pregnancy risk category C

How supplied
Available by prescription only
Capsules: 150 mg, 300 mg

Indications, route, and dosage
Refractory absence seizures
Adults and children: 10 mg/kg or 600 mg/m² P.O. daily. Maximum daily dosage is 1.2 g.

Pharmacodynamics
Anticonvulsant action: Methsuximide raises the seizure threshold; it suppresses characteristic spike-and-wave pattern by depressing neuronal transmission in the motor cortex and basal ganglia.

Pharmacokinetics
- *Absorption:* Methsuximide is absorbed from the GI tract; peak plasma concentrations occur in 1 to 4 hours.
- *Distribution:* Methsuximide is distributed widely throughout the body. Therapeutic plasma concentration levels appear to be 10 to 40 mcg/ml.
- *Metabolism:* Methsuximide is metabolized in the liver to several metabolites; N-demethyl methsuximide is a potent CNS depressant and may be the active metabolite.
- *Excretion:* Methsuximide is excreted in urine.

Contraindications and precautions
Methsuximide is contraindicated in patients with known hypersensitivity to succinimides and in patients with mixed forms of seizure disorders, because it may precipitate generalized tonic-clonic seizures.

Methsuximide should be used with caution in patients with hepatic or renal disease and in patients taking other CNS depressants or anticonvulsants. Abrupt withdrawal may precipitate absence seizures. Use of anticonvulsants during pregnancy has been associated with increased incidence of birth defects.

Interactions
Concomitant use of methsuximide with other CNS depressants (alcohol, narcotics, anxiolytics, antidepressants, antipsychotics, and other anticonvulsants) causes additive sedative and CNS depressant effects.

Effects on diagnostic tests
Methsuximide may elevate liver enzyme levels and cause abnormal renal function test results.

Adverse reactions
- CNS: drowsiness, ataxia, dizziness, irritability, nervousness, headache, insomnia, confusion, depression, aggressiveness, psychosis (rare).
- DERM: urticaria, pruritic and erythematous rashes, *Stevens-Johnson syndrome,* systemic lupus erythematosus.
- EENT: blurred vision, photophobia, periorbital edema.
- GI: nausea, vomiting, anorexia, diarrhea, weight loss, abdominal or epigastric pain, constipation.
- HEMA: eosinophilia, leukopenia, monocytosis, pancytopenia.

Note: Drug should be discontinued if signs of hypersensitivity, rash or unusual skin lesions, or any of the following signs of blood dyscrasia occur: joint pain, fever, sore throat, or unusual bleeding or bruising.

Overdose and treatment
Symptoms of overdose may include dizziness and ataxia (beginning within 1 hour after overdose); condition may progress to stupor and coma.

Treat overdose supportively. Monitor vital signs and fluid and electrolyte balance carefully. Charcoal hemoperfusion or hemodialysis may be used for severe cases.

▶ Special considerations
Besides those relevant to all *succinimide derivatives,* consider the following recommendations.
- Methsuximide is indicated for absence seizures refractory to other drugs.
- Methsuximide may be hemodialyzable. Dosage adjustments may be necessary in patients undergoing hemodialysis.
- Never change or withdraw drug suddenly. Abrupt withdrawal may precipitate absence seizures.
- Obtain complete blood count every 3 months; urinalysis and liver function tests every 6 months.

- Protect capsules from excessive heat (104° F [40° C]).
- When interviewing patients taking methsuximide, be aware that drug may cause irritability or nervousness.

Information for the patient
- Tell patient to take drug with milk or food if GI upset occurs.
- Warn patient not to use capsules that look like they aren't full or that contain contents that look melted.
- Tell patient to store capsules away from excessive heat and humidity to maintain effectiveness of drug. For example, tell patient not to store drug in a locked car.
- Tell patient to avoid alcoholic beverages.
- Warn patient not to discontinue medication abruptly or to change dosage unless prescribed.
- Advise patient to wear medical identification indicating medication and seizure disorder.
- Tell patient to promptly report skin rash, pregnancy, sore throat, joint pains, unexplained fever, or unusual bleeding or bruising.
- Warn patient to avoid activities that require alertness and good psychomotor coordination until CNS response to drug has been determined.

---

paraldehyde
Paral

- Pharmacologic classification: acetaldehyde polymer
- Therapeutic classification: anticonvulsant; sedative-hypnotic
- Controlled substance schedule IV
- Pregnancy risk category C

How supplied
Available by prescription only
Rectal or oral liquid: 1 g/ml

Indications, route, and dosage
Insomnia
Adults: 10 to 30 ml P.O. p.r.n.
Children: 0.3 ml/kg or 12 ml/m² P.O.
Sedation
Adults: 5 to 10 ml P.O. p.r.n.
Children: 0.15 ml/kg or 6 ml/m² P.O. p.r.n.
Management of seizures
Adults: Up to 12 ml (diluted 1:10) via gastric tube q 4 hours p.r.n. or 5 to 15 ml rectally delivered via gastric tube.

Status epilepticus
Children: 1 ml/year of age rectally. Do not exceed 5 ml; may repeat in 1 hour. Additional doses can be given by gastric tube. Administer 2 to 5 ml q 2 to 4 hours.
Management of alcohol withdrawal syndrome
Adults: 5 to 10 ml P.O. q 4 to 6 hours for the first 24 hours, then q 6 hours. Maximum dosage is 60 ml P.O. on day 1; 40 ml P.O. on subsequent days.

Pharmacodynamics
Anticonvulsant action: Paraldehyde depresses many levels of the CNS. Its actions are similar to barbiturates and alcohol. It exhibits anticonvulsant activity in doses that do not produce sleep, but the margin between these two effects is small.

Pharmacokinetics
- *Absorption:* Rapidly absorbed after oral administration. Maximum serum levels are reached within 1 hour.
- *Distribution:* CSF levels of the drug are about 30% lower than serum levels, but peak levels appear 30 to 60 minutes after administration. Paraldehyde crosses the placenta and appears in the fetal circulation.
- *Metabolism:* 80% to 90% of a dose is metabolized by the liver. The drug is probably depolymerized to acetaldehyde, which is oxidized by aldehyde dehydrogenase to acetic acid and eventually to carbon dioxide and water.
- *Excretion:* A substantial portion of the drug is excreted via the lungs. The remainder is utilized by the Krebs cycle. The average half-life is 7.5 hours.

Contraindications and precautions
Paraldehyde is contraindicated in gastroenteritis with ulceration. Use cautiously in patients with impaired hepatic function and asthma or other pulmonary disease.

Administration of decomposed paraldehyde has resulted in fatalities caused by metabolic acidosis or severe corrosion of the stomach (after oral administration) or rectum (after rectal administration). Always use a fresh supply of paraldehyde. Do not use if solution is brown or has a vinegary odor or if the container has been open longer than 24 hours.

Interactions
Concomitant use with alcohol or other CNS depressants can cause increased CNS depression. Use with caution.

Concomitant use with disulfiram may result in increased paraldehyde and acetaldehyde blood levels; possible toxic disulfiram reaction.

Effects on diagnostic tests
None reported.

Adverse reactions
- CNS: confusion, tremor, weakness, irritability, dizziness.
- CV: dilation of right side of heart, *circulatory collapse.*
- DERM: erythematous rash.
- GI: irritation, foul breath odor, gastric erosion.
- GU: nephrosis with prolonged use.
- Metabolic: metabolic acidosis.
- Other: *respiratory depression.*

Overdose and treatment
Paraldehyde overdose resembles chloral hydrate overdose: coma, severe hypotension, respiratory depression, pulmonary edema, and cardiac failure can occur. Because the rate of drug metabolism is slow, the drug-induced coma can last for several hours. Renal or hepatic failure may occur.

Diagnosis of overdose is facilitated by the characteristic breath odor caused by the drug.

Treat overdose supportively. Ensure adequate ventilation, maintain body temperature, and support circulation. Gastric lavage (if overdose was oral) or rectal lavage (if rectal route of administration) may be advantageous; some clinicians use a demulcent such as mineral oil to alleviate local irritation. Correct metabolic acidosis as needed.

▶ **Special considerations**
- Paraldehyde is a potentially toxic drug and many safer alternative agents are available.
- Always dilute before administration with iced juice or milk to mask taste and odor and to reduce GI distress.
- Dilute paraldehyde in olive oil or cottonseed oil 1:2 for rectal administration. Give as retention enema. May also use 200 ml normal saline solution to prepare enema.
- Keep patient's room well ventilated to remove exhaled paraldehyde.
- May cause drug dependence and severe withdrawal symptoms.
- Oral or rectal administration of decomposed paraldehyde may cause severe corrosion of stomach or rectum.

Information for the patient
- Always store the drug in its original container, tightly closed and away from heat. Do not use solutions that are discolored or smell like vinegar.
- Be sure to dilute well before taking.

Breast-feeding
It is not known if paraldehyde is excreted in breast milk. Because of the potential for severe respiratory depression in the neonate, avoid use in breast-feeding women.

---

paramethadione
Paradione

- Pharmacologic classification: oxazolidinedione derivative
- Therapeutic classification: anticonvulsant
- Pregnancy risk category D

How supplied
Available by prescription only
Capsules: 150 mg, 300 mg
Solution: 300 mg/ml (65% alcohol) with dropper

Indications, route, and dosage
Refractory absence seizures
Adults: Initially, 300 mg P.O. t.i.d; may increase by 300 mg weekly up to 600 mg q.i.d., if needed.
Children over age 6: 0.9 g P.O. daily in divided doses t.i.d. or q.i.d.
Children ages 2 to 6: 0.6 g P.O. daily in divided doses t.i.d. or q.i.d.
Children under age 2: 0.3 g P.O. daily in divided doses b.i.d.

Pharmacodynamics
Anticonvulsant action: Paramethadione raises the threshold for cortical seizures but does not modify the seizure pattern; it will not modify the maximal seizure pattern in patients undergoing electroconvulsive therapy. It decreases projection of focal activity and reduces both repetitive spinal cord transmission and spike-and-wave patterns of absence seizures.

Pharmacokinetics
- *Absorption:* Paramethadione is absorbed from the GI tract.
- *Distribution:* Paramethadione is distributed widely throughout the body.
- *Metabolism:* Paramethadione is demethylated in the liver to active metabolites.

• *Excretion:* Paramethadione is excreted in urine; it is unknown whether drug is excreted in breast milk.

Contraindications and precautions

Paramethadione is contraindicated during pregnancy and in patients with known hypersensitivity to oxazolidinedione derivatives; use paramethadione with extreme caution in patients with severe hepatic or renal disease, severe blood dyscrasia, or diseases of the retina or optic nerve because the drug may exacerbate diseases of the optic nerve. Preparation contains tartrazine; use with caution in patients with asthma or aspirin allergy because of possible allergic reactions.

Interactions

Concomitant use of paramethadione and mephenytoin or phenacemide may result in a high incidence of toxicity; such combinations should be avoided.

Effects on diagnostic tests

Paramethadione may cause abnormalities in liver function test results.

Adverse reactions

• CNS: drowsiness, sedation, fatigue, vertigo, headache, paresthesia, irritability.
• CV: hypertension, hypotension.
• DERM: acneiform or morbilliform rash, *exfoliative dermatitis, erythema multiforme,* petechiae, alopecia.
• EENT: hemeralopia, photophobia, diplopia, epistaxis, retinal hemorrhage.
• GI: nausea, vomiting, abdominal pain, weight loss, bleeding gums.
• GU: albuminuria, vaginal bleeding.
• HEMA: neutropenia, leukopenia, eosinophilia, thrombocytopenia, pancytopenia, *agranulocytosis, hypoplastic* and *aplastic anemia.*
• Hepatic: abnormal liver function test results.
• Other: lymphadenopathy, systemic lupus erythematosus.

Note: Drug should be discontinued if signs of hypersensitivity, any rash (even acneiform), or unusual skin lesions occur; if scotomata occur; if neutrophil count falls to or below 2,500/mm^3; if any of the following signs of blood dyscrasia occur: joint pain, fever, sore throat, or unusual bleeding or bruising; if patient has persistent or increasing albuminuria; if jaundice or other signs of hepatic dysfunction occur; or if syndromes resembling systemic lupus erythematosus, malignant lymphoma, or myasthenia gravis occur.

Overdose and treatment

Symptoms of overdose include nausea, drowsiness, ataxia, and visual disturbances; coma may follow massive overdose.

Treat overdose with immediate gastric lavage or emesis and with supportive measures. Monitor vital signs and fluid and electrolyte balance carefully. Alkalinization of urine may hasten renal excretion. Monitor blood counts and hepatic and renal function after recovery.

▶ **Special considerations**

Besides those relevant to all *oxazolidinedione derivatives,* consider the following recommendations.
• Paramethadione should be used only after less toxic alternative drugs have failed.
• Drug should not be withdrawn abruptly because this may precipitate seizures.

Information for the patient

• Emphasize need for close medical supervision.
• Advise women of childbearing age to use an effective contraceptive method and to notify physician promptly if they suspect pregnancy.
• Tell patient to take drug with food or milk to prevent GI distress.
• Urge patient to report the following reactions promptly: visual disturbance, excessive dizziness or drowsiness, sore throat, fever, bleeding or bruising, or skin rash.
• Inform patient that hemeralopia (day blindness) may be relieved with dark glasses.

Pediatric use

Dilute oral solution with water because of 65% alcohol content.

---

phenacemide
Phenurone

• Pharmacologic classification: substituted acetylurea derivative, open-chain hydantoin
• Therapeutic classification: anticonvulsant
• Pregnancy risk category D

How supplied

Available by prescription only
Tablets: 500 mg

Indications, route, and dosage
Refractory, complex-partial, generalized tonic-clonic, absence, and atypical absence seizures
Adults: 500 mg P.O. t.i.d; may increase by 500 mg weekly up to 5 g daily p.r.n.
Children ages 5 to 10: 250 mg P.O. t.i.d.; may increase by 250 mg weekly up to 1.5 g daily p.r.n.

Satisfactory seizure control may occur with dosages as low as 250 mg t.i.d.

Pharmacodynamics
Anticonvulsant action: Phenacemide elevates the seizure threshold by an unknown mechanism; it elevates the threshold for maximal seizures in patients undergoing electroconvulsive therapy and abolishes their tonic phase.

Pharmacokinetics
● *Absorption:* Phenacemide is absorbed well from the GI tract; duration of action is about 5 hours.
● *Distribution:* Unknown.
● *Metabolism:* Phenacemide is metabolized by the liver.
● *Excretion:* Phenacemide is excreted in urine. It is unknown whether drug is excreted in breast milk.

Contraindications and precautions
Phenacemide is contraindicated in patients with known hypersensitivity to phenacemide and in patients with jaundice or other signs of liver dysfunction because it may be hepatotoxic.

Use phenacemide with caution in patients with a history of drug allergy, especially to anticonvulsants, and in patients with personality disorders, as suicide attempts have occurred. Use phenacemide with extreme caution in patients taking other anticonvulsants. Paranoid symptoms have developed in patients receiving phenacemide and ethotoin concurrently.

Interactions
Concomitant use of phenacemide with ethotoin may cause paranoid symptoms; use with other anticonvulsants (mephenytoin, trimethadione, or paramethadione) may markedly increase toxicity.

Effects on diagnostic tests
Phenacemide may cause abnormalities in liver enzyme test results.

Adverse reactions
● CNS: drowsiness, dizziness, insomnia, headaches, paresthesia, *depression, suicidal tendencies,* aggressiveness, psychic changes.
● DERM: rashes.
● GI: anorexia, weight loss.
● GU: nephritis with marked albuminuria.
● HEMA: aplastic anemia, agranulocytosis, leukopenia.
● Hepatic: *hepatitis,* jaundice.
Note: Drug should be discontinued if signs of hypersensitivity, jaundice, or other hepatotoxicity occur; if marked depression of white blood cell (WBC) count (leukocyte level below 4,000/mm^3) occurs; if albumin, blood, casts, or leukocytes occur in urine; if rash occurs; or if patient shows new or exacerbated personality disorder.

Overdose and treatment
Symptoms of overdose include initial excitement followed by drowsiness, nausea, ataxia, and coma.

Treat overdose with gastric lavage or emesis and follow with supportive treatment. Monitor vital signs and fluid and electrolyte balance carefully. Hemodialysis or total exchange transfusion has been used for severe cases and pediatric patients. Careful evaluation of renal, hepatic, and hematologic status is crucial after recovery.

▶ Special considerations
Besides those relevant to all *hydantoin derivatives,* consider the following recommendations.
● This drug is extremely toxic and is usually reserved for patients with severe seizure disorders (especially mixed forms) resistant to other anticonvulsants.
● Obtain baseline liver function tests, complete blood counts, and urinalyses before and at monthly intervals during treatment; discontinue drug if a marked depression of blood count is observed.

Information for the patient
● Advise patient of potential serious toxicity with phenacemide. Urge patient to report any of the following immediately: pregnancy, jaundice, abdominal pain, pale stools, dark urine, fever, sore throat, mouth sores, rashes, unusual bleeding or bruising, or loss of appetite. All such reports mandate immediate review of laboratory studies.
● Inform patient about possible psychological reactions, and tell him to report immediately any changes in mood or affect, such as de-

creased interest in himself or his surroundings, depression, or aggression.

Pediatric use
Safety is not established for children under age 5.

Breast-feeding
Phenacemide is not known to be excreted in breast milk; however, because of potential for serious toxicity, alternate feeding method is recommended during phenacemide therapy.

phensuximide
Milontin

- Pharmacologic classification: succinimide derivative
- Therapeutic classification: anticonvulsant
- Pregnancy risk category D

How supplied
Available by prescription only
Capsules: 500 mg

Indications, route, and dosage
Absence seizures
Adults and children: 500 mg to 1 g P.O. b.i.d. or t.i.d.

Pharmacodynamics
Anticonvulsant action: Phensuximide raises the seizure threshold; it suppresses characteristic spike-and-wave pattern by depressing neuronal transmission in the motor cortex and basal ganglia.

Pharmacokinetics
- *Absorption:* Phensuximide is absorbed from the GI tract; peak plasma concentrations occur at 1 to 4 hours.
- *Distribution:* Phensuximide is distributed widely throughout the body.
- *Metabolism:* Little is known about phensuximide's metabolism; hydroxy metabolite has been isolated.
- *Excretion:* Excretion of phensuximide has not been studied; it is at least partially excreted in urine.

Contraindications and precautions
Phensuximide is contraindicated in patients with known hypersensitivity to succinimide derivatives. It should be use with caution in patients with hepatic or renal disease and in patients

taking other CNS depressants or anticonvulsants.

Phensuximide may increase the incidence of generalized tonic-clonic seizures if used alone to treat mixed seizures; abrupt withdrawal may precipitate absence seizures. Use of anticonvulsants during pregnancy has been associated with an increased incidence of birth defects.

Interactions
Concomitant use of phensuximide and other CNS depressants (alcohol, narcotics, anxiolytics, antidepressants, antipsychotics, and other anticonvulsants) may increase sedative effects.

Effects on diagnostic tests
None reported.

Adverse reactions
- CNS: muscular weakness, drowsiness, dizziness, ataxia, headache, insomnia, confusion, psychosis.
- DERM: pruritus, eruptions, erythema, *Stevens-Johnson syndrome.*
- GI: nausea, vomiting, anorexia, abdominal pain, diarrhea.
- GU: urinary frequency, renal damage, hematuria.
- HEMA: transient leukopenia, pancytopenia, *agranulocytosis,* eosinophilia.
- Other: periorbital edema.

Note: Drug should be discontinued if signs of hypersensitivity, rash, or unusual skin lesions occur or if any of the following signs of blood dyscrasia occur: joint pain, fever, sore throat, or unusual bleeding or bruising.

Overdose and treatment
Symptoms of overdose may include dizziness and ataxia, which may progress to stupor and coma. Treat overdose supportively. Carefully monitor vital signs and fluid and electrolyte balance. Charcoal hemoperfusion or hemodialysis may be used for severe cases.

▶ Special considerations
Besides those relevant to all *succinimide derivatives,* consider the following recommendations.
- Phensuximide is indicated for absence seizures refractory to other drugs.
- Patient should have periodic tests for hematologic and liver function. Complete blood counts are recommended every 3 months; urinalysis and liver function tests, every 6 months.
- Observe patient for signs of hematologic or

other severe adverse reactions. Drug can cause symptoms of systemic lupus erythematosus.
• Phensuximide may be removed by hemodialysis. Dosage adjustments may be necessary in patients undergoing dialysis.

Information for the patient
• Tell patient that drug may color urine pink, red, or brown. This is not harmful.
• Tell patient to take drug with food or milk to avoid GI upset, to avoid use of alcoholic beverages, and not to discontinue the drug abruptly or change dose except as directed.
• Encourage patient to report immediately skin rash, joint pain, fever, sore throat, bleeding, or bruising.

Breast-feeding
Excretion into breast milk unknown. Consider alternate feeding methods during therapy.

---

phenytoin, phenytoin sodium, phenytoin sodium (extended)
Dilantin

phenytoin sodium (prompt)
Diphenylan

• Pharmacologic classification: hydantoin derivative
• Therapeutic classification: anticonvulsant
• Pregnancy risk category D

How supplied
Available by prescription only
phenytoin
Tablets (chewable): 50 mg
Oral suspension: 30 mg/5 ml, 125 mg/5 ml
phenytoin sodium
Capsules: 30 mg, 100 mg
Injection: 50 mg/ml
phenytoin sodium (extended)
Capsules: 30 mg, 100 mg
phenytoin sodium (prompt)
Capsules: 30 mg, 100 mg

Indications, route, and dosage
Generalized tonic-clonic seizures, status epilepticus, seizures resulting from head trauma or metabolic abnormalities (Reye's syndrome)
Adults: Loading dosage is 10 to 15 mg/kg I.V. slowly, not to exceed 50 mg/minute; oral loading dosage consists of 1 g divided into three doses

(400 mg, 300 mg, 300 mg) given at 2-hour intervals. Maintenance dosage is 300 mg P.O. daily (extended only) or divided t.i.d. (extended or prompt).
Children: Loading dosage is 15 mg/kg I.V. at 50 mg/minute, or P.O. divided q 8 to 12 hours; then start maintenance dosage of 4 to 8 mg/kg P.O. or I.V. daily divided q 12 hours.
Seizures in patients who have been receiving phenytoin but who have missed one or more doses and have subtherapeutic levels
Adults: 100 to 300 mg I.V., not to exceed 50 mg/minute.
Children: 5 to 7 mg/kg I.V., not to exceed 50 mg/minute. May repeat lower dose in 30 minutes if needed.
†*Neuritic pain (migraine, trigeminal neuralgia, and Bell's palsy)*
Adults: 200 to 600 mg P.O. daily in divided doses.

Pharmacodynamics
Anticonvulsant action: Like other hydantoin derivatives, phenytoin stabilizes neuronal membranes and limits seizure activity by either increasing efflux or decreasing influx of sodium ions across cell membranes in the motor cortex during generation of nerve impulses. Phenytoin exerts its antiarrhythmic effects by normalizing sodium influx to Purkinje's fibers in patients with digitalis-induced arrhythmias.

Pharmacokinetics
• *Absorption:* Phenytoin is absorbed slowly from the small intestine; absorption is formulation-dependent and bioavailability may differ among products. Extended-release capsules give peak serum concentrations at 4 to 12 hours; prompt-release products peak at 1½ to 3 hours. I.M. doses are absorbed erratically; about 50% to 75% of I.M. dose is absorbed in 24 hours.
• *Distribution:* Phenytoin is distributed widely throughout the body; therapeutic plasma levels are 10 to 20 mcg/ml, although in some patients they occur at 5 to 10 mcg/ml. Lateral nystagmus may occur at levels above 20 mcg/ml; ataxia usually occurs at levels above 30 mcg/ml; significantly decreased mental capacity occurs at 40 mcg/ml. Phenytoin is about 90% protein-bound, less so in uremic patients.
• *Metabolism:* Phenytoin is metabolized by the liver to inactive metabolites.
• *Excretion:* Phenytoin is excreted in urine and exhibits dose-dependent (zero-order) elimination kinetics; above a certain dosage level, small

---

increases in dosage disproportionately increase serum levels.

Contraindications and precautions

Phenytoin is contraindicated in patients with hypersensitivity to hydantoins or phenacemide; I.V. phenytoin is contraindicated in patients with sinus bradycardia, sinoatrial or atrioventricular block, or Stokes-Adams syndrome.

Phenytoin should be used with caution in patients with acute intermittent porphyria, hepatic or renal dysfunction (especially in uremic patients, who have higher serum drug levels from decreased protein-binding), myocardial insufficiency, or respiratory depression; in elderly or debilitated patients; and in patients taking other hydantoin derivatives.

Interactions

Phenytoin interacts with many drugs. Diminished therapeutic effects and toxic reactions often are the result of recent changes in drug therapy. Phenytoin's therapeutic effects may be increased by concomitant use with allopurinol, chloramphenicol, cimetidine, diazepam, disulfiram, ethanol (acute), isoniazid, miconazole, phenacemide, phenylbutazone, succinimides, trimethoprim, valproic acid, salicylates, ibuprofen, chlorpheniramine, or imipramine.

Phenytoin's therapeutic effects may be decreased by barbiturates, carbamazepine, diazoxide, ethanol (chronic), folic acid, theophylline, antacids, antineoplastics, calcium gluconate, calcium, charcoal, loxapine, nitrofurantoin, or pyridoxine. Other drugs that lower the seizure threshold (such as antipsychotic agents) may alleviate phenytoin's therapeutic effects.

Phenytoin may decrease the effects of the following drugs by stimulating hepatic metabolism: corticosteroids, cyclosporine, dicumarol, digitoxin, meperidine, disopyramide, doxycycline, estrogens, haloperidol, methadone, metyrapone, quinidine, oral contraceptives, dopamine, furosemide, levodopa, or sulfonylureas.

Effects on diagnostic tests

Phenytoin may raise blood glucose levels by inhibiting pancreatic insulin release; it may decrease serum levels of protein-bound iodine and may interfere with the 1-mg dexamethasone suppression test.

Adverse reactions

- CNS: ataxia, slurred speech, confusion, dizziness, insomnia, nervousness, twitching, headache.
- CV: hypotension, *ventricular fibrillation.*

- DERM: scarlatiniform or morbilliform rash; bullous, exfoliative, or purpuric dermatitis; *Stevens-Johnson syndrome;* lupus erythematosus; hirsutism; *toxic epidermal necrolysis;* photosensitivity.
- EENT: nystagmus, diplopia, blurred vision.
- GI: nausea, vomiting, gingival hyperplasia (especially in children).
- HEMA: thrombocytopenia, leukopenia, *agranulocytosis,* pancytopenia, macrocytosis, megaloblastic anemia.
- Hepatic: *toxic hepatitis,* jaundice.
- Local: pain, necrosis, and inflammation at injection site; purple glove syndrome.
- Other: periarteritis nodosa, lymphadenopathy, hyperglycemia, osteomalacia, hypertrichosis.

Note: Drug should be discontinued if signs of hypersensitivity, hepatotoxicity, or blood dyscrasia occur or if lymphadenopathy or skin rash occurs.

Overdose and treatment

Early signs of overdose may include drowsiness, nausea, vomiting, nystagmus, ataxia, dysarthria, tremor, and slurred speech; hypotension, respiratory depression, and coma may follow. Death is caused by respiratory and circulatory depression. Estimated lethal dose in adults is 2 to 5 g.

Treat overdose with gastric lavage or emesis and follow with supportive treatment. Carefully monitor vital signs and fluid and electrolyte balance. Forced diuresis is of little or no value. Hemodialysis or peritoneal dialysis may be helpful.

▶ Special considerations

Besides those relevant to all *hydantoin derivatives,* consider the following recommendations.
- Phenytoin is indicated for generalized tonic-clonic and partial seizures.
- Monitoring of serum levels is essential because of dose-dependent excretion.
- Compliance in psychiatric patients may be problematic. Use serum levels to help monitor patient compliance.
- Only extended-release capsules are approved for once-daily dosing; all other forms are given in divided doses every 8 to 12 hours.
- Oral or nasogastric feeding may interfere with absorption of oral suspension; separate doses as much as possible from feedings. During continuous tube feeding, tube should be flushed before and after dose.
- If oral suspension is used, shake well.

• I.M. administration should be avoided; it is painful and drug absorption is erratic.

• Mix I.V. doses in normal saline solution and use within 1 hour; mixtures with dextrose 5% will precipitate. Do not refrigerate solution; do not mix with other drugs.

• When giving I.V., continuous monitoring of ECG, blood pressure, and respiratory status is essential.

• Abrupt withdrawal may precipitate status epilepticus.

• If using I.V. bolus, use slow (50 mg/minute) I.V. push or constant infusion; too-rapid I.V. injection may cause hypotension and circulatory collapse. Do not use I.V. push in veins on back of hand; larger veins are needed to prevent discoloration associated with purple glove syndrome.

• Phenytoin often is abbreviated as DPH (diphenylhydantoin), an older drug name.

Information for the patient

• Tell patient to use same brand of phenytoin consistently. Changing brands may change therapeutic effect.

• Tell patient to take drug with food or milk to minimize GI distress.

• Warn patient not to discontinue drug, except with medical supervision; to avoid hazardous activities that require alertness until CNS effect is determined; and to avoid alcoholic beverages, which can decrease effectiveness of drug and increase adverse reactions.

• Encourage patient to wear medical identification.

• Encourage good oral hygiene to minimize overgrowth and sensitivity of gums.

Geriatric use

Elderly patients metabolize and excrete phenytoin slowly; therefore, they may require lower doses.

Pediatric use

Special pediatric-strength oral suspension is available (30 mg/5 ml). Take extreme care to use correct strength. Do not confuse with adult strength (125 mg/5 ml).

Breast-feeding

Phenytoin is excreted into breast milk. Alternate feeding method is recommended during therapy.

primidone
Myidone, Mysoline

• Pharmacologic classification: barbiturate analogue
• Therapeutic classification: anticonvulsant
• Pregnancy risk category D

How supplied
Available by prescription only
Tablets: 50 mg, 250 mg
Oral suspension: 250 mg/5 ml

Indications, route, and dosage
Generalized tonic-clonic seizures, complex-partial seizures
Adults and children age 8 and over: 250 mg P.O. daily. Increase by 250 mg weekly up to a maximum of 2 g/day divided q.i.d.
Children under age 8: 10 to 25 mg/kg P.O. daily up to a maximum of 1 g/day divided q.i.d.
Benign familial tremor (essential tremor)
Adults: 750 mg/day P.O. divided t.i.d.

Pharmacodynamics
Anticonvulsant action: Primidone acts as a nonspecific CNS depressant used alone or with other anticonvulsants to control refractory generalized tonic-clonic seizures and to treat psychomotor or focal seizures. Mechanism of action is unknown; some activity may be from phenobarbital, an active metabolite.

Pharmacokinetics
• *Absorption:* Primidone is absorbed readily from the GI tract; serum concentrations peak at about 3 hours. Phenobarbital appears in plasma after several days of continuous therapy; most laboratory assays detect both phenobarbital and primidone. Therapeutic levels are 5 to 12 mcg/ml for primidone and 10 to 30 mcg/ml for phenobarbital.

• *Distribution:* Primidone is distributed widely throughout the body.

• *Metabolism:* Primidone is metabolized slowly by the liver to phenylethylmalonamide (PEMA) and phenobarbital; PEMA is the major metabolite.

• *Excretion:* Primidone is excreted in urine; substantial amounts are excreted in breast milk.

Contraindications and precautions
Primidone is contraindicated in patients with known hypersensitivity to barbiturates; in preg-

nancy because of hazard of respiratory depression and neonatal coagulation defects; in patients with severe respiratory disease or status asthmaticus because of respiratory depressant effects; in patients with porphyria because of potential for adverse hematologic effects; and in patients with markedly impaired hepatic function because of potential for enhanced hepatic impairment. Use drug with caution in patients taking alcohol and other CNS depressants.

Interactions
Alcohol and other CNS depressants, including narcotic analgesics, cause excessive depression in patients taking primidone. Carbamazepine and phenytoin may decrease effects of primidone and increase its conversion to phenobarbital; monitor serum levels to prevent toxicity.

Effects on diagnostic tests
Primidone may cause abnormalities in liver function test results.

Adverse reactions
- CNS: drowsiness, ataxia, emotional disturbances, vertigo, hyperirritability, fatigue.
- DERM: morbilliform rash, alopecia.
- EENT: diplopia, nystagmus, edema of the eyelids.
- GI: anorexia, nausea, vomiting.
- GU: impotence, polyuria.
- HEMA: leukopenia, eosinophilia.
- Other: edema, thirst.

Note: Drug should be discontinued if signs of hypersensitivity or hepatic dysfunction occur.

Overdose and treatment
Symptoms of overdose resemble those of barbiturate intoxication; they include CNS and respiratory depression, areflexia, oliguria, tachycardia, hypotension, hypothermia, and coma. Shock may occur.

Treat overdose supportively: in conscious patient with intact gag reflex, induce emesis with ipecac syrup; follow in 30 minutes with repeated doses of activated charcoal. Use lavage if emesis is not feasible. Alkalinization of urine and forced diuresis may hasten excretion. Hemodialysis may be necessary. Monitor vital signs and fluid and electrolyte balance.

▶ Special considerations
Besides those relevant to all *barbiturates,* consider the following recommendations.
- Patient should have review of complete blood count and liver function tests every 6 months.

- Abrupt withdrawal of primidone may cause status epilepticus; dosage should be reduced gradually.
- Barbiturates impair ability to perform tasks requiring mental alertness, such as driving a car.

Information for the patient
- Explain rationale for therapy and the potential risks and benefits.
- Teach patient signs and symptoms of adverse reactions.
- Tell patient to avoid alcohol and other sedatives to prevent added CNS depression.
- Tell patient not to discontinue drug or to alter dosage without medical approval.
- Explain that barbiturates may render oral contraceptives ineffective; advise patient to consider a different birth control method.
- Advise patient to avoid hazardous tasks that require mental alertness until degree of sedative effect is determined. Tell patient that ataxia and vertigo are common at first but disappear with continued therapy.
- Recommend that patient wear medical identification indicating medication and seizure disorder.

Geriatric use
Reduce dose in elderly patients; they often have decreased renal function.

Pediatric use
Primidone may cause hyperexcitability in children under age 6.

Breast-feeding
Considerable amounts of primidone are excreted in breast milk. Alternate feeding method is recommended during therapy.

---

trimethadione
Tridione

- Pharmacologic classification: oxazolidinedione derivative
- Therapeutic classification: anticonvulsant
- Pregnancy risk category D

How supplied
Available by prescription only
Capsules: 150 mg, 300 mg
Solution: 40 mg/ml

Indications, route, and dosage
Refractory absence seizures
Adults: Initially, 300 mg P.O. t.i.d.; may increase by 300 mg weekly up to 600 mg P.O. q.i.d.
Children: 20 to 50 mg/kg P.O. daily divided q 6 to 8 hours. Usual maintenance dosage is 40 mg/kg or 1 g/m^2 P.O. daily in divided doses t.i.d. or q.i.d., not to exceed 900 mg/day.

Pharmacodynamics
Anticonvulsant action: Trimethadione raises the threshold for cortical seizures but does not modify the seizure pattern. It decreases projection of focal activity and reduces both repetitive spinal cord transmission and spike-and-wave patterns of absence seizures.

Pharmacokinetics
- *Absorption:* Trimethadione is well and rapidly absorbed from the GI tract. Peak plasma concentrations occur in 30 minutes to 2 hours.
- *Distribution:* Trimethadione is distributed widely throughout the body; protein-binding is insignificant.
- *Metabolism:* Trimethadione is metabolized in the liver to an active metabolite.
- *Excretion:* Trimethadione is excreted slowly in urine.

Contraindications and precautions
Trimethadione is contraindicated in patients with known hypersensitivity to oxazolidinedione derivatives and in patients with renal or hepatic dysfunction. It should be used with caution in patients with severe blood dyscrasia, acute intermittent porphyria, or diseases of the retina or optic nerve.

Anticonvulsants have been associated with an increased incidence of birth defects. Trimethadione may cause fetal harm and is contraindicated during pregnancy.

Interactions
Concomitant use of trimethadione and mephenytoin or phenacemide may result in a high incidence of toxicity; such combinations should be avoided.

Effects on diagnostic tests
Trimethadione may elevate liver function test results.

Adverse reactions
- CNS: ataxia, drowsiness, fatigue, malaise, insomnia, dizziness, headache, paresthesia, irritability.
- CV: hypertension, hypotension.
- DERM: acneiform and morbilliform rash, *exfoliative dermatitis,* erythema multiforme, petechiae, alopecia.
- EENT: hemeralopia, diplopia, photophobia, epistaxis, retinal hemorrhage.
- GI: nausea, vomiting, anorexia, abdominal pain, bleeding gums.
- GU: nephrosis, albuminuria, vaginal bleeding.
- HEMA: neutropenia, leukopenia, eosinophilia, thrombocytopenia, pancytopenia, *agranulocytosis, hypoplastic and aplastic anemia.*
- Hepatic: abnormal liver function test results.
- Other: lymphadenopathy.

Note: Drug should be discontinued if signs of hypersensitivity, any rash (even acneiform), or unusual skin lesions occur; if scotomata occur; if neutrophil count falls to or below 2,500/mm^3; if any of the following signs of blood dyscrasia occur: joint pain, fever, sore throat, or unusual bleeding or bruising; if patient has persistent or increasing albuminuria; if jaundice or other signs of hepatic dysfunction occur; or if syndromes resembling systemic lupus erythematosus, malignant lymphoma, or myasthenia gravis occur.

Overdose and treatment
Symptoms of overdose include nausea, drowsiness, ataxia, and visual disturbances; coma may follow massive overdose. Treat overdose by immediate gastric lavage or emesis, with supportive measures. Monitor vital signs and fluid and electrolyte balance carefully. Alkalinization of urine may hasten renal excretion. Monitor blood counts and hepatic and renal function after recovery.

▶ Special considerations
Besides those relevant to all *oxazolidinedione derivatives,* consider the following recommendations.
- Trimethadione should not be withdrawn abruptly; this can precipitate absence seizures.
- Monitor complete blood counts and liver enzyme levels periodically during therapy.
- Trimethadione should be used only for absence seizures refractory to other anticonvulsants (such as ethosuximide). It is not effective for other types of seizure disorders and may precipitate a generalized tonic-clonic seizure.

Information for the patient
- Advise patient that follow-up laboratory tests are essential.
- Advise women of childbearing age to use an effective form of contraception and notify physician promptly if pregnancy is suspected.

• Tell patient to avoid ingesting alcoholic beverages.
• Tell patient to take drug with food or milk if GI upset occurs.
• Advise patient to wear medical identification indicating medication and seizure disorder.
• Explain that the drug may cause sensitivity to bright light. Sunscreens and protective clothing may be necessary.
• Warn that the drug may cause drowsiness or blurred vision. Patient should avoid hazardous tasks that require mental alertness until response to drug is determined.
• Advise patient to report the following: visual disturbances, excessive drowsiness, dizziness, sore throat, fever, unusual bleeding or bruising, or skin rash.
• Inform patient that hemeralopia (day blindness) may be relieved by wearing dark glasses.

Breast-feeding
Safety in breast-feeding has not been established. Alternate feeding method is recommended during therapy.

---

valproate sodium
Depakene Syrup, Myproic Acid Syrup

valproic acid
Depakene

divalproex sodium
Depakote

• Pharmacologic classification: carboxylic acid derivative
• Therapeutic classification: anticonvulsant
• Pregnancy risk category D

How supplied
Available by prescription only
valproate sodium
Syrup: 250 mg/5 ml
valproic acid
Capsules: 250 mg
divalproex sodium
Tablets (enteric-coated): 125 mg, 250 mg, 500 mg

Indications, route, and dosage
Simple and complex absence seizures and mixed seizures; investigationally in generalized tonic-clonic seizures
Adults and children: Initially, 15 mg/kg P.O. daily divided b.i.d. or t.i.d.; may increase by 5 to 10 mg/kg daily at weekly intervals up to a maximum of 60 mg/kg daily divided b.i.d. or t.i.d. The b.i.d. dosage is recommended for the enteric-coated tablets.
Note: Dosages of divalproex sodium are expressed as valproic acid.

Pharmacodynamics
Anticonvulsant action: Valproic acid's mechanism of action is unknown; effects may be from increased brain levels of gamma-aminobutyric acid (GABA), an inhibitory transmitter. Valproic acid also may decrease GABA's enzymatic catabolism.

Pharmacokinetics
• *Absorption:* Valproate sodium and divalproex sodium quickly convert to valproic acid after administration of oral dose; peak plasma concentrations occur in 1 to 4 hours (with uncoated tablets) and 3 to 5 hours (with enteric-coated tablets); bioavailability of drug is same for both dosage forms.
• *Distribution:* Valproic acid is distributed rapidly throughout the body; drug is 80% to 95% protein-bound.
• *Metabolism:* Valproic acid is metabolized by the liver.
• *Excretion:* Valproic acid is excreted in urine; some drug is excreted in feces and exhaled air. Breast milk levels are 1% to 10% of serum levels.

Contraindications and precautions
Valproic acid is contraindicated in patients with known hypersensitivity to valproic acid and in patients with a history of hepatic disease because valproic acid may be hepatotoxic. It should be used with caution in patients taking oral anticoagulants or multiple anticonvulsants. Patients with congenital metabolic or seizure disorders with mental retardation, especially in children under age 2, appear to be at increased risk of adverse reactions.

Interactions
Valproic acid may potentiate effects of MAO inhibitors and other CNS antidepressants and of oral anticoagulants. Besides additive sedative effects, valproic acid increases serum levels of primidone and phenobarbital; such combinations may cause excessive somnolence and re-

quire careful monitoring. Concomitant use with clonazepam may cause absence seizures and should be avoided.

Effects on diagnostic tests
Valproic acid may cause false-positive test results for urinary ketones; it also may cause abnormalities in liver function test results.

Adverse reactions
Because drug usually is used with other anticonvulsants, the adverse reactions reported may not be caused by valproic acid alone.
- CNS: sedation, emotional upset, depression, psychosis, aggression, hyperactivity, behavioral deterioration, muscle weakness, tremor, ataxia, headache, hallucinations.
- EENT: stomatitis, hypersalivation, nystagmus, diplopia, scotomata.
- GI: nausea, vomiting, indigestion, diarrhea, abdominal cramps, constipation, increased appetite and weight gain, anorexia, pancreatitis. *Note:* Lower incidence of GI effects occurs with divalproex.
- HEMA: inhibited platelet aggregation, *thrombocytopenia, increased bleeding time.*
- Hepatic: enzyme level elevations, *toxic hepatitis.*
- Metabolic: elevated serum ammonia levels.
- Other: alopecia, enuresis, curling or waving hair.
   Note: Drug should be discontinued if signs of hypersensitivity, hepatic dysfunction (markedly elevated liver enzyme levels or jaundice), or coagulation abnormalities (bruising or hemorrhage) occur.

Overdose and treatment
Symptoms of overdose include somnolence and coma.

   Treat overdose supportively: maintain adequate urine output, and monitor vital signs and fluid and electrolyte balance carefully. Naloxone reverses CNS and respiratory depression but also may reverse anticonvulsant effects of valproic acid. Valproic acid is not dialyzable.

▶ Special considerations
- Onset of therapeutic effects may require a week or more.
- Valproic acid may be used with other anticonvulsants.
- Patient should have review of liver function, platelet counts, and prothrombin times at baseline and at monthly intervals — especially during first 6 months.
- Therapeutic range is 50 to 100 mcg/ml.

- Drug should not be withdrawn abruptly.
- Tremor may indicate need for dosage reduction.
- Administer drug with food to minimize GI irritation. Enteric-coated formulation may be better tolerated.

Information for the patient
- Advise patient not to discontinue drug suddenly, not to alter dosage without medical approval, and to consult pharmacist before changing brand or using generic drug because therapeutic effect may change.
- Tell patient to swallow tablets whole to avoid local mucosal irritation and, if necessary, to take with food but not carbonated beverages because tablet may dissolve before swallowing, causing irritation and unpleasant taste.
- Tell patient not to use alcohol while taking drug; it may decrease drug's effectiveness and may increase adverse CNS effects.
- Advise patient to avoid tasks that require mental alertness until degree of CNS sedative effect is determined. Drug may cause drowsiness and dizziness.
- Teach patient signs and symptoms of hypersensitivity and adverse reactions and the need to report them.
- Encourage patient to wear medical identification indicating medication and seizure disorder while taking anticonvulsants.

Geriatric use
Elderly patients eliminate drug more slowly; lower dosages are recommended.

Pediatric use
Valproic acid is not recommended for use in children under age 2; this age-group is at highest risk for adverse reactions. Reportedly, hyperexcitability and aggressiveness have occurred in a few children.

Breast-feeding
Valproic acid appears in breast milk in concentration levels from 1% to 10% of serum concentrations. Alternate feeding method is recommended during therapy.

Antidepressants

amitriptyline hydrochloride
amoxapine
bupropion hydrochloride
clomipramine hydrochloride
desipramine hydrochloride
doxepin hydrochloride
fluoxetine hydrochloride
imipramine hydrochloride
imipramine pamoate
isocarboxazid
maprotiline hydrochloride
nortriptyline hydrochloride
phenelzine sulfate
protriptyline hydrochloride
tranylcypromine sulfate
trazodone hydrochloride
trimipramine maleate

Antidepressant drugs enhance alertness and may stimulate purposeful activity. Most of these agents fall into two pharmacologic groups: tricyclic antidepressants (TCAs) and monoamine oxidase (MAO) inhibitors. A third group, structurally and chemically unrelated to other known antidepressants, is now available and provides comparable results with fewer adverse effects.

Pharmacologic effects
● The *TCAs* (amitriptyline, amoxapine, clomipramine, desipramine, doxepin, imipramine, maprotiline, nortriptyline, protriptyline, trimipramine) are more effective and safer in moderate and severe depression than the MAO inhibitors; they also exert anxiolytic and sedative properties, which are beneficial in mild depression, and are used to treat enuresis.
● *MAO inhibitors* (isocarboxazid, phenelzine, tranylcypromine) provide symptomatic relief in severe reactive or endogenous depression.
● *Others* (bupropion, fluoxetine, trazodone) are also effective in various forms of depression.
● All three types of antidepressants potentiate noradrenergic function by different mechanisms and induce various adverse effects.

Mechanisms of action
Apparently the action of TCAs results from inhibition of the reuptake of norepinephrine and serotonin by neuron terminals. MAO inhibitors block intracellular metabolism of various amines, including epinephrine, norepinephrine, dopamine, and serotonin, increasing their concentrations in neuron terminals. The action of the newer antidepressants is unknown but presumed to be linked to inhibition of neuronal uptake of serotonin and other neurotransmitters.

Pharmacokinetics
● *Absorption and distribution:* TCAs, MAO inhibitors, and the newer agents are well absorbed after oral administration and widely distributed throughout the body. Except for fluoxetine, their bioavailability is affected by food.
● *Metabolism and excretion:* TCAs and the newer agents are extensively metabolized by hepatic microsomal enzymes and primarily excreted in urine, with a small fraction excreted in bile. Inactivation and elimination occur over several days, with half-lives that range from 16 to 80 hours. MAO inhibitors are thought to be cleaved, resulting in the release of active metabolites. They are inactivated by acetylation. All are metabolized rapidly by children and slowly by persons over age 60.

Adverse reactions and toxicity
The most common adverse reactions associated with antidepressants include dry mouth, excessive perspiration, constipation, blurred vision, hypotension, drowsiness, weight gain, palpitations, tachycardia, dizziness, metallic taste, and urine retention. MAO inhibitors can also produce paradoxical hypertension characterized by nausea, vomiting, headache, and palpitation. This reaction can be induced by foods containing tyramine. Significant and acute toxicity are not uncommon, and reversal of toxicity may be complicated by these agents' prolonged elimination.

Clinical considerations
● Safe use of antidepressants in pregnancy and lactation has not been established.
● Because antidepressants can cause numerous interactions, their use with other medications

---

ADVERSE REACTION POTENTIAL OF ANTIDEPRESSANTS

The chart below indicates the relative potential of tricyclic antidepressants and monoamine oxidase (MAO) inhibitors to produce specific adverse reactions.

CLASS AND DRUG	USUAL ADULT DOSAGE	ANTICHOLINERGIC EFFECTS	SEDATIVE EFFECTS	HYPOTENSIVE EFFECTS
Tricyclic antidepressants				
amitriptyline	50 to 100 mg/day	High	High	Moderate
clomipramine	250 mg/day	High	High	Moderate
desipramine	50 to 150 mg/day	Low	Low	Moderate
doxepin	50 to 150 mg/day	Moderate	High	High
imipramine	50 to 150 mg/day	Moderate	Moderate	High
nortriptyline	50 to 100 mg/day	Moderate	Moderate	Low
protriptyline	10 to 40 mg/day	Low	Low	Moderate
trimipramine	50 to 150 mg/day	Moderate	Moderate	Moderate
Monoamine oxidase inhibitors				
isocarboxazid	10 to 30 mg/day	Low	Low	Moderate
phenelzine	60 to 90 mg/day	Low	Moderate	Moderate
tranylcypromine	20 to 40 mg/day	Low	None	Moderate
Other				
amoxapine	150 to 300 mg/day	Low	Moderate	Low
bupropion	300 to 450 mg/day	None	None	Low
fluoxetine	20 to 60 mg/day	Very low	None	Low
maprotiline	50 to 150 mg/day	Low	Moderate	Low
trazodone	150 to 300 mg/day	None	High	Moderate

requires special precautions. (See individual drug entries.)
- TCAs have been used effectively in eating disorders (when weight gain is desired).
- After discontinuation of an MAO inhibitor, at least 14 days should elapse before another antidepressant including an MAO inhibitor is given and before elective surgery.
- Tolerance to these drugs' anticholinergic effects, such as dry mouth, tends to develop with continued use.
- Physical dependence may develop occasionally. Abrupt discontinuation of high dosage can result in withdrawal syndrome.
- Warn patients to avoid concomitant use of alcohol and products containing alcohol, such as some OTC cough preparations.
- Warn patients to avoid hazardous activities requiring mental alertness and physical coordination until drug's effects are known.
- Some patients may experience photosensitivity reactions. Advise patients to avoid prolonged exposure to sun and to use a sunscreeen during therapy.

amitriptyline hydrochloride
Amitril∗, Elavil, Emitrip, Endep, Enovil, Levate∗,
Mevaril∗, Novotriptyn∗

- Pharmacologic classification: tricyclic antidepressant
- Therapeutic classification: antidepressant
- Pregnancy risk category D

How supplied
Available by prescription only
Tablets: 10 mg, 25 mg, 50 mg, 75 mg, 100 mg,
150 mg
Injection: 10 mg/ml

Indications, route, and dosage
Depression; major depression with melancholia or psychotic symptoms; depressive phase of bipolar disorder; depression associated with organic disease, alcoholism, schizophrenia, or mental retardation; †***anorexia or bulimia associated with depression***
Adults: 50 to 100 mg P.O. daily divided t.i.d. or may be given h.s. In hospitalized patients, increase to 200 mg daily; maximum dosage is 300 mg daily; or 20 to 30 mg I.M. t.i.d. Change to oral route as soon as possible. Alternatively, the entire dosage can be given h.s. For maintenance therapy, reduce dosage as tolerated; most patients respond to 50 to 100 mg daily, but some will respond to doses as low as 25 to 40 mg daily.
Elderly patients and adolescents: 30 mg P.O. daily in divided doses; may be increased gradually as needed and tolerated to a maximum of 150 mg daily.
Parenteral therapy should be changed to oral route as soon as possible.
Prevention of cluster, migraine, and tension headaches
Adults: 25 mg P.O. h.s. Increase dosage at weekly intervals to a maximum of 150 mg daily. Average dose is 50 to 75 mg daily.
†***Adjunctive treatment of neurogenic pain***
Adults: 25 mg b.i.d. to q.i.d.

Pharmacodynamics
Antidepressant action: Amitriptyline is thought to exert its antidepressant effects by inhibiting reuptake of norepinephrine and serotonin in CNS nerve terminals (presynaptic neurons), resulting in increased concentrations and enhanced activity of these neurotransmitters in the synaptic cleft. Amitriptyline more actively inhibits reuptake of serotonin than norepinephrine; it carries a high incidence of undesirable sedation, but tolerance to this effect usually develops within a few weeks.

Pharmacokinetics
- *Absorption:* Amitriptyline is absorbed rapidly from the GI tract after oral administration and from muscle tissue after I.M. administration.
- *Distribution:* Amitriptyline is distributed widely into the body, including the CNS and breast milk. Drug is 96% protein-bound. Peak effect occurs 2 to 12 hours after a given dose, and steady state is achieved within 4 to 10 days; full therapeutic effect usually occurs in 2 to 4 weeks.
- *Metabolism:* Amitriptyline is metabolized by the liver to the active metabolite nortriptyline; a significant first-pass effect may account for variability of serum concentrations in different patients taking the same dosage. Therapeutic plasma levels are determined by taking the total levels of nortriptyline and amitriptyline; therapeutic levels are 75 to 225 mg/ml.
- *Excretion:* Most of drug is excreted in urine.

Contraindications and precautions
Amitriptyline is contraindicated in patients with known hypersensitivity to TCAs, trazodone, and related compounds; in the acute recovery phase of myocardial infarction because of its arrhythmogenic potential; in patients in coma or with severe respiratory depression because of additive CNS depressant effects; and during or within 14 days of therapy with MAO inhibitors.

Amitriptyline should be used with caution in patients with other cardiac disease (arrhythmias, CHF, angina pectoris, valvular disease, or heart block); respiratory disorders; alcoholism and seizure disorders; scheduled electroconvulsive therapy (ECT); bipolar disease; glaucoma; hyperthyroidism or in those taking thyroid hormone replacement; Type I and Type II diabetes; prostatic hypertrophy, paralytic ileus, or urine retention; hepatic or renal dysfunction; Parkinson's disease; and in those undergoing surgery with general anesthesia.

Interactions
Concomitant use of amitriptyline with sympathomimetics, including epinephrine, phenylephrine, phenylpropanolamine, and ephedrine (often found in nasal sprays) may increase blood pressure; use with warfarin may increase prothrombin time and cause bleeding.

Concomitant use with thyroid hormones, pimozide, or antiarrhythmic agents (quinidine, disopyramide, procainamide) may increase incidence of cardiac arrhythmias and conduction defects.

Amitriptyline may decrease hypotensive effects of centrally acting antihypertensive drugs, such as guanethidine, guanabenz, guanadrel, clonidine, methyldopa, and reserpine. Concomitant use with disulfiram or ethchlorvynol may cause delirium and tachycardia.

Additive effects are likely after concomitant use of amitriptyline with CNS depressants, including alcohol, analgesics, barbiturates, narcotics, tranquilizers, and anesthetics (oversedation); atropine or other anticholinergic drugs, including phenothiazines, antihistamines, meperidine, and antiparkinsonian agents (oversedation, paralytic ileus, visual changes, and severe constipation); or metrizamide (increased risk of seizures).

Barbiturates and heavy smoking induce amitriptyline metabolism and decrease therapeutic efficacy; phenothiazines and haloperidol decrease its metabolism, decreasing therapeutic efficacy; methylphenidate, cimetidine, oral contraceptives, propoxyphene, phenothiazines, haloperidol, and beta blockers may inhibit amitriptyline metabolism, increasing plasma levels and toxicity.

Effects on diagnostic tests

Amitriptyline may prolong conduction time (elongation of QT and PR intervals, flattened T waves on ECG); it also may elevate liver function test results, decrease WBC counts, and decrease or increase serum glucose levels.

Adverse reactions

● CNS: drowsiness, dizziness, sedation, excitation, tremors, weakness, headache, nervousness, *seizures,* peripheral neuropathy, extrapyramidal symptoms, anxiety, vivid dreams, decreased libido, confusion (more marked in elderly patients).
● CV: orthostatic hypotension, tachycardia, *arrhythmias, MI, stroke, heart block, CHF,* palpitations, hypertension, ECG changes.
● EENT: blurred vision, tinnitus, mydriasis, increased intraocular pressure.
● GI: dry mouth, constipation, abdominal cramping, nausea, vomiting, anorexia, diarrhea, paralytic ileus, jaundice.
● GU: urine retention.
● Other: sweating, photosensitivity, hypersensitivity (rash, urticaria, drug fever, edema).

After abrupt withdrawal of long-term therapy, nausea, headache, and malaise (does not indicate addiction) may occur.

Note: Drug should be discontinued (not abruptly) if signs of hypersensitivity occur. Reevaluate therapy if the following signs and symptoms occur: urine retention, extreme dry mouth, rash, excessive sedation, seizures, tachycardia, sore throat, fever, or jaundice.

Overdose and treatment

The first 12 hours after acute ingestion are a stimulatory phase characterized by excessive anticholinergic activity (agitation, irritation, confusion, hallucinations, hyperthermia, parkinsonian symptoms, seizure, urine retention, dry mucous membranes, pupillary dilation, constipation, and ileus). This is followed by CNS depressant effects, including hypothermia, decreased or absent reflexes, sedation, hypotension, cyanosis, and cardiac irregularities, including tachycardia, conduction disturbances, and quinidine-like effects on the ECG.

Severity of overdose is best indicated by widening of the QRS complex and usually represents a serum level in excess of 1,000 mg/ml. Metabolic acidosis may follow hypotension, hypoventilation, and seizures. Delayed cardiac anomalies and death may occur.

Treatment is symptomatic and supportive, including maintaining a patent airway, stable body temperature, and fluid and electrolyte balance. Monitor vital signs and ECG. Induce emesis with ipecac syrup if gag reflex is intact; follow with gastric lavage and activated charcoal to prevent further absorption. Dialysis is of little use. Treatment of seizures may include parenteral diazepam or phenytoin; treatment of arrhythmias, parenteral phenytoin or lidocaine; and treatment of acidosis, sodium bicarbonate. *Do not give barbiturates;* these may enhance CNS and respiratory depressant effects.

▶ Special considerations

Besides those relevant to all *TCAs,* consider the following recommendations.
● Amitriptyline may also be used to treat intractable hiccups and postherpetic neuralgia.
● When using to relieve cluster or migrane headache, allow a 6-week trial before concluding that the drug is ineffective.
● Amitriptyline causes a high incidence of sedation. Tolerance to sedative effects usually develops over several weeks.
● The full dose may be given at bedtime to help offset daytime sedation.
● Oral administration should be substituted for the parenteral route as soon as possible.

- I.M. administration may result in a more rapid onset of action than oral administration.
- The drug should not be withdrawn abruptly.
- The drug should be discontinued at least 48 hours before surgical procedures.
- Chewing gum, sugarless hard candy, or ice chips may alleviate dry mouth. Stress the importance of regular dental hygiene, as dry mouth can increase the incidence of dental caries.

Information for the patient
- Tell patient to take amitriptyline exactly as prescribed and not to double dose for missed ones.
- The full dose may be taken at bedtime to alleviate daytime sedation. Alternatively, it may be taken in the early evening to avoid morning "hangover."
- Explain that full effects of the drug may not become apparent for up to 4 weeks after initiation of therapy.
- Warn that drug may cause drowsiness or dizziness. Patient should avoid hazardous activities that require alertness until the full effects of the drug are known.
- Warn patient not to drink alcoholic beverages while taking this drug.
- Suggest taking drug with food or milk if it causes stomach upset and chewing gum or sucking hard candy to relieve dry mouth.
- After initial doses, patient should lie down for about 30 minutes and rise to upright position slowly to prevent dizziness or fainting.
- Warn patient not to stop taking drug abruptly.
- Encourage patient to report troublesome or unusual effects, especially confusion, movement disorders, rapid heartbeat, dizziness, fainting, or difficulty urinating.
- Because drug can cause photosensitivity, tell patient to wear protective clothing and use a suncreen to prevent sunburn.

Geriatric use
Elderly patients may be at greater risk for adverse cardiac effects.

Pediatric use
Drug is not recommended for children under age 12.

Breast-feeding
Amitriptyline is excreted in breast milk in concentrations equal to or greater than those in maternal serum. Approximately 1% of the ingested dose appears in the breast-feeding infant's serum. The potential benefit to the mother should outweigh the possible adverse reactions in the infant.

---

amoxapine
Asendin

- Pharmacologic classification: dibenzoxazepine, tricyclic antidepressant
- Therapeutic classification: antidepressant
- Pregnancy risk category C

How supplied
Available by prescription only
Tablets: 25 mg, 50 mg, 100 mg, 150 mg

Indications, route, and dosage
Depression associated with melancholia or psychotic symptoms; depressive phase of bipolar disorder; depression associated with organic disease or alcoholism; psychoneurotic anxiety; mixed symptoms of anxiety or depression
Adults: Initial dosage is 50 mg P.O. t.i.d; may increase to 100 mg t.i.d. on third day of treatment. Increases above 300 mg daily should be made only if this dosage has been ineffective during a trial period of at least 2 weeks. When effective dosage is established, entire dosage (not exceeding 300 mg) may be given h.s. Maximum dosage is 600 mg in hospitalized patients.
   Do not give more than 300 mg in a single dose.
Elderly patients: Initiate therapy at 25 mg P.O. b.i.d. or t.i.d. If necessary, dosage may be increased after the first week of therapy to 50 mg b.i.d. or t.i.d. Most patients respond to 100 to 150 mg daily, but some require up to 300 mg daily. For maintenance, reduce dosage to lowest effective level.

Pharmacodynamics
Antidepressant action: Amoxapine is thought to exert its antidepressant effects by inhibiting reuptake of norepinephrine and serotonin in CNS nerve terminals (presynaptic neurons), which results in increased concentrations and enhanced activity of these neurotransmitters in the synaptic cleft. Amoxapine has a greater inhibitory effect on norepinephrine reuptake than on serotonin. Amoxapine also blocks CNS dopamine receptors, which may account for the higher incidence of movement disorders during amoxapine therapy.

Pharmacokinetics

- *Absorption:* Amoxapine is absorbed rapidly and completely from the GI tract after oral administration.
- *Distribution:* Amoxapine is distributed widely into the body, including the CNS and breast milk. Drug is 92% protein-bound. Peak effect occurs in 8 to 10 hours; steady state, within 2 to 7 days. Proposed therapeutic plasma levels (parent drug and metabolite) range from 200 to 400 ng/ml.
- *Metabolism:* Amoxapine is metabolized by the liver to the active metabolite 8-hydroxyamoxapine; a significant first-pass effect may explain variability of serum concentrations in different patients taking the same dosage.
- *Excretion:* Amoxapine is excreted in urine and feces (7% to 18%); about 60% of a given dose is excreted as the conjugated form within 6 days.

Contraindications and precautions

Amoxapine is contraindicated in patients with known hypersensitivity to TCAs, trazodone, or related compounds; in the acute recovery phase of MI because of its potential arrhythmogenic effects; in patients in coma or severe respiratory depression because of additive CNS depression; and during or within 14 days of MAO therapy.

Amoxapine should be used cautiously in patients with other cardiac disease (arrhythmias, CHF, angina pectoris, valvular disease, or heart block); respiratory disorders; seizure disorders; scheduled electroconvulsive therapy; bipolar disease; glaucoma; hyperthyroidism or in those taking thyroid hormone replacement; Type I and Type II diabetes; prostatic hypertrophy, paralytic ileus, or urine retention; hepatic or renal dysfunction; Parkinson's disease; and in those undergoing surgery with general anesthesia. Caution also is recommended in patients with tardive dyskinesia, because amoxapine may induce or exacerbate this disorder.

Interactions

Concomitant use of amoxapine with sympathomimetics, including epinephrine, phenylephrine, phenylpropanolamine, and ephedrine (often found in nasal sprays) may increase blood pressure; use with warfarin may increase prothrombin time and cause bleeding.

Concomitant use with thyroid medication, pimozide, and antiarrhythmic agents (quinidine, disopyramide, procainamide) may increase the incidence of cardiac arrhythmias and conduction defects.

Amoxapine may decrease hypotensive effects of centrally acting antihypertensive drugs such as guanethidine, guanabenz, guanadrel, clonidine, methyldopa, and reserpine.

Concomitant use with disulfiram or ethchlorvynol may cause delirium and tachycardia.

Additive effects are likely after concomitant use of amoxapine with CNS depressants, including alcohol, analgesics, barbiturates, narcotics, tranquilizers, and anesthetics (oversedation); atropine or other anticholinergic drugs, including phenothiazines, antihistamines, meperidine, and antiparkinsonian agents (oversedation, paralytic ileus, visual changes, and severe constipation); or metrizamide (increased risk of seizures).

Barbiturates and heavy smoking induce amoxapine metabolism and decrease therapeutic efficacy; phenothiazines and haloperidol decrease its metabolism, decreasing therapeutic efficacy. Methylphenidate, cimetidine, oral contraceptives, propoxyphene, and beta blockers may inhibit amoxapine metabolism, increasing plasma levels and toxicity.

Effects on diagnostic tests

Amoxapine may prolong conduction time (elongation of QT and PR intervals, flattened T waves on ECG); it also may elevate liver function test results, decrease WBC counts, and decrease or increase serum glucose levels.

Adverse reactions

- CNS: drowsiness, dizziness, sedation, excitation, tremors, weakness, headache, nervousness, *seizures* (especially pronounced with this drug), peripheral neuropathy, extrapyramidal symptoms (numbness, tingling, ataxia, tardive dyskinesia, in 1% of patients), anxiety, vivid dreams, confusion (more marked in elderly patients).
- CV: orthostatic hypotension, tachycardia, *arrhythmias, MI, stroke, heart block, CHF,* palpitations, hypertension, ECG changes.
- EENT: blurred vision, tinnitus, mydriasis, increased intraocular pressure.
- Endocrine: breast enlargement or gynecomastia, testicular edema, sexual dysfunction.
- GI: dry mouth, constipation, nausea, vomiting, anorexia, diarrhea, paralytic ileus, jaundice.
- GU: urine retention.
- Other: sweating, photosensitivity, hypersensitivity (rash, urticaria, drug fever, edema).

After abrupt withdrawal of long-term therapy, nausea, headache, malaise (does not indicate addiction).

Note: Drug should be discontinued (not abruptly) if signs of hypersensitivity occur. Re-

---

evaluate therapy if the following reactions occur: urine retention, extreme dry mouth, rash, excessive sedation, seizures, tachycardia, sore throat, fever, tardive dyskinesia, or jaundice.

Overdose and treatment

The first 12 hours after acute ingestion are a stimulatory phase characterized by excessive anticholinergic activity (agitation, irritation, confusion, hallucinations, hyperthermia, parkinsonian symptoms, seizures, urine retention, dry mucous membranes, pupillary dilation, constipation, and ileus). This is followed by CNS depressant effects, including hypothermia, decreased or absent reflexes, sedation, hypotension, cyanosis, and cardiac irregularities, including tachycardia, conduction disturbances, and quinidine-like effects on the ECG.

Overdose with amoxapine produces a much higher incidence of CNS toxicity than do other antidepressants. Acute deterioration of renal function (evidenced by myoglobin in urine) occurs in 5% of overdosed patients; this is most likely to occur in patients with repeated seizures after the overdose. Seizures may progress to status epilepticus within 12 hours.

Severity of overdose is best indicated by widening of the QRS complex, which generally represents a serum level in excess of 1,000 ng/ml; serum concentrations are not usually helpful. Metabolic acidosis may follow hypotension, hypoventilation, and seizures.

Treatment is symptomatic and supportive, including maintaining a patent airway, stable body temperature, and fluid and electrolyte balance; monitoring vital signs and ECG; and monitoring renal status because of the risk of renal failure. Induce emesis with ipecac syrup if patient is conscious; follow with gastric lavage and activated charcoal to prevent further absorption. Dialysis is of little use. Treat seizures with parenteral diazepam or phenytoin; arrhythmias, with parenteral phenytoin or lidocaine; and acidosis, with sodium bicarbonate. *Do not give barbiturates;* these may enhance CNS and respiratory depressant effects.

▶ Special considerations

Besides those relevant to all *TCAs*, consider the following recommendations.
● Amoxapine is associated with a high incidence of seizures.
● The full dose may be given at bedtime to help reduce daytime sedation.
● The full dose should not be withdrawn abruptly.

● Tolerance to sedative effects usually develops over the first few weeks of therapy.
● The drug should be discontinued at least 48 hours before surgical procedures.
● Chewing gum, hard candy, or ice chips may alleviate dry mouth.
● Tardive dyskinesia and other extrapyramidal effects may occur because of amoxapine's dopamine-blocking activity. Elderly patients appear to be more susceptible to these effects.
● Watch for gynecomastia in males and females since amoxapine may increase cellular division in breast tissue.

Information for the patient

● Explain that the full effects of the drug may not become apparent for 2 to 4 weeks after initiation of therapy.
● Tell patient to take the medication exactly as prescribed; however, the full dose may be taken at bedtime to alleviate daytime sedation. Patient should not double dose for missed ones.
● Warn patient that drug may cause drowsiness or dizziness. Patient should avoid hazardous activities that require alertness until the full effects of the drug are known.
● Tell patient not to drink alcoholic beverages while taking this drug.
● Suggest taking drug with food or milk if it causes stomach upset and relieving dry mouth with ice chips, gum, or hard candy.
● After initial doses, patient should lie down for about 30 minutes and rise slowly to prevent dizziness.
● Warn patient not to stop taking drug abruptly.
● Encourage patient to report any unusual or troublesome reactions immediately, especially confusion, movement disorders, rapid heartbeat, dizziness, fainting, or difficulty urinating.
● Warn patient of the risks of tardive dyskinesia. Tell patient what symptoms to look for.
● Tell patient that exposure to sunlight, sunlamps, or tanning beds may cause burning of the skin or abnormal pigmentary changes. Advise patient to wear protective clothing and use a sunscreen.

Geriatric use

● Lower doses are indicated because older patients are more sensitive to the therapeutic and adverse effects of the drug. Recommended starting dose is 25 mg t.i.d.
● Elderly patients are much more susceptible to tardive dyskinesia and extrapyramidal symptoms.

Pediatric use
Not recommended for patients under age 16.

Breast-feeding
Amoxapine is excreted in breast milk in concentrations of 20% of maternal serum as parent drug and 30% as metabolites. The potential benefits to the mother should outweigh the possible adverse reactions in the infant.

---

bupropion hydrochloride
Wellbutrin

- Pharmacologic classification: aminoketone
- Therapeutic classification: antidepressant
- Pregnancy risk category B

How supplied
Available by prescription only
Tablets: 75 mg, 100 mg

Indications, route, and dosage
Depression
Adults: Initially, 100 mg P.O. b.i.d. If necessary, increase after 3 days to usual dosage of 100 mg P.O. t.i.d. If there is no response after several weeks of therapy, consider increasing dosage to 150 mg t.i.d.

Pharmacodynamics
Antidepressant action: The mechanism of action is unknown. Bupropion does not inhibit MAO; it is a weak inhibitor of norepinephrine, dopamine, and serotonin reuptake.

Pharmacokinetics
- *Absorption:* Animal studies indicate that only 5% to 20% of the drug is bioavailable. Peak plasma levels are achieved within 2 hours.
- *Distribution:* At plasma concentrations up to 200 mcg/ml, the drug appears to be about 80% bound to plasma proteins.
- *Metabolism:* Probably hepatic; several active metabolites have been identified. With prolonged use, the active metabolites are expected to accumulate in the plasma, and their concentration may exceed that of the parent compound. Bupropion appears to induce its own metabolism.
- *Excretion:* Primarily renal; elimination half-life of the parent compound in single-dose studies ranged from 8 to 24 hours.

Contraindications and precautions
Bupropion is contraindicated in patients who are allergic to the drug, patients who have taken MAO inhibitors within the previous 14 days, and patients with a seizure disorder. About 0.4% of patients treated at dosages up to 450 mg/day may experience seizures. If dosage increases to 600 mg/day, the incidence of seizures increases about tenfold.

Bupropion is also contraindicated in patients with a history of bulimia or anorexia nervosa because studies have revealed a higher incidence of seizures in these patients. Studies have also shown that patients who experience seizures often have predisposing factors (including histories of head trauma, prior seizure, or CNS tumors), or they may be taking a drug that lowers the seizure threshold.

Use cautiously in psychosis; in suicidal patients; patients with hepatic, renal or cardiac disease; and in elderly or debilitated patients.

Interactions
Concomitant administration with theophylline derivatives, levodopa, neuroleptics, MAO inhibitors, or TCAs or recent and rapid withdrawal of benzodiazepines may increase the risk of adverse reactions, including seizures. Animal studies suggest that bupropion may induce drug-metabolizing enzymes.

Effects on diagnostic tests
None reported.

Adverse reactions
- CNS: headache, akathisia, agitation, anxiety, confusion, decreased libido, delusions, euphoria, hostility, impaired sleep quality, insomnia, sedation, sensory disturbance, tremors.
- CV: arrhythmias, hypertension, hypotension, palpitations, syncope, tachycardia.
- DERM: pruritus, rash, cutaneous temperature disturbance.
- EENT: auditory disturbance, blurred vision.
- GI: appetite increase, constipation, dyspepsia, nausea, vomiting, dry mouth.
- GU: impotence, menstrual complaints, urinary frequency.
- Other: arthritis, fever and chills, excessive sweating, dysgeusia.
Note: In a controlled study, the above adverse reactions were reported more frequently in patients taking bupropion than in control subjects and reflect events reported by at least 1% of the study population.

Overdose and treatment

Signs of overdose include labored breathing, salivation, arched back, ptosis, ataxia, and seizures.

If the ingestion was recent, empty the stomach using gastric lavage or induce emesis with ipecac syrup, as appropriate; follow with activated charcoal. Treatment should be supportive. Monitor EEG and ECG for 48 hours after ingestion. Control seizures with I.V. benzodiazepines; stuporous, comatose, or convulsing patients may need intubation. There is no data to evaluate the benefits of dialysis, hemoperfusion, or diuresis.

▶ **Special considerations**
● Bupropion is usually reserved for use in patients who cannot tolerate or do not respond to other agents.
● Implement antiseizure precautions as necessary and appropriate.
● Periodically review usefulness of the drug during long-term therapy. Effectiveness of treatment of more than 6 weeks has not been evaluated.
● Many patients experience a period of increased restlessness, especially at initiation of therapy. This may include agitation, insomnia, and anxiety. In clinical studies, these symptoms required sedative-hypnotic agents in some patients; about 2% had to discontinue the drug.
● Antidepressants can cause manic episodes during the depressed phase in patients with bipolar disorder.
● Clinical trials revealed that 28% of the patients experienced a weight loss of 5 lb (2.3 kg) or more. This effect should be considered if weight loss is a major factor in the patient's depressive illness.

Information for the patient
● Advise the patient to take the drug regularly as scheduled and to take each day's dosage in three divided doses to minimize the risk of seizures.
● Warn patient to avoid the use of alcohol, which may contribute to the development of seizures.
● Advise the patient to avoid activities that require alertness and coordination until the CNS effects of the drug are known.
● Patient should not take any other medications, including OTC medications, without medical approval.
● Tell the patient that up to 4 weeks may be required before maximal clinical response is seen.
● Safe use during pregnancy has not been es-

tablished. Advise patient to report pregnancy to the physician immediately.

Geriatric use
No information available.

Pediatric use
Safety in children under age 18 has not been established.

Breast-feeding
Because of the potential for serious adverse reactions in the infant, breast-feeding during therapy is not recommended.

---

clomipramine hydrochloride
Anafranil

● Pharmacologic classification: tricyclic derivative
● Therapeutic classification: antiobsessional agent
● Pregnancy risk category C

How supplied
Available by prescription only
Capsules: 25 mg, 50 mg, 75 mg

Indications, route, and dosage
Treatment of obsessive-compulsive disorder (OCD)
Adults: Initially, 25 mg P.O. daily, gradually increasing to 100 mg P.O. daily (in divided doses, with meals) during the first 2 weeks. Maximum dosage is 250 mg daily. After titration, entire daily dose may be given h.s.
Children and adolescents: Initially, 25 mg P.O. daily, gradually increased to 3 mg/kg or 100 mg P.O. daily, whichever is smaller (in divided doses with meals) over the first 2 weeks. Maximum daily dosage is 3 mg/kg or 200 mg, whichever is smaller. After titration, entire dose may be given h.s.

Pharmacodynamics
Antiobsessional action: A selective inhibitor of serotonin (5-HT) reuptake into neurons within the CNS. It may also have some blocking activity at postsynaptic dopamine receptors. The exact mechanism by which clomipramine treats OCD is unknown.

Pharmacokinetics

- *Absorption:* Well-absorbed from the GI tract, but extensive first-pass metabolism limits bioavailability to about 50%.
- *Distribution:* Distributes well into lipophilic tissues; the volume of distribution is about 12 liters/kg. It is about 98% bound to plasma proteins.
- *Metabolism:* Primarily hepatic. Several metabolites have been identified; desmethylclomipramine is the primary active metabolite.
- *Excretion:* About 66% is excreted in the urine and the remainder in the feces. Mean elimination half-life of the parent compound is about 36 hours; the elimination half-life of desmethylclomipramine may be from 4.4 to 233 days.

Contraindications and precautions

Clomipramine is contraindicated in patients with a history of hypersensitivity to clomipramine or other tricyclic antidepressants (TCAs). It is also contraindicated in combination with an MAO inhibitor and in patients who have received an MAO inhibitor within the previous 2 weeks and during the acute recovery period after MI.

Use with caution in patients with a history of seizure disorders, in patients with brain damage, or in patients receiving other seizure threshold-lowering drugs. Use cautiously in patients who are at risk for suicide; in patients who are hyperthyroid or are receiving thyroid medication; in patients with urine retention; in patients with narrow-angle glaucoma or increased intraocular pressure, CV disease, impaired hepatic or renal function, tumors of the adrenal medulla, or acute intermittent porphyria; elderly or debilitated patients; and those who are receiving electroconvulsive therapy or electrocautery.

Safe use during pregnancy and lactation has not been established.

Interactions

Concomitant administration of MAO inhibitors with TCAs may cause hyperpyretic crisis, seizures, coma, and death.

Concurrent use of barbiturates increases the activity of hepatic microsomal enzymes with repeated doses and may decrease TCA blood levels. Monitor for decreased effectiveness. Barbiturates, alcohol, and other CNS depressants may cause an exaggerated depressant effect when used concomitantly with TCA derivatives.

Methylphenidate may increase TCA blood levels.

Epinephrine and norepinephrine may produce increased hypertensive effect in patients taking TCAs.

Effects on diagnostic tests

None reported.

Adverse reactions

- CNS: somnolence, tremors, headache, insomnia, libido change, nervousness, myoclonus, increased appetite, fatigue.
- CV: postural hypotension, palpitations, tachycardia.
- DERM: increased sweating, rash, pruritus.
- EENT: otitis media (children), blurred vision, pharyngitis, rhinitis.
- GI: dry mouth, constipation, nausea, dyspepsia, diarrhea, anorexia, abdominal pain.
- GU: micturition disorder, urinary tract infection, dysmenorrhea, impotence, ejaculation failure.
- Other: myalgia.

Overdose and treatment

Signs and symptoms of clomipramine overdose are similar to those of other TCAs and have included sinus tachycardia, intraventricular block, hypotension, irritability, fixed and dilated pupils, drowsiness, delirium, stupor, hyperreflexia, and hyperpyrexia. Monitor vital signs and ECG closely and protect the airway. Treatment for recent ingestion should include gastic lavage with large quantities of fluid followed by activated charcoal. Lavage should be continued for 12 hours because the anticholinergic effects of the drug slow gastric emptying. Hemodialysis, peritoneal dialysis, and forced diuresis are ineffective because of the high degree of plasma protein binding. Treat shock with plasma expanders or corticosteroids; treat seizures with diazepam. Some clinicians may cautiously use physostigmine to reverse the central anticholinergic effects.

▶ Special considerations

- Clomipramine may also be used by some clinicians in panic disorder or phobic disorder, but only if OCD is the primary diagnosis and dominates the clinical picture.
- To minimize the risk of overdose, this drug should be dispensed in small quantities.
- Monitor for urine retention and constipation. Suggest stool softener or high-fiber diet, as needed, and encourage adequate fluid intake.
- Do not withdraw drug abruptly.

Information for the patient

- Warn patient to avoid hazardous activities that require alertness or good psychomotor coordination until adverse CNS effects are known. This is especially important during initial titration when daytime sedation and dizziness may occur.
- Tell patient to avoid alcohol and other depressants during treatment.
- Patient may relieve dry mouth with ice chips, sugarless candy or gum, or saliva substitutes.
- Tell patient adverse GI effects can be minimize by taking the drug with meals during titration. Later, the entire daily dose may be taken at bedtime to limit daytime drowsiness.
- Tell patient to avoid using OTC medications, particularly antihistamines and decongestants, unless recommended by physician or pharmacist.
- Emphasize the importance of taking the drug as prescribed even if feeling better. Tell patient not to discontinue the drug abruptly but to contact physician if adverse reactions become troublesome.
- Tell patient to wear protective clothing and use a sunscreen to protect from sunburn.
- Advise patient to report the following adverse reactions immediately: sore throat, fever, malaise, unusual bleeding, easy bruising, persistent nausea or vomiting, or difficulty in urinating.

Breast-feeding

It is not known if the drug is excreted in breast milk. Use with caution in breast-feeding women.

---

desipramine hydrochloride
Norpramin, Pertofrane

- Pharmacologic classification: dibenzazepine tricyclic antidepressant
- Therapeutic classification: antidepressant, anxiolytic
- Pregnancy risk category C

How supplied

Available by prescription only
Tablets: 10 mg, 25 mg, 50 mg, 75 mg, 100 mg, 150 mg
Capsules: 25 mg, 50 mg

Indications, route, and dosage

Endogenous depression; major depression with melancholia or psychotic symptoms; depression associated with organic disease, alcoholism, schizophrenia, or mental retardation; depressive phase of bipolar disorder
Adults: 75 to 150 mg P.O. daily in divided doses, increasing to a maximum of 300 mg daily. Alternatively, the entire dosage can be given h.s.
Elderly patients and adolescents: 25 to 50 mg P.O. daily, increasing gradually to a maximum of 100 mg daily. Give in divided doses throughout the day or as a single dose h.s.
†*Attention deficit disorder*
Children: 1 to 6 mg/kg P.O. daily; usual dose is 3.5 mg/kg daily.

Pharmacodynamics

Antidepressant action: Desipramine is thought to exert its antidepressant effects by inhibiting reuptake of norepinephrine and serotonin in CNS nerve terminals (presynaptic neurons), which results in increased concentrations and enhanced activity of these neurotransmitters in the synaptic cleft. Desipramine more strongly inhibits reuptake of norepinephrine than serotonin; it has a lesser incidence of sedative effects and less anticholinergic and hypotensive activity than its parent compound, imipramine.

Pharmacokinetics

- *Absorption:* Desipramine is absorbed rapidly from the GI tract after oral administration.
- *Distribution:* Desipramine is distributed widely into the body, including the CNS and breast milk. Drug is 90% protein-bound. Peak effect occurs in 4 to 6 hours; steady state, within 2 to 11 days, with full therapeutic effect in 2 to 4 weeks.
- *Metabolism:* Desipramine is metabolized by the liver; a significant first-pass effect may explain variability of serum concentrations in different patients taking the same dosage.
- *Excretion:* Drug is excreted primarily in urine.

Contraindications and precautions

Desipramine is contraindicated in patients with known hypersensitivity to TCAs, trazodone, and related compounds; in the acute recovery phase of MI because of its potential arrhythmogenic effects and ECG changes; in patients in coma or severe respiratory depression because of added CNS depressant effects; and during or within 14 days of therapy with MAO inhibitors.
Desipramine should be used cautiously in patients with other cardiac disease (arrhythmias,

---

CHF, angina pectoris, valvular disease, or heart block); respiratory disorders; seizure disorders; scheduled electroconvulsive therapy; bipolar disease, glaucoma, hyperthyroidism, or patients taking thyroid hormone replacement; Type I and Type II diabetes; prostatic hypertrophy, paralytic ileus, or urine retention; hepatic or renal dysfunction; Parkinson's disease; and in those undergoing surgery with general anesthesia.

Use cautiously in pregnant and lactating patients because safety has not been established. Although the drug has been used for attention deficit disorder, it should be used cautiously in children because limited studies have not established safety and efficacy.

If product contains tartrazine, drug may precipitate asthma in patients with aspirin allergy.

Interactions
Concomitant use of desipramine with sympathomimetics, including epinephrine, phenylephrine, phenylpropanolamine, and ephedrine (often found in nasal sprays) may increase blood pressure; use with warfarin may increase prothrombin time and cause bleeding.

Concomitant use with thyroid medication, pimozide, or antiarrhythmic agents (quinidine, disopyramide, procainamide) may increase incidence of cardiac arrhythmias and conduction defects.

Desipramine may decrease hypotensive effects of centrally acting antihypertensive drugs, such as guanethidine, guanabenz, guanadrel, clonidine, methyldopa, and reserpine. Concomitant use with disulfiram or ethchlorvynol may cause delirium and tachycardia. Additive effects are likely after concomitant use of desipramine and CNS depressants, including alcohol, analgesics, barbiturates, narcotics, tranquilizers, and anesthetics (oversedation); atropine and other anticholinergic drugs, including phenothiazines, antihistamines, meperidine, and antiparkinsonian agents (oversedation, paralytic ileus, visual changes, and severe constipation); and metrizamide (increased risk of seizures).

Barbiturates and heavy smoking induce desipramine metabolism and decrease therapeutic efficacy; phenothiazines and haloperidol decrease its metabolism, decreasing therapeutic efficacy. Methylphenidate, cimetidine, oral contraceptives, propoxyphene, and beta blockers may inhibit desipramine metabolism, increasing plasma levels and toxicity.

Effects on diagnostic tests
Desipramine may prolong conduction time (elongation of QT and PR intervals, flattened T waves on ECG); it also may elevate liver function test results, decrease WBC counts, and decrease or increase serum glucose levels.

Adverse reactions
● CNS: drowsiness, dizziness, sedation, excitation, tremors, weakness, headache, nervousness, *seizures,* peripheral neuropathy, extrapyramidal symptoms, anxiety, vivid dreams, confusion (more marked in elderly patients).
● CV: orthostatic hypotension, tachycardia, *arrhythmias, MI, stroke, heart block, CHF,* palpitations, hypertension (including some surgical patients), ECG changes.
● EENT: blurred vision, tinnitus, mydriasis, increased intraocular pressure.
● GI: dry mouth, constipation, nausea, vomiting, anorexia, diarrhea, paralytic ileus, jaundice.
● GU: urine retention.
● Other: sweating, photosensitivity, hypersensitivity (rash, urticaria, drug fever, edema).

After abrupt withdrawal of long-term therapy, nausea, headache, and malaise (does not indicate addiction) may occur.

Note: Drug should be discontinued (not abruptly) if signs of hypersensitivity occur. Monitor carefully for the following: urine retention, extreme dry mouth, rash, excessive sedation, seizures, tachycardia, sore throat, fever, or jaundice. Dizziness, fatigue, or orthostatic hypotension may indicate need for reduced dosage.

Overdose and treatment
The first 12 hours after acute ingestion are a stimulatory phase characterized by excessive anticholinergic activity (agitation, irritation, confusion, hallucinations, parkinsonian symptoms, hyperthermia, seizures, urine retention, dry mucous membranes, pupillary dilation, constipation, and ileus). This is followed by CNS depressant effects, including hypothermia, decreased or absent reflexes, sedation, hypotension, cyanosis, and cardiac irregularities, including tachycardia, conduction disturbances, and quinidine-like effects on the ECG.

Severity of overdose is best indicated by widening of the QRS complex, which usually represents a serum level in excess of 1,000 ng/ml; serum levels are generally not helpful. Metabolic acidosis may follow hypotension, hypoventilation, and seizures.

Treatment is symptomatic and supportive, including maintaining a patent airway, stable body temperature, and fluid and electrolyte balance. Closely monitor vital signs and ECG. Induce emesis with ipecac syrup if patient is conscious;

follow with gastric lavage and activated charcoal to prevent further absorption. Dialysis is of little use. Treat seizures with parenteral diazepam or phenytoin; arrhythmias, with parenteral phenytoin or lidocaine; and acidosis, with sodium bicarbonate. *Do not give barbiturates;* these may enhance CNS and respiratory depressant effects. Hyperpyrexia may be controlled with cooling measures such as ice packs or cold baths.

Monitor cardiac function for at least 5 days.

▶ **Special considerations**
Besides those relevant to all *TCAs,* consider the following recommendations.
● Check standing and sitting blood pressure to assess orthostasis before administering desipramine.
● Desipramine has a lesser incidence of sedative effects and less anticholinergic and hypotensive effects than its parent compound imipramine.
● The full dose may be given at bedtime to help offset daytime sedation.
● Tolerance usually develops to the sedative effects of the drug during the initial weeks of therapy.
● The drug should not be withdrawn abruptly, but tapered gradually over time.
● The drug should be discontinued at least 48 hours before surgical procedures.

Information for the patient
● Tell patient that full dose may be taken at bedtime to alleviate daytime sedation.
● Explain that the full effects of the drug may not become apparent for 4 weeks or more after initiation of therapy.
● Tell patient to take the medication exactly as prescribed and not to double dose for missed ones.
● Tell patient that heavy smoking may decrease the effectiveness of the drug.
● To prevent dizziness, advise patient to lie down for about 30 minutes after each dose at start of therapy and to avoid sudden postural changes, especially when rising to upright position.
● Warn patient not to stop taking drug abruptly.
● Encourage patient to report any unusual or troublesome effects, especially confusion, movement disorders, rapid heartbeat, dizziness, fainting, or difficulty urinating.
● Tell patient to wear protective clothing and use a sunscreen to minimize risk of sunburn.
● Tell patient chewing gum, sugarless hard candy, or ice chips may alleviate dry mouth.
● Stress importance of regular dental hygiene to avoid caries.

● Warn patient to avoid alcohol while taking this medication.
● Warn patient to notify physician promptly if she suspects pregnancy.

Geriatric use
Elderly patients may be more susceptible to adverse cardiac reactions.

Pediatric use
Drug is not routinely recommended for patients under age 12. However, some clinicians may use it for attention deficit disorder in younger children.

Breast-feeding
Desipramine is excreted in breast milk in concentrations equal to those in maternal serum. The potential benefit to the mother should outweigh the possible adverse reactions in the infant.

---

doxepin hydrochloride
Adapin, Sinequan, Triadapin∗

● Pharmacologic classification: tricyclic antidepressant
● Therapeutic classification: antidepressant
● Pregnancy risk category C

How supplied
Available by prescription only
Tablets: 10 mg, 25 mg, 50 mg, 75 mg, 100 mg, 150 mg
Oral concentrate: 10 mg/ml

Indications, route, and dosage
Endogenous depression; major depression with melancholia or psychotic symptoms; depression associated with organic disease, alcoholism, schizophrenia, or mental retardation; depressive phase of bipolar disorder; moderate to severe anxiety
Adults: Initially, 50 to 75 mg P.O. daily in divided doses to a maximum of 300 mg daily. Up to 150 mg may be taken h.s.
Mild to moderate anxiety or depression
Adults: Initially, 10 to 25 mg P.O. t.i.d.; adjust dosage according to patient response. Usual optimal dose is 75 to 150 mg daily. After adjustment, total dose may be taken h.s.

Pharmacodynamics

Antidepressant action: Doxepin is thought to exert its antidepressant effects by inhibiting reuptake of norepinephrine and serotonin in CNS nerve terminals (presynaptic neurons), which results in increased levels and enhanced activity of these neurotransmitters in the synaptic cleft. Doxepin more actively inhibits reuptake of serotonin than norepinephrine. Anxiolytic effects of this drug usually precede antidepressant effects. Doxepin also may be used as an anxiolytic. Doxepin has the greatest sedative effect of all TCAs; tolerance to this effect usually develops in a few weeks.

Pharmacokinetics

● *Absorption:* Doxepin is absorbed rapidly from the GI tract after oral administration.
● *Distribution:* Doxepin is distributed widely into the body, including the CNS and breast milk. Drug is 90% protein-bound. Peak effect occurs in 2 to 4 hours; steady state is achieved within 7 days. Therapeutic concentrations (parent drug and metabolite) are thought to range from 150 to 250 ng/ml.
● *Metabolism:* Doxepin is metabolized by the liver to the active metabolite desmethyldoxepin. A significant first-pass effect may explain variability of serum concentrations in different patients taking the same dosage.
● *Excretion:* Most of drug is excreted in urine.

Contraindications and precautions

Doxepin is contraindicated in patients with known hypersensitivity to TCAs, trazodone, and related compounds; in the acute recovery phase of MI because of its potential arrhythmogenic effects and ECG changes; in patients in coma or severe respiratory depression because of additive CNS depression; and during or within 14 days of therapy with MAO inhibitors. Doxepin is also contraindicated in breast-feeding women because of the hazard of respiratory depression in the infant.

Doxepin should be used cautiously in elderly or debilitated patients; patients with other cardiac disease (arrhythmias, CHF, angina pectoris, valvular disease, or heart block); respiratory disorders; alcoholism and seizure disorders; scheduled electroconvulsive therapy; bipolar disease; glaucoma; hyperthyroidism or in those taking thyroid hormone replacement; Type I and Type II diabetes; prostatic hypertrophy, paralytic ileus, or urine retention; hepatic or renal dysfunction; or Parkinson's disease; and in those undergoing surgery with general anesthesia.

Interactions

Concomitant use of doxepin with sympathomimetics, including epinephrine, phenylephrine, phenylpropanolamine, and ephedrine (often found in nasal sprays) may increase blood pressure; use with warfarin may increase prothrombin time and cause bleeding.

Concomitant use with thyroid medication, pimozide, and antiarrhythmic agents (quinidine, disopyramide, procainamide) may increase incidence of cardiac arrhythmias and conduction defects.

Doxepin may decrease hypotensive effects of centrally acting antihypertensive drugs, such as guanethidine, guanabenz, guanadrel, clonidine, methyldopa, and reserpine. Concomitant use with disulfiram or ethchlorvynol may cause delirium and tachycardia. Additive effects are likely after concomitant use of doxepin with CNS depressants, including alcohol, analgesics, barbiturates, narcotics, tranquilizers, and anesthetics (oversedation); atropine and other anticholinergic drugs, including phenothiazines, antihistamines, meperidine, and antiparkinsonian agents (oversedation, paralytic ileus, visual changes, and severe constipation); and metrizamide (increased risk of seizures).

Barbiturates and heavy smoking induce doxepin metabolism and decrease therapeutic efficacy; phenothiazines and haloperidol decrease its metabolism, decreasing therapeutic efficacy; methylphenidate, cimetidine, oral contraceptives, propoxyphene, and beta blockers may inhibit doxepin metabolism, increasing plasma levels and toxicity.

Effects on diagnostic tests

Doxepin may prolong conduction time (elongation of QT and PR intervals, flattened T waves on ECG); it also may elevate liver function test results, decrease WBC counts, and decrease or increase serum glucose levels.

Adverse reactions

● CNS: drowsiness, dizziness, sedation, excitation, tremors, weakness, headache, nervousness, *seizures,* peripheral neuropathy, extrapyramidal symptoms, anxiety, vivid dreams, decreased libido, confusion (more marked in elderly patients).
● CV: orthostatic hypotension, tachycardia, arrhythmias, *MI, stroke, heart block, CHF,* palpitations, hypertension, ECG changes.
● EENT: blurred vision, tinnitus, mydriasis, increased intraocular pressure.
● GI: dry mouth, constipation, nausea, vomiting, anorexia, diarrhea, paralytic ileus, jaundice.

● GU: urine retention.
● Other: sweating, photosensitivity, hypersensitivity (rash, urticaria, drug fever, edema).

After abrupt withdrawal of long-term therapy, nausea, headache, and malaise (does not indicate addiction) may occur.

Note: Drug should be discontinued (not abruptly) if signs of hypersensitivity occur, and the following reactions reported: urine retention, extreme dry mouth, rash, excessive sedation, seizures, tachycardia, sore throat, fever, or jaundice.

Overdose and treatment
The first 12 hours after acute ingestion are a stimulatory phase characterized by excessive anticholinergic activity (agitation, irritation, confusion, hallucinations, hyperthermia, parkinsonian symptoms, seizure, urine retention, dry mucous membranes, pupillary dilation, constipation, and ileus). This is followed by CNS depressant effects, including hypothermia, decreased or absent reflexes, sedation, hypotension, cyanosis, and cardiac irregularities, including tachycardia, conduction disturbances, and quinidine-like effects on the ECG.

Severity of overdose is best indicated by widening of QRS complex. Usually, this represents a serum concentration in excess of 1,000 ng/ml. Serum concentrations are usually not helpful. Metabolic acidosis may follow hypotension, hypoventilation, and seizures.

Treatment is symptomatic and supportive, including maintaining a patent airway, stable body temperature, and fluid and electrolyte balance. Induce emesis with ipecac syrup if patient is conscious; follow with gastric lavage and activated charcoal to prevent further absorption. Dialysis is of little use. Treat seizures with parenteral diazepam or phenytoin; arrhythmias, with parenteral phenytoin or lidocaine; and acidosis, with sodium bicarbonate. *Do not give barbiturates;* these may enhance CNS and respiratory depressant effects.

▶ Special considerations
● Periodically assess CBC and liver function tests during long-term therapy.
● Check patient's sitting and supine blood pressure to establish baseline before administering drug.

Information for the patient
● Teach patient to dilute oral concentrate with 120 ml water, milk, or juice (grapefruit, orange, pineapple, prune, or tomato). Drug is incompatible with carbonated beverages.

● Advise patient to avoid alcohol or other sedative drugs while taking doxepin. Drug has a strong sedative effect and such combinations can cause excessive sedation.
● Warn patient to avoid taking any other drugs while taking doxepin unless they have been prescribed.
● Instruct patient to take full dose at bedtime.
● Tell the patient that therapeutic effects may not be seen for as long as 4 weeks after initiation of therapy. Encourage patient to continue compliance.

Geriatric use
Elderly patients are more likely to develop adverse CNS reactions.

Breast-feeding
Patient should not breast-feed while taking doxepin; doxepin is excreted in breast milk, especially if taken in high doses.

---

fluoxetine hydrochloride
Prozac

● Pharmacologic classification: serotonin uptake inhibitor
● Therapeutic classification: antidepressant
● Pregnancy risk category B

How supplied
Available by prescription only
Pulvules: 20 mg

Indications, route, and dosage
Endogenous depression, major depressive illness
Adults: 20 mg P.O. daily in the morning. Increase dosage after several weeks to 40 mg daily with a dose in the morning and at noon. Do not exceed 80 mg daily.
†*Obsessive-compulsive disorder*
Adults: Initially, 20 mg daily. Titrate dosage as required; most patients need 60 to 80 mg daily.
†*Adjunctive treatment of exogenous obesity*
Adults: Initially, 20 mg P.O. daily; titrate dosage as necessary. Most clinicians have repeated dosage of 60 mg daily or less for periods up to 8 weeks.

Pharmacodynamics
Antidepressant action: The antidepressant action of fluoxetine is purportedly related to its

---

inhibition of CNS neuronal uptake of serotonin. Fluoxetine blocks uptake of serotonin, but not of norepinephrine, into human platelets. Animal studies suggest it is a much more potent uptake inhibitor of serotonin than of norepinephrine.

Pharmacokinetics

● *Absorption:* Fluoxetine is well absorbed after oral administration. Its absorption is not altered by food.
● *Distribution:* Fluoxetine is apparently highly protein-bound (about 95%). Steady-state plasma levels range from 47 to 469 ng/ml, but may not correlate well with therapeutic response.
● *Metabolism:* Fluoxetine is metabolized primarily in the liver to active metabolites.
● *Excretion:* Drug is excreted by the kidneys. Elimination half-life is 2 to 3 days. Norfluoxetine (the primary active metabolite) has an elimination half-life of 7 to 9 days.

Contraindications and precautions

Contraindicated in patients hypersensitive to the drug. In early trials, about 4% of all patients taking the drug developed a rash or urticaria, and all recovered after the drug was discontinued. Because a substantial percentage of patients taking fluoxetine may experience anxiety, nervousness, and insomnia, administer this drug early in the day to avoid sleep disturbance. Monitor changes in weight during therapy because significant weight loss may occur, especially in underweight patients.

Interactions

Concomitant use with diazepam may prolong the half-life of diazepam. Concomitant use with tryptophan may lead to increased adverse CNS effects (agitation, restlessness) and GI distress. Avoid concomitant administration with other highly protein-bound drugs (such as warfarin). Avoid concomitant administration with other psychoactive drugs (MAO inhibitors, antipsychotics).

Effects on diagnostic tests

None reported.

Adverse reactions

● CNS: headache, nervousness, insomnia, drowsiness, sedation, anxiety, tremor, dizziness, fatigue, diminished concentration, abnormal dreams, agitation.
● CV: hot flushes, palpitations.
● DERM: sweating, rash, pruritus.
● GI: nausea, diarrhea, dry mouth, anorexia, dyspepsia, constipation, abdominal pain, vomiting, taste change, flatulence, gastroenteritis.
● GU: sexual dysfunction, urinary tract infection, frequent micturition, painful menstruation.
● Musculoskeletal: back, joint, limb, or muscle pain.
● Respiratory: flulike syndrome, upper respiratory infection, pharyngitis, nasal congestion, sinusitis, cough, dyspnea, bronchitis, rhinitis.
● Other: asthenia, fever, chest pain, allergy, viral infection, limb pain, weight loss.

Overdose and treatment

Symptoms of overdose include agitation, restlessness, hypomania, and other signs of CNS excitation; and, in patients who took higher doses of fluoxetine, nausea and vomiting. Among approximately 38 reports of acute overdose with fluoxetine, two fatalities involved plasma concentrations of 4.57 mg/liter and 1.93 mg/liter. One involved 1.8 g of fluoxetine with an undetermined amount of maprotiline; another death involved combined ingestion of fluoxetine, codeine, and temazepam. One other patient developed two tonic-clonic seizures after taking 3 g of fluoxetine; these seizures remitted spontaneously and did not require treatment with anticonvulsants.

To treat fluoxetine overdose, establish and maintain a patent airway; ensure adequate oxygenation and ventilation. Activated charcoal, which may be used with sorbitol, may be as effective as emesis or lavage.

Monitor cardiac and vital signs, and provide usual supportive measures. Fluoxetine-induced seizures that do not subside spontaneously may respond to diazepam. Forced diuresis, dialysis, hemoperfusion, and exchange transfusion are unlikely to be of benefit.

▶ Special considerations

● Consider the inherent risk of suicide until significant improvement of depressive state occurs. High-risk patients should have close supervision during initial drug therapy. To reduce risk of suicidal overdose, prescribe the smallest quantity of pulvules consistent with good management.
● Full antidepressant effect may be delayed until 4 weeks of treatment or longer.
● Treatment of acute depression usually requires at least several months of continuous drug therapy; optimal duration of therapy has not been established.
● Impaired hepatic function can delay the elimination of fluoxetine and its metabolite norfluoxetine, prolonging the drug's elimination half-life.

Therefore, use fluoxetine with caution in patients with liver disease.

● In patients with severely impaired renal function, chronic administration of fluoxetine is associated with significant accumulation of this drug or its metabolites.

● Prescribe lower or less frequent dosage in patients with renal or hepatic impairment. Also consider lower or less frequent dosage in elderly patients and others with concurrent disease or multiple drug therapy.

● Because of its long elimination half-life, changes in fluoxetine dosage will not be reflected in plasma for several weeks, affecting titration to final dose and withdrawal from treatment.

Information for the patient

● Tell patient drug may cause dizziness or drowsiness. Patient should avoid hazardous tasks that require alertness until CNS response to drug is established.

● Tell patient to avoid ingestion of alcohol and to seek medical approval before taking other drugs.

● Tell patient to promptly report rash or hives, anxiety or nervousness, anorexia (especially in underweight patients), suspicion of pregnancy, or intent to become pregnant.

● Tell patient to notify physician of sexual dysfunction. Dosage adjustment may correct this problem.

---

imipramine hydrochloride
Apo-Imipramine∗, Impril∗, Janimine, Novopramine∗, Tofranil

imipramine pamoate
Tofranil-PM

● Pharmacologic classification: dibenzazepine tricyclic antidepressant
● Therapeutic classification: antidepressant
● Pregnancy risk category D

How supplied
Available by prescription only
Tablets: 10 mg, 25 mg, 50 mg
Capsules: 75 mg, 100 mg, 125 mg, 150 mg
Injection: 12.5 mg/ml

Indications, route, and dosage
Depression, †*anxiety,* †*neurogenic pain,* †*panic disorder,* †*chronic pain syndromes*
Adults: Initially, 75 to 100 mg P.O. or I.M. daily in divided doses, with 25- to 50-mg increments, up to 200 mg. Alternatively, some patients can start with lower doses (25 mg P.O.) and titrate slowly in 25-mg increments every other day. Maximum dosage is 300 mg daily. Alternatively, the entire dosage may be given h.s. (I.M. route rarely used.) Maximum dosage: 200 mg daily for outpatients, 300 mg daily for inpatients, and 100 mg daily for elderly patients.
†*Attention deficit disorder*
Children: 2.5 to 5 mg/kg P.O. daily.

Pharmacodynamics
Antidepressant action: Imipramine is thought to exert its antidepressant effects by inhibiting reuptake of norepinephrine and serotonin in CNS nerve terminals (presynaptic neurons), which results in increased concentrations and enhanced activity of these neurotransmitters in the synaptic cleft. Imipramine also has anticholinergic activity and is used to treat nocturnal enuresis in children over age 6.

Pharmacokinetics
● *Absorption:* Imipramine is absorbed rapidly from the GI tract and muscle tissue after oral and I.M. administration.
● *Distribution:* Imipramine is distributed widely into the body, including the CNS and breast milk. Drug is 90% protein-bound. Peak effect occurs in ½ to 2 hours; steady state is achieved within 2 to 5 days. Therapeutic plasma levels (parent drug and metabolite) are thought to range from 150 to 300 ng/ml.
● *Metabolism:* Imipramine is metabolized by the liver to the active metabolite desipramine. A significant first-pass effect may explain variability of serum concentrations in different patients taking the same dosage.
● *Excretion:* Most of drug is excreted in urine.

Contraindications and precautions
Imipramine is contraindicated in patients with known hypersensitivity to TCAs, trazodone, and related compounds; in the acute recovery phase of MI because of its arrhythmogenic potential; in patients in coma or severe respiratory depression because of additive CNS depression; and during or within 14 days of therapy with MAO inhibitors.

Imipramine should be used cautiously in patients with other cardiac disease (arrhythmias,

---

CHF, angina pectoris, valvular disease, increased QRS intervals, or heart block); respiratory disorders; seizure disorders; scheduled electroconvulsive therapy; bipolar disease; glaucoma; hyperthyroidism or in those taking thyroid hormone replacement; Type I and Type II diabetes; prostatic hypertrophy, paralytic ileus, or urine retention; hepatic or renal dysfunction; Parkinson's disease; and in those undergoing surgery with general anesthesia.

Some formulations contain tartrazine and may provoke asthma in patients with aspirin allergy.

Interactions

Concomitant use of imipramine with sympathomimetics, including epinephrine, phenylephrine, phenylpropanolamine, and ephedrine (often found in nasal sprays) may increase blood pressure; use with warfarin may increase prothrombin time and cause bleeding. Concomitant use with thyroid medication, pimozide, and antiarrhythmic agents (quinidine, disopyramide, procainamide) may increase incidence of cardiac arrhythmias and conduction defects.

Imipramine may decrease hypotensive effects of centrally acting antihypertensive drugs, such as guanethidine, guanabenz, guanadrel, clonidine, methyldopa, and reserpine. Concomitant use with disulfiram or ethchlorvynol may cause delirium and tachycardia.

Additive effects are likely after concomitant use of imipramine with CNS depressants, including alcohol, analgesics, barbiturates, narcotics, tranquilizers, and anesthetics (oversedation); atropine or other anticholinergic drugs, including phenothiazines, antihistamines, meperidine, and antiparkinsonian agents (oversedation, paralytic ileus, visual changes, and severe constipation); or metrizamide (increased risk of seizures).

Barbiturates and heavy smoking induce imipramine metabolism and decrease therapeutic efficacy; phenothiazines and haloperidol decrease its metabolism, decreasing therapeutic efficacy. Methylphenidate, cimetidine, oral contraceptives, propoxyphene, and beta blockers may inhibit imipramine metabolism, increasing plasma levels and toxicity.

Effects on diagnostic tests

Imipramine may prolong conduction time (elongation of QT and PR intervals, flattened T waves on ECG); it also may elevate liver function test results, decrease WBC counts, and decrease or increase serum glucose levels.

Adverse reactions

● CNS: drowsiness, dizziness, sedation, excitation, tremor, weakness, headache, nervousness, *seizures*, peripheral neuropathy, extrapyramidal symptoms, anxiety, vivid dreams, confusion (more marked in elderly patients), decreased libido, sexual dysfunction.
● CV: orthostatic hypotension, tachycardia, arrhythmias, *MI, stroke, heart block, CHF*, palpitations, hypertension, ECG changes.
● EENT: blurred vision, tinnitus, mydriasis, increased intraocular pressure.
● GI: dry mouth, constipation, nausea, vomiting, anorexia, diarrhea, paralytic ileus, jaundice.
● GU: urine retention.
● Other: sweating, photosensitivity, hypersensitivity (rash, urticaria, drug fever, edema).

After abrupt withdrawal of long-term therapy, nausea, headache, or malaise (does not indicate addiction) may occur.

Note: Drug should be discontinued (not abruptly) if signs of hypersensitivity occur such as urine retention, extreme dry mouth, rash, excessive sedation, seizures, tachycardia, sore throat, fever, or jaundice.

Overdose and treatment

Imipramine overdose is frequently life-threatening, particularly when combined with alcohol. The first 12 hours after acute ingestion are a stimulatory phase characterized by excessive anticholinergic activity (agitation, irritation, confusion, hallucinations, hyperthermia, parkinsonian symptoms, seizure, urine retention, dry mucous membranes, pupillary dilation, constipation, and ileus). This is followed by CNS depressant effects, including hypothermia, decreased or absent reflexes, sedation, hypotension, cyanosis, and cardiac irregularities, including tachycardia, conduction disturbances, and quinidine-like effects on the ECG.

Severity of overdose is best indicated by widening of the QRS complex, which usually represents a serum level in excess of 1,000 ng/ml; serum concentrations are usually not helpful. Metabolic acidosis may follow hypotension, hypoventilation, and seizures.

Treatment is symptomatic and supportive, including maintaining a patent airway, stable body temperature, and fluid or electrolyte balance. Monitor vital signs and ECG. Induce emesis with ipecac syrup if patient is conscious; follow with gastric lavage and activated charcoal to prevent further absorption. Dialysis is of little use. Treat seizures with parenteral diazepam or phenytoin; arrhythmias, with parenteral phenytoin or lidocaine; and acidosis, with sodium bicarbonate. *Do not give barbiturates;* these may enhance CNS and respiratory depressant effects.

► **Special considerations**
Besides those relevant to all *TCAs,* consider the following recommendations.
• Imipramine may be used to treat nocturnal enuresis in children.
• Imipramine is associated with a high incidence of orthostatic hypotension. Check sitting and standing blood pressures after initial dose.
• Do not give the full daily dosage at one time.
• I.M. administration may result in a more rapid onset of action than that with oral administration. However, oral therapy should be substituted for parenteral therapy as soon as possible.
• Drug should not be withdrawn abruptly, but tapered gradually over time.
• Do not give drug I.V.
• Tolerance to the sedative effects of this drug usually develops over several weeks.
• Drug should be discontinued at least 48 hours before surgical procedures.

Information for the patient
• Tell patient to take the medication exactly as prescribed, not to take the full daily dosage at one time, and not to double dose for missed doses.
• Explain that the full effects of the drug may not become apparent for up to 4 to 6 weeks after initiation of therapy.
• Warn patient not to discontinue drug abruptly, not to share drug with others, and not to drink alcoholic beverages while taking this drug.
• Suggest taking drug with food or milk if it causes stomach upset.
• Suggest relieving dry mouth with ice chips, chewing gum, or sugarless hard candy. Encourage good dental prophylaxis since persistent dry mouth may lead to increased incidence of dental caries.
• Encourage patient to report any unusual or troublesome effects immediately, including confusion, movement disorders, rapid heartbeat, dizziness, fainting, or difficulty urinating.
• Advise patient to wear protective clothing and use a sunscreen to prevent sunburn.
• Tell patient to notify physician immediately about suspected pregnancy.

Geriatric use
Recommended dosage, 30 to 40 mg P.O. daily, not to exceed 100 mg daily. Initiate therapy at low doses (10 mg) and titrate slowly. Elderly patients may be at greater risk for adverse cardiac reactions.

Pediatric use
Not recommended for treating depression in patients younger than age 12. Do not use pamoate salt for enuresis in children.

Breast-feeding
Imipramine is excreted in breast milk in low concentrations. The potential benefit to the mother should outweigh possible risks to the infant.

<hr>

isocarboxazid
Marplan

• Pharmacologic classification: monoamine oxidase inhibitor
• Therapeutic classification: antidepressant
• Pregnancy risk category C

How supplied
Available by prescription only
Tablets: 10 mg

Indications, route, and dosage
Severe depression unresponsive to other antidepressants or electroconvulsive therapy (ECT) and in patients who cannot take TCAs
Adults: 10 mg P.O. t.i.d.; reduce to 10 to 20 mg daily in divided doses when condition improves (usually in 1 to 4 weeks).
†*Bulimia with depression*
Adults: 10 to 50 mg P.O. daily. Adjust dosage to lowest effective level based on patient tolerance and response.

Pharmacodynamics
Antidepressant action: Depression is thought to result from low CNS concentrations of neurotransmitters, including norepinephrine and serotonin. Isocarboxazid inhibits MAO, an enzyme that normally inactivates amine-containing substances, thus increasing the concentration and activity of norepinephrine and dopamine in the synaptic cleft.

Pharmacokinetics
• *Absorption:* Isocarboxazid is absorbed rapidly and completely from the GI tract.
• *Distribution:* Not yet determined; dosage adjustments are determined by therapeutic response and adverse reaction profile. The drug probably crosses the placenta and enters breast milk.

<hr>

*Canada only   †Unlabeled clinical use   Italicized adverse reactions are life-threatening.

● *Metabolism:* Hepatic.
● *Excretion:* Isocarboxazid is excreted primarily in urine within 24 hours; some is excreted in feces via the biliary tract. Half-life is 2½ hours (relatively short), but enzyme inhibition is prolonged and unrelated to half-life.

Contraindications and precautions

Isocarboxazid is contraindicated in patients with uncontrolled hypertension and seizure disorders because the drug may precipitate hypertensive reactions and lower the seizure threshold.

Isocarboxazid should be used cautiously in patients with a history of severe headaches, angina pectoris or other cardiovascular diseases, Type I and Type II diabetes, Parkinson's disease and other motor disorders, hyperthyroidism, pheochromocytoma, renal or hepatic insufficiency, and bipolar disease (reduce dosage during manic phase).

Interactions

Foods containing high concentrations of tyramine or other pressor amines may precipitate hypertensive crisis. Isocarboxazid enhances pressor effects of amphetamines, ephedrine, phenylephrine, phenylpropanolamine, and related drugs and may result in serious CV toxicity; most OTC cold, hay fever, and weight-reduction products contain these drugs.

Concomitant use of isocarboxazid with disulfiram may cause tachycardia, flushing, or palpitations. Concomitant use with general or spinal anesthetics, which are normally metabolized by MAO, may cause severe hypotension and excessive CNS depression; isocarboxazid should be discontinued for at least 1 week before using these agents. Isocarboxazid decreases effectiveness of local anesthetics (for example, procaine and lidocaine), resulting in poor nerve block. Use cautiously and in reduced dosage with alcohol, barbiturates and other sedatives, narcotics, dextromethorphan, and TCAs. Cocaine and vasoconstrictors in local anesthetics may precipitate a hypertensive response.

Effects on diagnostic tests

Isocarboxazid therapy elevates liver function test results and urinary catecholamine levels.

Adverse reactions

● CNS: dizziness, vertigo, weakness, headache, overactivity, hyperreflexia, tremor, muscle twitching, mania, insomnia, confusion, memory impairment, fatigue, agitation, nervousness.
● CV: orthostatic hypotension, arrhythmias, *paradoxical hypertension,* palpitations, tachycardia, *fatal intracranial hemorrhage during hypertensive crisis.*
● EENT: blurred vision.
● GI: dry mouth, anorexia, nausea, diarrhea, constipation, abdominal pain.
● GU: urine retention, dysuria, discolored urine.
● Hepatic: jaundice.
● Other: peripheral edema, sweating, weight changes, hypersensitivity (rash), altered libido.
Note: Drug should be discontinued if signs of hypersensitivity occur; if rash or jaundice occurs; or if severe headache, palpitations, or fainting spells occur, indicating impending hypertensive crisis.

Overdose and treatment

Signs of overdose include exacerbations of adverse reactions or exaggerated responses to normal pharmacologic activity; such symptoms become apparent slowly (in 24 to 48 hours) and may persist up to 2 weeks. Agitation, flushing, tachycardia, hypotension, hypertension, palpitations, motor activity, twitching, increased deep tendon reflexes, seizures, hyperpyrexia, cardiorespiratory arrest, and coma may occur.

Treat symptomatically and supportively: give 5 to 10 mg phentolamine I.V. push for hypertensive crisis; treat seizures, agitation, or tremor with I.V. diazepam; tachycardia with beta-blockers; and fever with cooling blankets. Monitor vital signs and fluid and electrolyte balance. Use of sympathomimetics (such as norepinephrine and phenylephrine) is contraindicated in hypotension caused by MAO inhibitors.

▶ Special considerations

Besides those relevant to all *MAO inhibitors,* consider the following recommendations.
● Isocarboxazid is an MAO inhibitor and is generally less effective than TCAs. Avoid combining with alcohol or other depressant.
● Recommended only when TCAs or ECT is ineffective or contraindicated.
● Watch for suicidal tendencies.
● Dose is usually reduced to maintenance level as soon as possible.
● Do not withdraw drug abruptly.
● Weigh patient biweekly; check for edema and urine retention.
● Have phentolamine (Regitine) available to counteract severe hypertension.
● Continue precautions 10 days after stopping drug because of long-lasting effects.
● Expect time lag of 1 to 4 weeks before noticeable effect.
● Obtain baseline blood pressure readings,

complete blood count, and liver function test results before beginning therapy, and continue to monitor throughout treatment.

● During hypertensive crisis, immediately discontinue drug. Monitor vital signs and institute therapy to lower blood pressure. Administer antihypertensives slowly to prevent excessive hypotension.

● Assess for symptoms of abrupt withdrawal of long-term therapy, including headache, excitability, depression, and hallucinations.

Information for the patient

● Warn patient to avoid foods high in tyramine or tryptophan (aged hard cheese, Chianti wine, beer, hard liquor aged in wooden casks [such as whiskey], avocados, chicken livers, chocolate, bananas, soy sauce, meat tenderizers, salami, bologna, preserved meats), large amounts of caffeine, and self-medication with OTC drugs, especially cold, hay fever, or diet preparations.

● Warn patient about dizziness. Tell patient to get out of bed slowly, sitting up first for 1 minute.

● Tell patient that severe headaches may be a symptom of a serious complication and must be evaluated by a physician immediately.

● Tell patient not to discontinue the drug abruptly.

● Advise patient to rise slowly from sitting or lying position to prevent a sudden drop in blood pressure, which may cause fainting.

Geriatric use

Isocarboxazid is contraindicated in elderly or debilitated patients.

Pediatric use

Isocarboxazid is not recommended for children under age 16.

Breast-feeding

Isocarboxazid may be excreted in breast milk. Use with caution in breast-feeding women.

---

maprotiline hydrochloride
Ludiomil

● Pharmacologic classification: tricyclic antidepressant
● Therapeutic classification: antidepressant
● Pregnancy risk category B

How supplied
Available by prescription only
Tablets: 25 mg, 50 mg, 75 mg

Indications, route, and dosage
Depression with melancholia or psychotic symptoms; dysthymic disorders; depressive phase of bipolar disorder; mixed symptoms of anxiety and depression
Adults: Initial dosage is 75 mg P.O. daily for patients with mild to moderate depression. The dosage may be increased, as required, to 150 mg daily. Maximum daily dosage is 225 mg in patients who are hospitalized. Usually given t.i.d.; may be given in a single daily dose. Maintain initial dosage for 1 week before increasing; increase by 25-mg increments. For maintenance therapy, use lowest effective level. Most adults respond to 75 to 150 mg daily; elderly patients usually respond to 50 to 75 mg daily.

Pharmacodynamics
Antidepressant action: Maprotiline is thought to exert its antidepressant effects by inhibiting reuptake of norepinephrine and serotonin in CNS nerve terminals (presynaptic neurons), which results in increased concentration and enhanced activity of these neurotransmitters in the synaptic cleft. Maprotiline has minimal inhibitory effect on serotonin reuptake. Maprotiline is also anxiolytic.

Pharmacokinetics
● *Absorption:* Maprotiline is absorbed slowly but completely from the GI tract after oral administration.
● *Distribution:* Maprotiline is distributed widely into the body, including the CNS and breast milk. Drug is 88% protein-bound. Peak serum concentration levels occur 8 to 24 hours after oral dose; steady-state plasma levels and peak therapeutic effect usually occur within 2 weeks. Proposed therapeutic serum levels range between 200 and 300 ng/ml.
● *Metabolism:* Maprotiline is metabolized slowly by the liver to the active metabolite desme-

---

thylmaprotiline; a significant first-pass effect may account for variability of serum concentrations in different patients taking the same dosage.
• *Excretion:* Most of drug is excreted in urine as metabolites within 3 weeks. About 30% is excreted in feces via the biliary tract.

Contraindications and precautions

Maprotiline is contraindicated in patients with known hypersensitivity to TCAs, trazodone, and related compounds; in the acute recovery phase of MI because of its arrhythmogenic potential; in coma or severe respiratory depression because of additive CNS depression; and during or within 14 days of therapy with MAO inhibitors because the combination can precipitate hyperpyrexia, hypertension, and seizures.

Use maprotiline cautiously in patients with other cardiac disease (arrhythmias, CHF, angina pectoris, valvular disease, or heart block); respiratory disorders; alcoholism and seizure disorders; scheduled electroconvulsive therapy; bipolar disease; glaucoma; hyperthyroidism or in those taking thyroid hormone replacement; Type I and Type II diabetes; prostatic hypertrophy, paralytic ileus, or urine retention; hepatic or renal dysfunction; Parkinson's disease; and in those undergoing surgery with general anesthesia.

Interactions

Concomitant use of maprotiline with sympathomimetics, including epinephrine, phenylephrine, phenylpropanolamine, and ephedrine (often found in nasal sprays), may increase blood pressure; use with warfarin may increase prothrombin time and cause bleeding. Concomitant use with thyroid hormones, pimozide, and antiarrhythmic agents (quinidine, disopyramide, procainamide) may increase incidence of cardiac arrhythmias and conduction defects. Maprotiline may decrease hypotensive effects of centrally acting antihypertensive drugs, such as guanethidine, guanabenz, guanadrel, clonidine, methyldopa, and reserpine. Concomitant use with disulfiram or ethchlorvynol may cause delirium and tachycardia.

Additive effects are likely after concomitant use of maprotiline with CNS depressants, including alcohol, analgesics, barbiturates, narcotics, tranquilizers, and anesthetics (oversedation); atropine and other anticholinergic drugs, including phenothiazines, antihistamines, meperidine, and antiparkinsonian agents (oversedation, paralytic ileus, visual changes,

and severe constipation); and metrizamide (increased risk of seizures).

Barbiturates and heavy smoking induce maprotiline metabolism and decrease therapeutic efficacy; phenothiazines and haloperidol decrease its metabolism, decreasing therapeutic efficacy; methylphenidate, cimetidine, oral contraceptives, propoxyphene, and beta blockers may inhibit maprotiline metabolism, increasing plasma levels and toxicity.

Effects on diagnostic tests

Maprotiline may prolong conduction time (elongation of QT and PR intervals, flattened T waves on ECG); it also may elevate liver function test results, decrease WBC counts, and decrease or increase serum glucose levels.

Adverse reactions

• CNS: drowsiness, dizziness, sedation, excitation, tremor, weakness, headache, nervousness, *seizures* (high incidence), peripheral neuropathy, extrapyramidal symptoms, anxiety, vivid dreams, confusion (more marked in elderly patients).
• CV: orthostatic hypotension, tachycardia, arrhythmias, *stroke, heart block, CHF,* palpitations, hypertension, ECG changes.
• EENT: blurred vision, tinnitus, mydriasis, increased intraocular pressure.
• GI: dry mouth, constipation, nausea, vomiting, anorexia, diarrhea, paralytic ileus, jaundice.
• GU: urine retention.
• Other: sweating, photosensitivity, hypersensitivity (rash, urticaria, drug fever, edema).

After abrupt withdrawal of long-term therapy, nausea, headache, and malaise (does not indicate addiction) may occur.

Note: Drug should be discontinued (not abruptly) if signs of hypersensitivity occur. Monitor for urine retention, extreme dry mouth, skin rash, excessive sedation, seizures, tachycardia, sore throat, fever, or jaundice.

Overdose and treatment

The first 12 hours after acute ingestion are a stimulatory phase characterized by excessive anticholinergic activity (agitation, irritation, confusion, hallucinations, hyperthermia, parkinsonian symptoms, seizure, urine retention, dry mucous membranes, pupillary dilation, constipation, and ileus). This is followed by CNS depressant effects, including hypothermia, decreased or absent reflexes, sedation, hypotension, cyanosis, and cardiac irregularities, including tachycardia, conduction disturbances, and quinidine-like effects on the ECG.

Severity of overdose is best indicated by prolongation of QRS complex beyond 100 milliseconds; this usually indicates a serum level in excess of 1,000 ng/ml. Metabolic acidosis may follow hypotension, hypoventilation, and seizures.

Treatment is symptomatic and supportive, including maintaining a patent airway, stable body temperature, and fluid and electrolyte balance. Monitor vital signs and ECG. Induce emesis with ipecac syrup if patient is conscious; follow with gastric lavage and activated charcoal to prevent further absorption. Dialysis is of little use. Treat seizures with parenteral diazepam or phenytoin; arrhythmias, with parenteral phenytoin or lidocaine; and acidosis, with sodium bicarbonate. *Do not give barbiturates;* these may enhance CNS and respiratory depressant effects.

▶ **Special considerations**
Besides those relevant to all *TCAs,* consider the following recommendations.
● Maprotiline may possess a greater potential to induce seizures than other TCAs. Patients with abnormal EEGs should be watched closely.
● To minimize risk of seizures, total daily dosage should be less than 200 mg.

Information for the patient
● Tell patient not to take the full daily dosage at one time and not to double dose for missed doses.
● Explain that the full effects of the drug may not become apparent for up to 4 weeks after initiation of therapy. Patient should take the medication exactly as prescribed.
● Warn patient not to discontinue drug abruptly, not to share drug with others, and not to drink alcoholic beverages while taking the drug.
● Encourage patient to report any unusual or troublesome effects immediately, including confusion, movement disorders, rapid heartbeat, dizziness, fainting, or difficulty urinating.

Geriatric use
Patients over age 60 should be given lower than average doses; 25 to 50 mg daily is usually satisfactory. Maintenance dosage should be lower than standard adult dosage.

Pediatric use
Maprotiline is not recommended for children under age 18.

Breast-feeding
Maprotiline is excreted in breast milk in concentrations equal to or greater than those in

patient's serum; potential benefit to mother must outweigh possible hazard to infant.

---

nortriptyline hydrochloride
Aventyl, Pamelor

● Pharmacologic classification: tricyclic antidepressant
● Therapeutic classification: antidepressant
● Pregnancy risk category D

How supplied
Available by prescription only
Capsules: 10 mg, 25 mg, 50 mg, 75 mg
Oral solution: 10 mg/5ml (4% alcohol)

Indications, route, and dosage
Depression with melancholia or psychotic symptoms; depression associated with organic disease, alcoholism, schizophrenia, or mental retardation; depressive phase of bipolar disorder
Adults: 25 mg P.O. t.i.d. or q.i.d., gradually increasing to a maximum of 150 mg daily. Alternatively, entire dosage may be given h.s. Reduce dosage to lowest possible effective dose. Most patients respond to 30 to 50 mg daily.

Pharmacodynamics
Antidepressant action: Nortriptyline is thought to exert its antidepressant effects by inhibiting reuptake of norepinephrine and serotonin in CNS nerve terminals (presynaptic neurons), which results in increased concentrations and enhanced activity of these neurotransmitters in the synaptic cleft. Nortriptyline inhibits reuptake of serotonin more actively than norepinephrine; it is less likely than other TCAs to cause orthostatic hypotension.

Pharmacokinetics
● *Absorption:* Nortriptyline is absorbed rapidly from the GI tract after oral administration.
● *Distribution:* Nortriptyline is distributed widely into the body, including the CNS and breast milk. Drug is 95% protein-bound. Peak plasma levels occur within 8 hours after a given dose; steady-state serum levels are achieved within 2 to 4 weeks. Therapeutic serum level ranges from 50 to 150 ng/ml.
● *Metabolism:* Nortriptyline is metabolized by the liver; a significant first-pass effect may account for variability of serum concentrations in different patients taking the same dosage.

• *Excretion:* Most of drug is excreted in urine; some is excreted in feces via the biliary tract.

Contraindications and precautions

Nortriptyline is contraindicated in patients with known hypersensitivity to TCAs, trazodone, and related compounds; in the acute recovery phase of MI because it can cause arrhythmias and depress cardiac function; in patients in coma or severe respiratory depression because of additive CNS depression; and during or within 14 days of therapy with MAO inhibitors because this combination may cause excessive sympathetic stimulation with hypertensive crisis, high fevers, and seizures.

Nortriptyline should be used cautiously in patients with other cardiac disease (arrhythmias, CHF, angina pectoris, valvular disease, or heart block) and in patients with respiratory disorders; alcoholism and seizure disorders because this drug may lower the seizure threshold; bipolar disease; glaucoma because drug may increase intraocular pressure, even in normal doses; hyperthyroidism or hypothyroidism treated with thyroid hormone replacement; Type I and Type II diabetes; prostatic hypertrophy, paralytic ileus, or urine retention because drug may worsen these conditions. Also use with caution in patients with hepatic or renal dysfunction because impaired metabolism and excretion may result in drug accumulation; in patients receiving electroconvulsive therapy because of added risk of hypomania and delirium; with Parkinson's disease; and in those undergoing surgery with general anesthesia.

Interactions

Concomitant use of nortriptyline with sympathomimetics, including epinephrine, phenylephrine, phenylpropanolamine, and ephedrine (often found in nasal sprays), may increase blood pressure; use with warfarin may increase prothrombin time and cause bleeding. Concomitant use with thyroid medication, pimozide, or antiarrhythmic agents (quinidine, disopyramide, procainamide) may increase incidence of cardiac arrhythmias and conduction defects.

Nortriptyline may decrease hypotensive effects of centrally acting antihypertensive drugs, such as guanethidine, guanabenz, guanadrel, clonidine, methyldopa, and reserpine.

Concomitant use with disulfiram or ethchlorvynol may cause delirium and tachycardia.

Additive effects are likely after concomitant use of nortriptyline with CNS depressants, including alcohol, analgesics, barbiturates, narcotics, tranquilizers, and anesthetics (oversedation); atropine and other anticholinergic drugs, including phenothiazines, antihistamines, meperidine, and antiparkinsonian agents (oversedation, paralytic ileus, visual changes, and severe constipation); and metrizamide (increased risk of seizures).

Barbiturates and heavy smoking induce nortriptyline metabolism and decrease therapeutic efficacy; phenothiazines and haloperidol decrease its metabolism, decreasing therapeutic efficacy; methylphenidate, cimetidine, oral contraceptives, propoxyphene, and beta blockers may inhibit nortriptyline metabolism, increasing plasma levels and toxicity.

Effects on diagnostic tests

Nortriptyline may prolong conduction time (elongation of QT and PR intervals, flattened T waves on ECG); it also may elevate liver function test results, decrease WBC count, and decrease or increase serum glucose levels.

Adverse reactions

• CNS: drowsiness, dizziness, sedation, excitation, tremor, weakness, headache, nervousness, seizures, peripheral neuropathy, extrapyramidal symptoms, anxiety, vivid dreams, confusion (more marked in elderly patients).
• CV: orthostatic hypotension, tachycardia, *arrhythmias, MI, stroke, heart block, CHF,* palpitations, hypertension, ECG changes.
• DERM: rash, urticaria, drug fever, edema.
• EENT: blurred vision, tinnitus, mydriasis, increased intraocular pressure.
• GI: dry mouth, constipation, nausea, vomiting, anorexia, diarrhea, paralytic ileus, jaundice.
• GU: urine retention.
• Other: sweating, photosensitivity, hypersensitivity (rash, urticaria, drug fever, edema).

After abrupt withdrawal of long-term therapy, nausea, headache, and malaise (does not indicate addiction) may occur.

Note: Drug should be discontinued (not abruptly) if signs of hypersensitivity occur. Monitor for urine retention, extreme dry mouth, rash, excessive sedation, seizures, tachycardia, sore throat, fever, or jaundice.

Overdose and treatment

The first 12 hours after acute ingestion are a stimulatory phase characterized by excessive anticholinergic activity (agitation, irritation, confusion, hallucinations, hyperthermia, parkinsonian symptoms, seizures, urine retention, dry mucous membranes, pupillary dilation, constipation, and ileus). This is followed by CNS depressant effects, including hypothermia, decreased or absent reflexes, sedation, hypotension, cyanosis, and cardiac irregularities, including tachycardia, conduction disturbances, and quinidine-like effects on the ECG.

Severity of overdose is best indicated by prolonging QRS complex beyond 100 milliseconds, which usually indicates a serum level above 1,000 ng/ml. Metabolic acidosis may follow hypotension, hypoventilation, and seizures.

Treatment is symptomatic and supportive, including maintaining a patent airway, stable body temperature, and fluid and electrolyte balance. Monitor vital signs and ECG. Induce emesis with ipecac syrup if patient is conscious; follow with gastric lavage and activated charcoal to prevent further absorption. Dialysis is usually ineffective. Treat seizures with parenteral diazepam or phenytoin; arrhythmias, with parenteral phenytoin or lidocaine; and acidosis, with sodium bicarbonate. *Do not give barbiturates;* these may enhance CNS and respiratory depressant effects.

▶ **Special considerations**
Besides those relevant to all *TCAs,* consider the following recommendations.
● Nortriptyline may be administered at bedtime to reduce daytime sedation. Tolerance to sedative effects usually develops over the initial weeks of therapy.
● Drug should be withdrawn gradually over a few weeks; however, it should be discontinued at least 48 hours before surgical procedures.

Information for the patient
● Explain that patient may not see full effects of drug therapy for up to 4 weeks after start of therapy.
● Warn patient about sedative effects.
● Suggest taking full daily dose at bedtime to prevent daytime sedation.
● Tell patient not to drink alcoholic beverages, not to double dose after missing doses, and not to discontinue the drug abruptly, except as instructed.
● Warn patient about possible dizziness. Tell patient to lie down for about 30 minutes after each dose at start of therapy and to avoid sudden postural changes, to avoid dizziness. Postural hypotension is usually less severe than with amitriptyline.
● Urge patient to report unusual reactions promptly: confusion, movement disorders, fainting, rapid heartbeat, or difficulty urinating.

Geriatric use
Lower dosages may be indicated. Elderly patients are at greater risk for adverse cardiac reactions.

Pediatric use
Not recommended for children. Lower dosages may be indicated for adolescents.

Breast-feeding
Nortriptyline is excreted in breast milk in low concentrations; potential benefit to mother should outweigh potential harm to infant.

---

phenelzine sulfate
Nardil

● Pharmacologic classification: monoamine oxidase inhibitor
● Therapeutic classification: antidepressant
● Pregnancy risk category C

How supplied
Available by prescription only
Tablets: 15 mg

Indications, route, and dosage
Severe depression; depression accompanied by anxiety; neurotic depression; patients unresponsive to other therapies (TCAs or electroconvulsive therapy)
Adults: 15 mg P.O. t.i.d. Increase rapidly to 60 mg daily; as soon as response occurs, reduce dose to 15 mg daily. Maximum daily dose is 90 mg. Onset of maximum therapeutic effect is 2 to 6 weeks. Slowly reduce dosage to lowest effective level over several weeks. Many patients respond to 15 mg P.O. daily or every other day.
†*Migraine headache prophylaxis*
Adults: 45 to 60 mg P.O. daily in divided doses.
†*Bulimia with characteristics of atypical depression*
Adults: 60 to 90 mg P.O. daily in divided doses; adjust dosage according to patient response.

Pharmacodynamics
Antidepressant action: Depression is thought to result from low CNS concentrations of neurotransmitters, including norepinephrine and serotonin. Phenelzine inhibits MAO, an enzyme that normally inactivates amine-containing substances, thus increasing the concentration and activity of these agents.

Pharmacokinetics

- *Absorption:* Phenelzine is absorbed rapidly and completely from the GI tract.
- *Distribution:* Not well understood.
- *Metabolism:* Hepatic.
- *Excretion:* Phenelzine is excreted primarily in urine within 24 hours; some drug is excreted in feces via the biliary tract. Half-life is relatively short, but enzyme inhibition is prolonged and unrelated to drug half-life.

Contraindications and precautions

Phenelzine is contraindicated in patients with uncontrolled hypertension and seizure disorders because it may provoke hypertensive crisis and lowers the seizure threshold, even in patients controlled with anticonvulsant therapy.

Phenelzine should be used cautiously in patients with angina pectoris and other CV disease; in patients with Type I and Type II diabetes; in patients with Parkinson's disease and other motor disorders or hyperthyroidism because it may worsen these conditions; in patients with pheochromocytoma because of risk of hypertensive crisis; in patients with renal or hepatic insufficiency because diminished metabolism and excretion can cause drug accumulation; and in patients with bipolar illness because drug may provoke sudden mood change from depression to mania (reduce dosage during manic phase).

Interactions

Phenelzine enhances pressor effects of amphetamines, ephedrine, phenylephrine, phenylpropanolamine, and related drugs and may result in serious CV toxicity; most OTC cold, hay fever, and weight-reduction products contain these drugs.

Concomitant use of phenelzine with disulfiram may cause tachycardia, flushing, or palpitations. Concomitant use with general or spinal anesthetics, which are normally metabolized by MAO, may cause severe hypotension and excessive CNS depression. Phenelzine decreases effectiveness of local anesthetics (for example, procaine and lidocaine), resulting in poor nerve block, and should be discontinued for at least 1 week before use of these agents.

Use cautiously and in reduced dosage with alcohol, barbiturates and other sedatives, narcotics, dextromethorphan, and TCAs.

Effects on diagnostic tests

Phenelzine therapy elevates liver function test results and urinary catecholamine levels and may elevate WBC count.

Adverse reactions

- CNS: dizziness, vertigo, headache, overactivity, hyperreflexia, tremor, muscle twitching, mania, jitters, agitation, nervousness, insomnia, confusion, memory impairment, drowsiness, weakness, fatigue.
- CV: palpitations, tachycardia, *fatal intracranial hemorrhage during hypertensive crisis,* paradoxical hypertension, orthostatic hypotension, arrhythmias.
- GI: dry mouth, anorexia, nausea, constipation, abdominal pain.
- GU: urine retention, dysuria, discolored urine.
- Hepatic: jaundice.
- Other: peripheral edema, sweating, weight changes.

Note: Drug should be discontinued if any of the following occurs: signs of hypersensitivity, rash, jaundice, or severe headache, palpitations, or fainting spells, indicating impending hypertensive crisis.

Overdose and treatment

Signs of overdose include exacerbations of adverse reactions or exaggerated responses to normal pharmacologic activity; such symptoms become apparent slowly (within 24 to 48 hours) and may persist for up to 2 weeks. Agitation, flushing, tachycardia, hypotension, hypertension, palpitations, increased motor activity, twitching, increased deep tendon reflexes, seizures, hyperpyrexia, cardiorespiratory arrest, and coma may occur. Doses of 375 mg to 1.5 g have been ingested with fatal and nonfatal results.

Treat symptomatically and supportively: give 5 to 10 mg phentolamine I.V. push for hypertensive crisis; treat seizures, agitation, or tremor with I.V. diazepam; tachycardia with beta blockers; and fever with cooling blankets. Monitor vital signs and fluid and electrolyte balance; maintain a patent airway. Supplemental oxygen and mechanical ventilation should be provided, as needed. Use of sympathomimetics (such as norepinephrine or phenylephrine) is contraindicated in hypotension caused by MAO inhibitors.

▶ Special considerations

Besides those relevant to all *MAO inhibitors,* consider the following recommendations.

- At start of therapy, patient should lie down for about 1 hour after taking phenelzine; to prevent dizziness from orthostatic blood pressure changes, patient should avoid sudden changes to standing position.
- Unlike that with other MAO inhibitors, com-

bination therapy with phenelzine and TCAs is generally well tolerated.

Information for the patient
● Warn patient not to take alcohol, other CNS depressants, or any self-prescribed medications (such as cold, hay fever, or diet preparations) without medical approval.
● Explain that many foods and beverages – such as wine, beer, cheeses, preserved fruits, meats, and vegetables – may interact with this drug. A list of foods to avoid can usually be obtained from the dietary department or pharmacy at most hospitals.
● Tell patient to avoid hazardous activities that require alertness until the drug's full effect on the CNS is known. Suggest taking drug at bedtime to minimize daytime sedation.
● Tell patient to take the drug exactly as prescribed and not to double dose if a dose is missed.
● Tell patient not to stop taking the drug abruptly and to report any problems; dosage reduction can relieve most adverse reactions.
● Tell patient that severe headaches may indicate a complication and must be evaluated by a physician immediately.
● Tell patient to rise slowly from a sitting or lying position to prevent a sudden drop in blood pressure, which may cause fainting.

Geriatric use
Phenelzine is not recommended for patients over age 60.

Pediatric use
Not recommended for use in children under age 16.

---

protriptyline hydrochloride
Triptil, Vivactil

● Pharmacologic classification: tricyclic antidepressant
● Therapeutic classification: antidepressant
● Pregnancy risk category C

How supplied
Available by prescription only
Tablets: 5 mg, 10 mg

Indications, route, and dosage
Major depression with melancholia or psychotic symptoms
Adults: 15 to 40 mg P.O. daily in divided doses, increasing gradually to a maximum of 60 mg daily.
Adolescent and elderly patients: Initially, 5 mg P.O. t.i.d. Increase gradually if necessary, then reduce dosage to lowest effective level.
†*Obstructive sleep apnea*
Adults: 10 to 60 mg P.O. daily in divided doses.

Pharmacodynamics
Antidepressant action: Protriptyline is thought to exert its antidepressant effects by inhibiting reuptake of norepinephrine and serotonin in CNS nerve terminals (presynaptic neurons), which results in increased concentrations of these neurotransmitters in the synaptic cleft. Protriptyline inhibits reuptake of serotonin and norepinephrine equally. Protriptyline has CNS stimulatory effects and may be most useful in treating withdrawn, depressed patients.

Pharmacokinetics
● *Absorption:* Protriptyline is absorbed slowly from the GI tract after oral administration. Peak plasma levels occur in 24 to 30 hours.
● *Distribution:* Protriptyline is distributed widely into the body and crosses the placenta. Drug is 90% protein-bound. Proposed therapeutic drug levels range from 70 to 170 ng/ml. Steady-state plasma levels and peak therapeutic effect are achieved within 2 weeks.
● *Metabolism:* Protriptyline is metabolized by the liver; a significant first-pass effect may account for variability of serum concentrations in different patients taking the same dosage.
● *Excretion:* Most of drug is excreted slowly in urine; some is excreted in feces via the biliary tract. About 50% of a given dose is excreted as metabolites within 16 days. It is unknown if the drug is excreted in breast milk.

Contraindications and precautions
Protriptyline is contraindicated in patients with known hypersensitivity to TCAs, trazodone, and related compounds; in the acute recovery phase of MI because of potential for cardiac arrhythmias; in coma or severe respiratory depression because of additive CNS depression; and during or within 14 days of therapy with MAO inhibitors because this combination may result in hypertensive response.
   Protriptyline should be used cautiously in patients with other cardiac disease (arrhythmias, CHF, angina pectoris, valvular disease, or heart

---

block) because of additive antiarrhythmic effects; in patients with respiratory disorders because of additive respiratory depression; in patients with alcoholism and seizure disorders or during scheduled electroconvulsive therapy because drug lowers seizure threshold; in patients with bipolar disease because drug may induce or worsen manic phase; in patients with glaucoma; in patients with hyperthyroidism or in those taking thyroid hormone replacement; in patients with Type I and Type II diabetes; in patients with prostatic hypertrophy, paralytic ileus, or urine retention because drug may worsen these conditions; in patients with hepatic or renal dysfunction because diminished metabolism and excretion cause drug to accumulate; in patients with Parkinson's disease because drug may exacerbate tremors, especially at high doses; and in patients undergoing surgery with general anesthesia, because of increased sensitivity to cardiac effects of general anesthetics or pressor agents.

Interactions

Concomitant use of protriptyline with sympathomimetics, including epinephrine, phenylephrine, phenylpropanolamine, and ephedrine (often found in nasal sprays), may increase blood pressure; use with warfarin may increase prothrombin time and cause bleeding. Concomitant use with thyroid medication, pimozide, and antiarrhythmic agents (quinidine, disopyramide, procainamide) may increase incidence of cardiac arrhythmias and conduction defects.

Protriptyline may decrease hypotensive effects of centrally acting antihypertensive drugs, such as guanethidine, guanabenz, guanadrel, clonidine, methyldopa, and reserpine.

Concomitant use with disulfiram or ethchlorvynol may cause delirium.

Additive effects are likely after concomitant use of protriptyline with CNS depressants, including alcohol, analgesics, barbiturates, narcotics, tranquilizers, and anesthetics (oversedation); atropine and other anticholinergic drugs, including phenothiazines, antihistamines, meperidine, and antiparkinsonian agents (oversedation, paralytic ileus, visual changes, and severe constipation); and metrizamide (increased risk of seizures).

Barbiturates and heavy smoking induce protriptyline metabolism and decrease therapeutic efficacy; phenothiazines and haloperidol decrease protriptyline's metabolism, decreasing its therapeutic efficacy; methylphenidate, cimetidine, oral contraceptives, propoxyphene,

and beta blockers may inhibit protriptyline metabolism, increasing plasma levels and toxicity.

Effects on diagnostic tests

Protriptyline may prolong conduction time (elongation of QT and PR intervals, flattened T waves on ECG); it also may elevate liver enzyme levels, decrease WBC counts, and decrease or increase serum glucose levels.

Adverse reactions

● CNS: drowsiness, dizziness, sedation, excitation, tremor, weakness, headache, nervousness, seizures, peripheral neuropathy, extrapyramidal symptoms, anxiety, vivid dreams, manic behavior; exacerbation of symptoms; confusion (more marked in elderly patients).
● CV: orthostatic hypotension, tachycardia, *arrhythmias, MI, stroke, heart block, CHF,* palpitations, hypertension, ECG changes.
● EENT: blurred vision, tinnitus, mydriasis, increased intraocular pressure.
● GI: dry mouth, constipation, nausea, vomiting, anorexia, diarrhea, paralytic ileus, jaundice.
● GU: urine retention.
● Other: sweating, photosensitivity, hypersensitivity (rash, urticaria, drug fever, edema, weight gain, hypothermia).

After abrupt withdrawal of long-term therapy, nausea, headache, and malaise (does not indicate addiction) may occur.

Note: Drug should be discontinued (not abruptly) if signs of hypersensitivity occur, such as urine retention, extreme dry mouth, skin rash, excessive sedation, seizures, tachycardia, sore throat, fever, or jaundice.

Overdose and treatment

The first 12 hours after acute ingestion are a stimulatory phase characterized by excessive anticholinergic activity (agitation, irritation, confusion, hallucinations, parkinsonism symptoms, seizures, urine retention, dry mucous membranes, pupillary dilation, constipation, and ileus). This is followed by CNS depressant effects, including hypothermia, decreased or absent reflexes, sedation, hypotension, cyanosis, and cardiac irregularities, including tachycardia, conduction disturbances, and quinidine-like effects on the ECG.

Severity of overdose is best indicated by prolongation of QRS complex beyond 100 milliseconds, which usually represents a serum level in excess of 1,000 ng/ml; serum levels are usually not helpful. Metabolic acidosis may follow hypotension, hypoventilation, and seizures.

Treatment is symptomatic and supportive, including maintaining a patent airway, stable body temperature, and fluid and electrolyte balance. Monitor vital signs and ECG closely. Induce emesis with ipecac syrup if gag reflex is intact; follow with gastric lavage and activated charcoal to prevent further absorption. Dialysis is usually ineffective. Treat seizures with parenteral diazepam or phenytoin; arrhythmias, with parenteral phenytoin or lidocaine; and acidosis, with sodium bicarbonate. *Do not give barbiturates*; these may enhance CNS and respiratory depressant effects.

▶ **Special considerations**
Besides those relevant to all *TCAs*, consider the following recommendations.
● Protriptyline has a stimulatory effect on the CNS and may be better suited for withdrawn patients. It also has less sedative effect and a lower incidence of orthostatic hypotension.
● Because of protriptyline's stimulant effect, increased dosage should be administered in the morning.
● Protriptyline should be withdrawn gradually over a period of a few weeks; never abruptly.
● The drug should be discontinued at least 48 hours before surgical procedures.
● Chewing gum, hard candy, or ice chips may alleviate dry mouth.

Information for the patient
● Explain that patient may not experience full effects of the drug for up to 4 weeks after therapy begins.
● Tell patient to take the medication exactly as prescribed, not to double dose for missed doses, and to avoid alcoholic beverages while taking the drug.
● Warn patient that drug may cause stimulation or dizziness. Patient should avoid hazardous activities that require alertness until the drug's full effects are known.
● Tell patient not to share drug with others and to store it safely away from children.
● Suggest taking protriptyline with food or milk if it causes stomach upset and relieving dry mouth with chewing gum or sugarless candy.
● To prevent dizziness or fainting at start of therapy, patient should lie down for about 30 minutes after taking each dose and should avoid sudden postural changes, especially when rising to upright position.
● Advise patient not to stop taking drug suddenly and to report adverse reactions promptly, especially confusion, movement disorders, rapid heartbeat, dizziness, fainting, or difficulty urinating.

● To relieve insomnia with this drug, patient should take dose as early in the day as possible.

Geriatric use
Elderly patients are more sensitive to therapeutic effects and more prone to adverse cardiac reactions. Monitor cardiovascular reactions in patients receiving more than 20 mg daily.

Pediatric use
Protriptyline is not recommended for children under age 12.

Breast-feeding
Protriptyline may be excreted in breast milk. The potential benefit to the mother should outweigh the possible adverse reactions in the infant.

⬛⬛⬛⬛⬛⬛⬛⬛⬛⬛⬛⬛⬛⬛⬛⬛

tranylcypromine sulfate
Parnate

● Pharmacologic classification: monoamine oxidase inhibitor
● Therapeutic classification: antidepressant
● Pregnancy risk category C

How supplied
Available by prescription only
Tablets: 10 mg

Indications, route, and dosage
Severe depression; major depressive illness without melancholia in closely supervised patients unresponsive to other therapies (TCAs or electroconvulsive therapy [ECT])
Adults: 10 mg P.O. b.i.d. Increase to maximum of 30 mg daily after 2 weeks, if necessary, and reduce to 10 to 20 mg daily when response occurs.

During ECT, maintain current dosage; reduce to 10 mg daily thereafter.

Therapeutic effects of tranylcypromine begin earlier than those of other monoamine oxidase (MAO) inhibitors—7 to 10 days vs. 21 to 30 days; MAO activity also returns to pretreatment values more rapidly.
†*Bulimia with characteristics of atypical depression*
Adults: 30 to 40 mg P.O. daily.

Pharmacodynamics

Antidepressant action: Endogenous depression is thought to result from low CNS concentrations of neurotransmitters, including norepinephrine and serotonin. Tranylcypromine acts by inhibiting effects of MAO, an enzyme that normally inactivates amine-containing substances, thus increasing synaptic levels of norepinephrine and dopamine.

Pharmacokinetics

● *Absorption:* Tranylcypromine is absorbed rapidly and completely from the GI tract. Peak serum levels occur at 1 to 3 hours; onset of therapeutic activity may not occur for 3 to 4 weeks.

● *Distribution:* Tranylcypromine's distribution is not fully understood. Dosage adjustments are determined by therapeutic response and adverse reaction profile.

● *Metabolism:* Tranylcypromine is metabolized in the liver.

● *Excretion:* Tranylcypromine is excreted primarily in urine within 24 hours; some drug is excreted in feces via the biliary tract. Half-life is 2½ hours (relatively short); enzyme inhibition is prolonged and unrelated to half-life.

Contraindications and precautions

Tranylcypromine is contraindicated in patients with uncontrolled hypertension, because it may precipitate hypertensive crisis; and in patients with seizure disorders because it lowers the seizure threshold, even in patients controlled on anticonvulsant therapy.

Tranylcypromine should be used cautiously in patients with angina pectoris and other cardiovascular disease, Type I and Type II diabetes, Parkinson's disease and other motor disorders, hyperthyroidism, pheochromocytoma (drug may worsen these conditions); in patients with renal or hepatic insufficiency (reduced metabolism and excretion may cause drug to accumulate); and in patients with manic-depressive illness (drug may provoke or worsen manic phase; reduce dosage during manic phase).

Interactions

Concomitant use of tranylcypromine with amphetamines, ephedrine, phenylephrine, phenylpropanolamine, or related drugs may result in serious cardiovascular toxicity; most nonprescription cold, hay fever, and weight-reduction products contain these drugs. Circulatory collapse and death have occurred after administration of meperidine. Concomitant use with disulfiram may cause tachycardia, flushing, or palpitations. Foods containing high concentrations of tyramine, tryptophan, or other vasopressors should be avoided.

Concomitant use with general or spinal anesthetics, which are normally metabolized by MAO, may cause severe hypotension and excessive CNS depression. Tranylcypromine should be discontinued for at least 1 week before using these agents.

Tranylcypromine decreases effectiveness of local anesthetics (for example, procaine and lidocaine), resulting in poor nerve block. Cocaine or local anesthetics containing vasoconstrictors should be avoided. Use cautiously and in reduced dosage with alcohol, barbiturates and other sedatives, narcotics, and dextromethorphan. Wait at least 2 weeks before switching to TCAs.

Effects on diagnostic tests

Tranylcypromine therapy elevates liver function test results and urinary catecholamine levels.

Adverse reactions

● CNS: dizziness, vertigo, headache, overactivity, hyperreflexia, tremor, muscle twitching, mania, jitters, confusion, memory impairment, fatigue, agitation, nervousness.

● CV: orthostatic hypotension, *arrhythmias,* paradoxical hypertension, palpitations, tachycardia, *fatal intracranial hemorrhage during hypertensive crisis.*

● EENT: blurred vision.

● GI: dry mouth, anorexia, nausea, diarrhea, constipation, abdominal pain.

● GU: changed libido, impotence, urine retention, dysuria, discolored urine.

● Hepatic: jaundice.

● Other: hypersensitivity (rash), peripheral edema, sweating, weight changes, chills.

Note: Drug should be discontinued if patient develops signs of hypersensitivity, severe headache, palpitations, or fainting spells (which could indicate impending hypertensive crisis).

Overdose and treatment

Signs and symptoms of tranylcypromine overdose include exacerbations of adverse reactions or an exaggerated response to normal pharmacologic activity; such signs and symptoms become apparent slowly (24 to 48 hours) and may persist for up to 2 weeks. Agitation, flushing, tachycardia, hypotension, hypertension, palpitations, increased motor activity, twitching, increased deep tendon reflexes, seizures, hyperpyrexia, cardiorespiratory arrest, or coma may occur. Deaths have occurred with doses of 350 mg.

Treat symptomatically and supportively: give 5 to 10 mg of phentolamine I.V. push for hypertensive crisis; treat seizures, agitation, or tremor with I.V. diazepam, tachycardia with beta blockers, and fever with cooling blankets. Monitor vital signs and fluid and electrolyte balance. Sympathomimetics (such as norepinephrine and phenylephrine) are contraindicated in hypotension produced by MAO inhibitors.

▶ Special considerations
Besides those relevant to all *MAO inhibitors,* consider the following recommendations.
● To prevent dizziness induced by orthostatic blood pressure changes, patient should lie down after taking the drug and avoid abrupt postural changes, especially when arising.
● Tranylcypromine has a more rapid onset of antidepressant effect than other MAO inhibitors (7 to 10 days vs. 21 to 30 days). MAO activity also returns rapidly to pretreatment values.

Information for the patient
● Warn patient to avoid taking alcohol and other CNS depressants or any OTC medications such as cold, hay fever, or diet preparations without medical approval.
● To minimize daytime sedation, patient can take medication at bedtime.
● Explain that many foods and beverages containing tyramine or tryptophan, such as wines, beer, cheeses, preserved fruits, meats, and vegetables, may interact with this drug. Patient can usually obtain list of foods to avoid from the hospital dietary department or pharmacy.
● Tell patient that sudden severe headaches may indicate a complication and must be evaluated by a physician immediately.
● Tell patient to avoid hazardous activities that require alertness until the full effect of the drug on the CNS is known.
● Tell patient to take drug exactly as prescribed, not to double dose if a dose is missed, and not to stop taking the drug abruptly. Patient should promptly report any adverse reactions. Dosage reduction can relieve most adverse reactions.
● Tell patient to rise slowly from a sitting or lying position to prevent a sudden drop in blood pressure, which may cause fainting.
● Advise patient to store drug safely away from children.

Geriatric use
Drug is not recommended for patients over age 60.

Pediatric use
Drug is not recommended for children under age 16.

Breast-feeding
Safety has not been established. Drug should be used with caution.

---

trazodone hydrochloride
Desyrel, Trialodine

● Pharmacologic classification: triazolopyridine derivative
● Therapeutic classification: antidepressant
● Pregnancy risk category C

How supplied
Available by prescription only
Tablets: 50 mg, 100 mg, 150 mg

Indications, route, and dosage
Major depression with or without anxiety
Adults: Initial dosage is 150 mg daily in divided doses, which can be increased by 50 mg daily q 3 to 4 days. Average dosage ranges from 150 to 400 mg daily. Maximum dosage is 400 mg daily in outpatients; 600 mg daily in hospitalized patients.
†*Schizophrenia*
Adults: 150 to 600 mg daily in divided doses; usual dose is 300 mg daily.
†*Alcohol dependence*
Adults: 50 to 75 mg P.O. daily.
†*Anxiety status*
Adults: 25 to 150 mg P.O. daily in divided doses.

Pharmacodynamics
Antidepressant action: Trazodone is thought to exert its antidepressant effects by inhibiting reuptake of serotonin (and to a lesser extent norepinephrine) in CNS nerve terminals (presynaptic neurons), which results in increased concentration and enhanced activity of these neurotransmitters in the synaptic cleft. Trazodone shares some properties with TCAs; it has antihistaminic, alpha blocking, analgesic, and sedative effects, and relaxant effects on skeletal muscle. Unlike TCAs, however, trazodone counteracts the pressor effects of norepinephrine, has limited effects on the CV system, and, in particular, has no direct quinidine-like effects on cardiac tissue; it also causes relatively few anticholinergic effects. Trazodone has been used in patients with alcohol dependence to

decrease tremors and to alleviate anxiety and depression. Adverse reactions are somewhat dose-related; incidence increases with higher dosage levels.

Pharmacokinetics

• *Absorption:* Trazodone is well absorbed from the GI tract after oral administration. Peak effect occurs in 1 hour. Concomitant ingestion of food delays absorption, extends peak effect of drug to 2 hours, and increases amount of drug absorbed by 20%.

• *Distribution:* Trazodone is distributed widely in the body; it does not concentrate in any particular tissue. Drug is 90% protein-bound. Proposed therapeutic drug levels have not been established. Steady-state plasma levels are reached in 3 to 7 days, and onset of therapeutic activity occurs in 7 days.

• *Metabolism:* Trazodone is metabolized by the liver; over 75% of metabolites are excreted within 3 days.

• *Excretion:* Majority of drug (75%) is excreted in urine; small amounts, in breast milk. The rest is excreted in feces via the biliary tract.

Contraindications and precautions

Trazodone is contraindicated in patients with known hypersensitivity to TCAs, trazodone, and related compounds; and in the acute recovery phase of MI. It should be used with great caution in patients with other cardiac disease (arrhythmias, CHF, angina pectoris, valvular disease, or heart block) because similar drugs have adversely affected cardiac function.

Trazodone should be used cautiously in patients with priapism or ejaculatory disorders because drug may cause or exacerbate such disorders; surgical correction is necessary (and not always successful) in as many as 30% of patients who experience priapism (prolonged, painful erections). It also should be used with caution in patients receiving electroconvulsive therapy and in patients with hepatic or renal dysfunction.

Interactions

Additive effects are likely after concomitant use of trazodone with antihypertensive drugs, such as guanethidine, guanabenz, guanadrel, clonidine, methyldopa, and reserpine (hypotension); and with CNS depressants, such as alcohol, analgesics, barbiturates, narcotics, tranquilizers, and anesthetics (oversedation).

Trazodone may increase serum levels of phenytoin and digoxin.

Effects on diagnostic tests

Trazodone may prolong conduction time (elongation of QT and PR intervals, flattened T waves on ECG); it also may elevate liver function test results, decrease WBC counts, and alter serum glucose levels.

Adverse reactions

• CNS: drowsiness, dizziness, sedation (in 20% to 50% of patients), anxiety, tremor, weakness, headache, nervousness, fatigue, vivid dreams and nightmares, confusion, anger, hostility, impaired speech, peripheral neuropathies.

• CV: orthostatic hypotension, tachycardia, *arrhythmias, MI, stroke, heart block, CHF,* palpitations, hypertension, shortness of breath, fainting.

• EENT: blurred vision, tinnitus, mydriasis, increased intraocular pressure.

• GI: dry mouth (in 15% to 30% of patients), constipation, nausea, vomiting, anorexia, bad taste in mouth.

• GU: urine retention, priapism possibly leading to impotence, retrograde ejaculation, amenorrhea, hematuria.

• Other: sweating, hypersensitivity (rash, urticaria, drug fever, edema), sexual dysfunction.

   Note: Drug should be discontinued (not abruptly) if signs of hypersensitivity occur or if urine retention, hematuria, extreme dry mouth, rash, excessive sedation, seizures, tachycardia or other arrhythmias, fainting spells, or priapism or other sexual dysfunction occurs.

Overdose and treatment

The most common signs and symptoms of trazodone overdose are drowsiness and vomiting; other signs and symptoms include orthostatic hypotension, tachycardia, headache, shortness of breath, dry mouth, and incontinence. Coma, respiratory arrest, seizures, and ECG changes may occur.

Treatment is symptomatic and supportive and includes maintaining a patent airway, stable vital signs, and fluid and electrolyte balance. Monitor ECG closely. Treat seizures with anticonvulsants. Induce emesis with ipecac syrup if gag reflex is intact; follow with gastric lavage (begin with lavage if emesis is unfeasible) and activated charcoal to prevent further absorption. Forced diuresis may aid elimination. Dialysis is usually ineffective.

▶ **Special considerations**
- Administering trazodone with food helps to prevent GI upset and increases absorption by 20%.
- Adverse reactions appear more frequently when dosages exceed 300 mg daily.
- 150-mg tablet may be broken on the scoring to obtain doses of 50, 75, or 100 mg.
- Tolerance to adverse reactions (especially sedative effects) usually develops after 1 to 2 weeks of treatment.
- Trazodone has been used in alcohol dependence to decrease tremor and relieve anxiety and depression. Dosages range from 50 to 75 mg daily.
- This drug has fewer adverse cardiac and anticholinergic effects than TCAs.
- Drug may cause prolonged, painful erections that may require surgical correction. Consider carefully before prescribing for male patients, especially those who are sexually active.
- Trazodone should not be withdrawn abruptly. However, it should be discontinued at least 48 hours before surgical procedures.
- Sugarless chewing gum or hard candy, or ice chips may relieve dry mouth.
- Hypotension may occur; monitor blood pressure.

Information for the patient
- Tell patient that full effects of the drug may not become apparent for up to 2 weeks after therapy begins.
- Tell patient to take drug exactly as prescribed and not to double dose for missed ones, not to share drug with others, and not to discontinue drug abruptly.
- Inform patient that drug may cause drowsiness or dizziness; instruct patient not to drive or participate in other activities that require mental alertness until the full effects of the drug are known.
- Tell patient to avoid alcoholic beverages or medicinal elixirs while taking this drug.
- Warn patient to store drug safely away from children.
- Suggest taking drug with food or milk if it causes stomach upset.
- To prevent dizziness, patient should lie down for about 30 minutes after taking the medication and avoid sudden postural changes, especially rising to upright position.
- Suggest chewing ice chips, sugarless chewing gum, or sugarless hard candy to relieve dry mouth.
- Advise patient to report any unusual effects immediately and to report prolonged, painful

erections; sexual dysfunction; dizziness; fainting; or rapid heartbeat.

Geriatric use
Elderly patients usually require lower initial dosages; they are more likely to develop adverse reactions. However, trazodone may be preferred in elderly patients because it has fewer adverse cardiac reactions.

Pediatric use
Drug is not recommended for children under age 18.

---

trimipramine maleate
Surmontil

- Pharmacologic classification: tricyclic antidepressant
- Therapeutic classification: antidepressant, anxiolytic
- Pregnancy risk category C

How supplied
Available by prescription only
Capsules: 25 mg, 50 mg, 100 mg

Indications, route, and dosage
Major depression, depression with melancholia or psychotic symptoms
Adults: 75 mg daily in divided doses, increased to 200 mg daily. Dosages over 300 mg daily are not recommended.
For maintenance therapy, reduce dosage to lowest effective level (range 50 to 150 mg daily). Administer as a single dose h.s. Continue therapy for at least 3 months to minimize risk of relapse.
Adolescents and elderly patients: Begin therapy at 50 mg daily, and gradually increase as needed to 100 mg daily.

Pharmacodynamics
Antidepressant action: Trimipramine is thought to exert its antidepressant effects by equally inhibiting reuptake of norepinephrine and serotonin in CNS nerve terminals (presynaptic neurons), which results in increased concentration and enhanced activity of these neurotransmitters in the synaptic cleft. Trimipramine also has anxiolytic effects and inhibits gastric acid secretion.

Pharmacokinetics
- *Absorption:* Trimipramine is absorbed rapidly from the GI tract after oral administration.
- *Distribution:* Trimipramine is distributed widely in the body; it crosses the placenta and may enter breast milk. Drug is 90% protein-bound. Peak effect occurs in 2 hours; steady state within 7 days.
- *Metabolism:* Trimipramine is metabolized by the liver; a significant first-pass effect may explain variability of serum levels in different patients taking the same dosage.
- *Excretion:* Most of drug is excreted in urine; some is excreted in feces via the biliary tract.

Contraindications and precautions
Trimipramine is contraindicated in patients with known hypersensitivity to TCAs, trazodone, and related compounds; in the acute recovery phase of MI because drug depresses cardiac function and causes arrhythmias; in patients in coma or severe respiratory depression (additive CNS and respiratory depression); and during or within 14 days of therapy with MAO inhibitors.

Trimipramine should be used cautiously in patients with other cardiac disease (arrhythmias, CHF, angina pectoris, valvular disease, or heart block), respiratory disorders, seizure disorders, scheduled electroconvulsive therapy, bipolar disease, glaucoma, hyperthyroidism, and parkinsonism; in patients taking thyroid hormone replacement; in patients with Type I and Type II diabetes; in patients with prostatic hypertrophy, paralytic ileus, or urine retention because drug may worsen these conditions; in patients with hepatic or renal dysfunction because diminished metabolism and excretion causes the drug to accumulate; and in patients undergoing surgery with general anesthesia because drug may increase cardiac sensitivity to the effects of general anesthetics or pressor agents.

Interactions
Concomitant use of trimipramine with sympathomimetics, including epinephrine, phenylephrine, phenylpropanolamine, and ephedrine (often found in nasal sprays) may increase blood pressure; use with warfarin may increase prothrombin time and cause bleeding.

Concomitant use with thyroid medication, pimozide, and antiarrhythmic agents (quinidine, disopyramide, procainamide) may increase incidence of cardiac arrhythmias and conduction defects.

Trimipramine may decrease hypotensive effects of centrally acting antihypertensive drugs, such as guanethidine, guanabenz, guanadrel, clonidine, methyldopa, and reserpine.

Concomitant use with disulfiram or ethchlorvynol may cause delirium and tachycardia.

Additive effects are likely after concomitant use of trimipramine with CNS depressants, including alcohol, analgesics, barbiturates, narcotics, tranquilizers, and anesthetics (oversedation); atropine and other anticholinergic drugs, including phenothiazines, antihistamines, meperidine, and antiparkinsonian agents (oversedation, paralytic ileus, visual changes, and severe constipation); and metrizamide (increased risk of seizures).

Barbiturates and heavy smoking induce trimipramine metabolism and decrease therapeutic efficacy; phenothiazines and haloperidol decrease its metabolism, decreasing therapeutic efficacy; methylphenidate, cimetidine, oral contraceptives, propoxyphene, and beta blockers may inhibit trimipramine metabolism, increasing plasma levels and toxicity.

Effects on diagnostic tests
Trimipramine may prolong conduction time (elongation of QT and PR intervals, flattened T waves on ECG); it also may elevate liver function test levels, decrease WBC counts, and alter serum glucose levels. Trimipramine may alter prothrombin time.

Adverse reactions
- CNS: drowsiness, dizziness, sedation, excitation, tremor, weakness, headache, nervousness, *seizures,* peripheral neuropathy, extrapyramidal symptoms, anxiety, vivid dreams, confusion (more marked in elderly patients).
- CV: orthostatic hypotension, tachycardia, *arrhythmias, MI, stroke, heart block, CHF,* palpitations, hypertension, ECG changes.
- EENT: blurred vision, tinnitus, mydriasis, increased intraocular pressure.
- GI: dry mouth, constipation, nausea, vomiting, anorexia, diarrhea, paralytic ileus, jaundice.
- GU: urine retention.
- Other: sweating, photosensitivity, hypersensitivity (rash, urticaria, drug fever, edema).

After abrupt withdrawal of long-term therapy, nausea, headache, and malaise (does not indicate addiction) may occur.

Note: Drug should be discontinued (not abruptly) if signs of hypersensitivity occur; dosage adjustment or discontinuation may be required if any of the following occur: urine retention, extreme dry mouth, skin rash, excessive sedation, seizures, tachycardia, sore throat, fever, or jaundice.

Overdose and treatment
The first 12 hours after acute ingestion are a stimulatory phase characterized by excessive anticholinergic activity (agitation, irritation, confusion, hallucinations, parkinsonian symptoms, seizures, urine retention, dry mucous membranes, pupillary dilation, constipation, and ileus). This is followed by CNS depressant effects, including hypothermia, decreased or absent reflexes, sedation, hypotension, cyanosis, and cardiac irregularities (including tachycardia, conduction disturbances, and quinidine-like effects on the ECG).

Severity of overdose is best indicated by prolongation of QRS interval beyond 100 milliseconds, which usually represents a serum level in excess of 1,000 ng/ml; serum levels are generally not helpful. Metabolic acidosis may follow hypotension, hypoventilation, and seizures.

Treatment is symptomatic and supportive and includes monitoring vital signs and ECG and maintaining a patent airway, stable body temperature, and fluid and electrolyte balance. Induce emesis with ipecac syrup if patient is conscious; follow with gastric lavage and activated charcoal to prevent further absorption. Dialysis is of little use. Treat seizures with parenteral diazepam or phenytoin; arrhythmias, with parenteral phenytoin or lidocaine; and acidosis, with sodium bicarbonate. *Do not give barbiturates;* these may enhance CNS and respiratory depressant effects.

▶ **Special considerations**
Besides those relevant to all *TCAs,* consider the following recommendations.
● The full dosage may be given at bedtime to help offset daytime sedation.
● Trimipramine also has been used to decrease gastric acid secretion in peptic ulcer disease; however, safety and efficacy for this use have not been established.
● Watch for bleeding because the drug may cause alterations in prothrombin time.
● The drug should not be withdrawn abruptly. However, it should be discontinued at least 48 hours before surgical procedures.
● Tolerance generally develops to the sedative effects of this drug.
● Observe patient for suicidal ideation.

Information for the patient
● Advise patient to take full dosage at bedtime to minimize daytime sedation.
● Explain that full effects of the drug may not become apparent for up to 4 to 6 weeks after therapy begins.

● Tell patient to take the drug exactly as prescribed, not to double dose for missed ones; not to discontinue drug suddenly, and not to share drug with others.
● Warn patient that drug may cause drowsiness or dizziness. Patient should avoid hazardous activities that require alertness until the full effects of the drug are known.
● Warn patient not to drink alcoholic beverages or medicinal elixirs while taking this drug.
● Tell patient to store drug safely away from children.
● Suggest taking drug with food or milk if it causes stomach upset and to ease dry mouth with sugarless chewing gum, hard candy, or ice chips.
● To prevent dizziness, advise patient to lie down for about 30 minutes after each dose and to avoid abrupt postural changes, especially when rising to an upright position.
● Tell patient to report adverse reactions promptly, especially confusion, movement disorders, rapid heartbeat, dizziness, fainting, or difficulty urinating.

Geriatric use
Recommended starting dose for elderly patients is 25 mg. Such patients may be more vulnerable to adverse cardiac reactions.

Breast-feeding
Trimipramine may enter breast milk. Use with caution in breast-feeding women.

Antimanic agents

lithium carbonate
lithium citrate
verapamil hydrochloride

Lithium salts have been known to treat manic episodes since 1949; however, this practice was not accepted in the United States until 1970 because of concerns about safety. Lithium is used to treat mania and recurrent attacks of manic-depressive illness. Alternative therapies for patients who don't respond to lithium include anticonvulsants (such as carbamazepine or valproic acid) or the calcium channel blocker verapamil.

Pharmacologic effects
● *Lithium* is not a sedative, depressant, or euphoriant and has almost no discernible psychotropic effect in persons who are not manic.
● *Verapamil* blocks slow calcium channels in nerve cells, as well as cardiac and vascular smooth muscle. It is used primarily as an antihypertensive, antianginal, and antiarrhythmic.

Mechanism of action
● *Lithium* is suspected to produce its antimanic effects through action on biological membranes. Lithium can replace sodium in supporting a single-cell action potential but is an inadequate substrate for the sodium pump and cannot maintain membrane potential. It is also associated with increased neuronal tryptophan uptake and serotonin synthesis.
● *Verapamil* blocks slow calcium channels. It may interfere with neuronal sodium-calcium exchange mechanisms.

Pharmacokinetics
● *Absorption and distribution:* Lithium is readily absorbed after oral administration, and absorption is complete in about 8 hours. Peak plasma concentrations occur in 2 to 4 hours. Slow or extended-release products provide a slower rate of absorption and minimize fluctuations in blood levels. There is no evidence of protein binding. Food does not appear to adversely affect bioavailability. Lithium is widely distributed throughout body tissues and fluids. Concentrations in bone, thyroid, and brain tissue are often 50% greater than corresponding serum concentrations. Distribution to heart, lungs, kidneys, and muscles is slower and less complete. Lithium is distributed in saliva and readily crosses the placenta; maternal and fetal serum concentrations are about equal. Lithium is found in breast milk at 33% to 50% of concentrations found in serum.

Verapamil is well absorbed after oral administration, but a significant amount of the drug is lost to first-pass hepatic biotransformation. Peak levels occur within 2 hours after regular tablets and 6 to 8 hours after extended-release tablets.
● *Metabolism and excretion:* Lithium is not metabolized and is excreted almost entirely in the urine. Elimination appears to be biphasic, with ⅓ to ⅔ of an acute dose excreted during the first 6- to 12-hour initial phase, followed by a slower excretion phase over the next 10 to 14 days. Repeated administration results in increased lithium excretion over the first 5 to 6 days until equilibrium between ingestion and excretion is reached.

Verapamil is extensively metabolized in the liver and excreted in the urine. Its elimination half-life is 6 to 12 hours.

Adverse reactions and toxicity
Adverse reactions to lithium are usually dose-dependent and involve the CNS, GI, and renal systems. Such reactions commonly include lethargy, fatigue, muscle weakness, tremor, nausea, diarrhea, bloating, polyuria, and polydipsia, which usually occur during initial treatment and subside with continued therapy.

Lithium intoxication is usually associated with high-dose or prolonged administration and is characterized by CNS effects, including drowsiness, confusion, giddiness, apathy, and coarse hand tremor. Toxicity may also develop as a result of water loss in patients with fever, decreased fluid or food intake, vomiting, diarrhea, or pyelonephritis and in those receiving treatment with diuretics.

Adverse reactions to verapamil relate to the drug's action on the CV system. Hypotension,

---

*Canada only　　　　†Unlabeled clinical use　　　　Italicized adverse reactions are life-threatening.

bradycardia, and orthostatic hypotension may occur, especially early in therapy. Constipation and nausea may also occur. High doses can lead to AV block, ventricular asystole, or heart failure.

Clinical considerations
● Because lithium can cause fetal toxicity, it should not be used in pregnant women except in life-threatening situations or severe disease.
● Use with caution in patients with preexisting CV or thyroid dysfunction.
● Elderly patients are more likely to develop lithium intoxication.
● In 1% to 4% of patients, clinically significant hypothyroidism may develop and require supplemental thyroid therapy.
● Monitor renal function before and regularly during lithium therapy.
● Monitor serum lithium concentrations carefully and adjust dose as necessary.
● When drugs with high-sodium content are used concomitantly, monitor serum lithium concentrations because sodium intake can influence renal elimination of lithium.
● Instruct patients to avoid dehydration and to promptly report prolonged nausea, vomiting, diarrhea, and polyuria to their physicians.
● Teach patients and their families how to recognize the signs and symptoms of lithium toxicity. Advise them to promptly report such symptoms to their physicians, who will probably direct them to discontinue lithium therapy immediately.
● The clinical effectiveness of verapamil in treating manic-depressive illness is still being evaluated.

---

lithium carbonate
Carbolith∗, Duralith∗, Eskalith, Eskalith CR, Lithane, Lithizine∗, Lithobid, Lithonate, Lithotabs

lithium citrate
Cibalith-S

● Pharmacologic classification: alkali metal
● Therapeutic classification: antimanic, antipsychotic
● Pregnancy risk category D

How supplied
Available by prescription only
Capsules: 300 mg
Tablets: 300 mg (300 mg = 8.12 mEq lithium)
Tablets (sustained-release): 300 mg, 450 mg
Syrup (sugarless): 300 mg/5 ml (0.3% alcohol)

Indications, route, and dosage
Prevention or control of mania; prevention of depression in patients with bipolar illness
Adults: 300 to 600 mg or 5 to 10 ml lithium citrate (each 5 ml lithium citrate contains 8 mEq lithium, equivalent to 300 mg lithium carbonate) P.O. up to q.i.d, increasing on the basis of blood levels and clinical response to achieve optimal dosage. Dosages to a maximum of 2.7 g daily divided t.i.d. or q.i.d. may be required in the acute manic phase of bipolar illness; for maintenance therapy, the usual dosage is 900 mg to 1.2 g of lithium carbonate or 15 to 20 ml lithium citrate (about 24 to 32 mEq) in two to four divided doses daily. Recommended therapeutic lithium blood levels: 1 to 1.5 mEq/liter for acute mania; 0.6 to 1 mEq/liter for maintenance therapy; and 2 mEq/liter as maximum. Dosage should be decreased rapidly when the acute attack has subsided.
†Major depression, †schizoaffective disorder, †schizophrenic disorder, †alcohol dependence
Adults: 300 mg lithium carbonate P.O. t.i.d. to q.i.d.
Apparent mixed bipolar disorder in children
Children: Initially, 15 to 60 mg/kg or 0.5 to 1.5 g/m² lithium carbonate P.O. daily in three divided doses. Do not exceed usual adult dosage. Adjust dosage based on patient response and serum lithium levels; usual dosage range is 150 to 300 mg daily in divided doses.

Pharmacodynamics
Antimanic action: Lithium is thought to exert its antipsychotic and antimanic effects by competing with other cations for exchange at the sodium-potassium ionic pump, thus altering cationic exchange at the tissue level. It also inhibits adenyl cyclase, reducing intracellular levels of the secondary messengers cyclic adenosine monophosphate (cAMP) and, to a lesser extent, cyclic guanosine monophosphate (cGMP).

Pharmacokinetics
● *Absorption:* Rate and extent of absorption vary with dosage form: absorption is complete within 6 hours of oral administration.
● *Distribution:* Distributed widely into the body, including breast milk; concentrations in thyroid gland, bone, and brain tissue exceed serum lev-

---

els. Peak effects occur at 30 minutes to 3 hours; liquid peaks at 15 minutes to 1 hour. Steady-state serum level is achieved in 12 hours, at which time trough levels should be drawn: therapeutic effect begins in 5 to 10 days and is maximal within 3 weeks. Therapeutic and toxic serum levels and therapeutic effects show good correlation. Therapeutic range is 0.6 to 1.2 mEq/liter; adverse reactions increase as level reaches 1.5 to 2 mEq/liter – such concentrations may be necessary in acute mania. Toxicity usually occurs at levels above 2 mEq/liter.

● *Metabolism:* Not metabolized.

● *Excretion:* 95% of dose is excreted unchanged in urine; about 50% to 80% of a given dose is excreted within 24 hours. Level of renal function determines elimination rate.

Contraindications and precautions

Lithium is contraindicated in patients with known hypersensitivity to lithium.

Lithium should be used cautiously in patients with CV disease because drug causes ECG changes (including T wave depression in 20% to 30% of patients), heart block, and premature ventricular contractions; in patients with renal dysfunction, because delayed elimination may induce lithium toxicity and diabetes insipidus (characterized by extreme thirst and excessive urination in 30% to 50% of patients); in patients with hypovolemia, sodium depletion, or dehydration, which increase drug's effects; in patients with hypothyroidism because of risk of disease exacerbation or goiter formation; in patients with psoriasis, because lithium may exacerbate condition; and in patients with seizure disorders, because drug may induce seizures. Many oral lithium products contain tartrazine, which may exacerbate asthma or respiratory disorders in aspirin-allergic patients.

Lithium has caused pseudotumor cerebri with papilledema and increased ICP in some patients. If this occurs, the drug should be discontinued, if possible. Some clinicians may elect to treat the patient with acetazolamide.

Interactions

Concomitant use of lithium with thiazide diuretics may decrease renal excretion and enhance lithium toxicity; diuretic dosage may need to be reduced by 30%. Indomethacin, phenylbutazone, piroxicam, and other nonsteroidal anti-inflammatory agents also decrease renal excretion of lithium and may require a 30% reduction in lithium dosage.

Mazindol, tetracyclines, phenytoin, carbamazepine, and methyldopa may increase lith-

ium toxicity. Antacids and other drugs containing sodium, calcium, theophylline, aminophylline, or caffeine may increase lithium excretion by renal competition for elimination, thus decreasing lithium's therapeutic effect.

Lithium may interfere with pressor effects of sympathomimetic agents, especially norepinephrine; may potentiate the effects of neuromuscular blocking agents (such as succinylcholine, pancuronium, and atracurium); and may decrease the effects of chlorpromazine.

Concomitant use with haloperidol may result in severe encephalopathy characterized by confusion, tremor, extrapyramidal effects, and weakness. Use this combination with caution.

Dietary sodium may alter the renal elimination of lithium. Increased sodium intake may increase elimination of drug, whereas decreased intake may decrease its elimination.

Effects on diagnostic tests

Lithium causes false-positive test results for thyroid function tests; drug also elevates neutrophil count.

Adverse reactions

● CNS: tremor, drowsiness, headache, confusion, restlessness, dizziness, psychomotor retardation, stupor, lethargy, coma, blackouts, *epileptiform seizures,* EEG changes, worsened organic brain syndrome, impaired speech, ataxia, muscle weakness, incoordination, hyperexcitability, exacerbation of psychotic symptoms, pseudotumor cerebri.

● CV: reversible ECG changes, *arrhythmias,* hypotension, *peripheral circulatory collapse,* allergic vasculitis, ankle and wrist edema, bradycardia.

● DERM: pruritus, rash, diminished or lost sensation, drying and thinning of hair.

● EENT: tinnitus, impaired vision.

● GI: nausea, vomiting, anorexia, diarrhea, dry mouth, thirst, metallic taste.

● GU: polyuria, glycosuria, incontinence, *nephrotoxicity with long-term use,* decreased renal concentrating capacity.

● Metabolic: transient hyperglycemia, goiter, hypothyroidism (lowered triiodothyronine, thyroxine, and protein-bound iodine levels; elevated ^{131}I uptake), hyponatremia.

● Other: weight gain (25%).

The severity of lithium toxicity parallels serum concentration:

Less than 1.5 mEq/liter – thirst, nausea, vomiting, diarrhea, polyuria, slurred speech, hand tremors, weakness.

1.5 to 2 mEq/liter – GI distress, hand tremors,

---

confusion, muscle twitching, ECG changes, incoordination.

2 to 2.5 mEq/liter—ataxia, polyuria, large volume of dilute urine, ECG changes, seizures, abnormal motor activity, tinnitus, hypotension, coma.

Note: Drug should be discontinued if any of the following occurs—hypersensitivity, severe hypothyroidism or goiter, slurred speech, ataxia, incoordination, arrhythmias, seizures, decreased renal function, or rash.

Overdose and treatment

Vomiting and diarrhea occur within 1 hour of acute ingestion (induce vomiting in noncomatose patients if it is not spontaneous). Death has occurred in patients ingesting 10 to 60 g of lithium; patients have ingested 6 g with minimal toxic effects. Serum lithium levels above 3.4 mEq/liter are potentially fatal.

Overdose with chronic lithium ingestion may follow altered pharmacokinetics, drug interactions, or volume or sodium depletion; sedation, confusion, hand tremors, joint pain, ataxia, muscle stiffness, increased deep tendon reflexes, visual changes, and nystagmus may occur. Symptoms may progress to coma, movement abnormalities, tremor, seizures, and CV collapse.

Treatment is symptomatic and supportive; closely monitor vital signs. If emesis is not feasible, treat with gastric lavage. Monitor fluid and electrolyte balance; correct sodium depletion with normal saline solution. Institute hemodialysis if serum level is above 3 mEq/liter, and in severely symptomatic patients unresponsive to fluid and electrolyte correction, or if urine output decreases significantly. Serum rebound of tissue lithium stores (from high volume distribution) commonly occurs after dialysis and may necessitate prolonged or repeated hemodialysis. Peritoneal dialysis may help but is less effective.

▶ Special considerations

• Use cautiously with haloperidol, other antipsychotics, neuromuscular blocking agents, and diuretics; in elderly or debilitated persons; and in thyroid disease, brain damage, severe debilitation or dehydration, and sodium depletion.
• Lithium should be discontinued before electroconvulsive therapy.
• Determination of lithium blood concentration is crucial to the safe use of the drug. Lithium shouldn't be used in patients who can't have regular lithium blood level checks. Be sure patient or responsible family member can comply with instructions.
• Shake syrup formulation before administration.
• Patient should take drug with food or milk to reduce GI upset.
• Monitor baseline ECG, thyroid, and renal studies, and electrolyte levels. Monitor lithium blood levels 8 to 12 hours after first dose, usually before morning dose, two or three times weekly first month, then weekly to monthly on maintenance therapy.
• Monitor serum levels and watch for signs of impending toxicity. When lithium blood levels are below 1.5 mEq/liter, adverse reactions are usually mild.
• Monitor fluid intake and output, especially when surgery is scheduled.
• Adjust fluid and sodium ingestion to compensate if excessive loss occurs through protracted sweating or diarrhea. Under normal conditions, patients should have fluid intake of 2,500 to 3,000 ml daily and a balanced diet with adequate sodium intake.
• Monitor for signs of edema or sudden weight gain.
• Check urine for specific gravity level below 1.015, which may indicate diabetes insipidus.
• Lithium may alter glucose tolerance in diabetic patients. Monitor blood glucose levels closely.
• Expect lag of 1 to 3 weeks before drug's beneficial effects are noticed. Other psychotropic medications (for example, chlorpromazine) may be necessary during this interim period.
• Arrange for outpatient follow-up of thyroid and renal functions every 6 to 12 months. Thyroid should be palpated to check for enlargement.
• Lithium is used investigationally to increase WBC count in patients undergoing cancer chemotherapy. It is also used investigationally to treat cluster headaches, aggression, organic brain syndrome, tardive dyskinesia, and syndrome of inappropriate antidiuretic hormone secretion.
• Lithane tablets contain tartrazine, a dye that may precipitate an allergic reaction in certain individuals, particularly asthmatics sensitive to aspirin.

Information for the patient

• Explain to patient that lithium has a narrow therapeutic margin of safety. A blood level that is even slightly too high can be dangerous.
• Advise patient to carry an identification/

---

instruction card (available from pharmacy) with toxicity and emergency information.

● Warn patient and family to watch for signs of toxicity (diarrhea, vomiting, dehydration, drowsiness, muscle weakness, tremor, fever, and ataxia) and to expect transient nausea, polyuria, thirst, and discomfort during first few days. If toxic symptoms occur, patient should withhold one dose and call physician promptly.

● Warn ambulatory patient to avoid hazardous activities that require alertness and good psychomotor coordination until CNS response to drug is determined.

● Advise patient to maintain adequate water intake and adequate — but not excessive — sodium in diet.

● Explain importance of regular follow-up visits to measure lithium serum levels.

● Tell patient to avoid large amounts of caffeine, which will interfere with drug's effectiveness.

● Advise patient to seek medical approval before initiating weight-loss program.

● Tell patient not to switch brands of lithium or take other drugs (prescription or OTC) without medical approval. Different brands may not provide equivalent effect.

● Warn patient against stopping drug abruptly.

● Tell patient to explain to close friend or family members the signs of lithium overdose, in case emergency aid is needed.

Geriatric use
Elderly patients are more susceptible to chronic overdose and toxic effects, especially dyskinesia. These patients usually respond to a lower dosage.

Pediatric use
Lithium is not recommended for use in children under age 12.

Breast-feeding
Lithium level in breast milk is 33% to 50% that of maternal serum level. Breast-feeding should be avoided during treatment with lithium.

---

verapamil hydrochloride
Calan, Isoptin

● Pharmacologic classification: calcium channel blocker
● Therapeutic classification: antianginal, antiarrhythmic, antihypertensive
● Pregnancy risk category C

How supplied
Available by prescription only
Tablets: 80 mg, 120 mg
Tablets (extended-release): 240 mg
Injection: 2.5 mg/ml

Indications, route, and dosage
†*Bipolar disorder*
Adults: 80 mg P.O. t.i.d. or q.i.d.
†*Migraine headache*
Adults: Initial dose 80 mg P.O. t.i.d. Dosage may be increased gradually to a maximum of 450 mg/day continued at least 5 weeks before concluding therapy is ineffective.

Pharmacodynamics
● *Psychotropic action:* The exact mechanism by which verapamil acts in bipolar disorder is unknown. It may be related to the drug's effect on sodium-calcium counterexchange.

● *Migraine prophylaxis action:* The mechanism by which the drug acts to prevent migraine headache is unkown. It may act by restoring normal inhibitory tone to the pain modulating pathways in the trigeminal vascular system.

Pharmacokinetics
● *Absorption:* Absorbed rapidly and completely from the GI tract after oral administration; however, only about 20% to 35% of the drug reaches systemic circulation because of first-pass effect. When administered orally, peak effects occur within 1 to 2 hours with conventional tablets and within 4 to 8 hours with sustained-release preparations. When administered I.V., effects occur within minutes after injection and usually persist about 30 to 60 minutes (although they may last up to 6 hours).

● *Distribution:* Steady-state distribution volume in healthy adults ranges from about 4.5 to 7 liters/kg but may increase to 12 liters/kg in patients with hepatic cirrhosis. Approximately 90% of circulating drug crosses placental barrier. Therapeutic plasma level range is 80 to 300 mg/ml.

• *Metabolism:* Metabolized in the liver.
• *Excretion:* Excreted in the urine as unchanged drug and active metabolites. Elimination half-life is normally 6 to 12 hours and increases to as much as 16 hours in patients with hepatic cirrhosis. In infants, elimination half-life may be 5 to 7 hours.

Contraindications and precautions
Verapamil is contraindicated in patients with severe hypotension (systolic blood pressure below 90 mm Hg) or cardiogenic shock because of the drug's hypotensive effect; in patients with second- or third-degree AV block or sick sinus syndrome (unless a functioning artificial ventricular pacemaker is in place) because of the drug's effects on the cardiac conduction system; in patients with severe left ventricular dysfunction (indicated by pulmonary wedge pressure above 20 mm Hg and left ventricular ejection fraction below 20%), unless heart failure results from supraventricular tachycardia, because the drug may worsen the condition; in patients with ventricular dysfunction or AV abnormalities who are receiving beta-adrenergic blockers because of the drug's negative inotropic effect and inhibition of the cardiac conduction system; and in patients with known hypersensitivity to the drug.

Verapamil should be used with caution in patients with moderately severe ventricular dysfunction or heart failure because the drug may precipitate or worsen the condition; in patients with hypertrophic cardiomyopathy because the drug may cause serious and sometimes fatal adverse CV effects (pulmonary edema, hypotension, heart block, or sinus arrest); in patients with hepatic or renal impairment because the drug may accumulate (generally, the dose should be reduced and the patient carefully monitored); in patients with sick sinus syndrome (with a functioning artificial ventricular pacemaker), atrial flutter, or fibrillation with an accessory bypass tract (such as Wolff-Parkinson-White or Lown-Ganong-Levine syndrome) because the drug may precipitate life-threatening adverse effects (ventricular fibrillation or cardiac arrest); in patients with wide-complex ventricular tachycardia because the drug may cause marked hemodynamic deterioration and ventricular fibrillation; and in patients receiving the drug I.V. because of possible adverse hemodynamic effects (hypotension) and adverse ECG effects (such as bradycardia and heart block).

Interactions
Concomitant use of verapamil with beta blockers may cause additive effects leading to CHF, conduction disturbances, arrhythmia, and hypotension, especially if high beta blocker doses are used, if the drugs are administered I.V., or if the patient has moderately severe to severe CHF, severe cardiomyopathy, or recent MI.

Concomitant use of oral verapamil with digoxin may increase serum digoxin concentration by 50% to 75% during the first week of therapy. Concomitant use with antihypertensives may lead to combined antihypertensive effects, resulting in clinically significant hypotension. Concomitant use with drugs that attenuate alpha-adrenergic response (such as prazosin and methyldopa) may cause excessive blood pressure reduction. Concomitant use with disopyramide may cause combined negative inotropic effects; with quinidine to treat hypertrophic cardiomyopathy, may cause excessive hypotension; with carbamazepine, may cause increased serum carbamazepine levels and subsequent toxicity; with rifampin, may substantially reduce verapamil's oral bioavailability; with lithium, may decrease plasma lithium levels; with calcium salts and vitamin D, may decrease effectiveness of verapamil.

Effects on diagnostic tests
None reported.

Adverse reactions
• CNS: dizziness, headache, fatigue, mental depression, confusion, psychotic symptoms.
• CV: transient hypotension, *heart failure,* bradycardia, AV block, *ventricular asystole,* peripheral edema.
• GI: constipation, nausea (primarily with oral form).
• Hepatic: elevated liver enzyme levels.
Note: Drug should be discontinued if systolic pressure falls below 90 mm Hg, if heart failure worsens, or if arrhythmia, hemodynamically significant bradycardia, or second- or third-degree heart block occurs.

Overdose and treatment
Clinical effects of overdose are primarily extensions of adverse reactions. Heart block, asystole, and hypotension are the most serious reactions and require immediate attention.

Treatment may include administering I.V. isoproterenol, norepinephrine, epinephrine, atropine, or calcium gluconate in usual doses. Adequate hydration should be ensured. Monitor cardiac and respiratory function.

---

*Canada only   †Unlabeled clinical use   Italicized adverse reactions are life-threatening.

In patients with hypertrophic cardiomyopathy, alpha-adrenergic agents, including methoxamine, phenylephrine, and metaraminol, should be used to maintain blood pressure. (Isoproterenol and norepinephrine should be avoided.) Inotropic agents, including dobutamine and dopamine, may be used if necessary.

If severe conduction disturbances, such as heart block and asystole, occur with hypotension that does not respond to drug therapy, cardiac pacing should be initiated immediately, with cardiopulmonary resuscitation measures as indicated.

In patients with Wolff-Parkinson-White or Lown-Ganong-Levine syndrome and a rapid ventricular rate caused by hemodynamically significant antegrade conduction, synchronized cardioversion may be used. Lidocaine and/or procainamide may be used as adjuncts.

▶ **Special considerations**
● If verapamil is initiated in patient receiving carbamazepine, a 40% to 50% reduction in carbamazepine dosage may be necessary. Monitor patient closely for signs of toxicity.
● Reduce dosage in patients with renal or hepatic impairment.
● If verapamil is added to therapy of patient receiving digoxin, digoxin dose should be reduced by half with subsequent monitoring of serum drug levels.
● Obtain periodic liver function tests.
● Weigh patient daily.

Information for the patient
Urge patient to report signs of CHF, such as swelling of hands and feet or shortness of breath.

Geriatric use
Elderly patients may require lower doses.

Breast-feeding
Verapamil is excreted in breast milk. To avoid possible adverse effects in infants, breast-feeding should be discontinued during verapamil therapy.

Antiparkinsonian agents

amantadine hydrochloride
benztropine mesylate
biperiden hydrochloride
biperiden lactate
bromocriptine mesylate
diphenhydramine hydrochloride
levodopa
levodopa-carbidopa
orphenadrine citrate
pergolide mesylate
procyclidine hydrochloride
selegiline hydrochloride
trihexyphenidyl hydrochloride

The goal of therapy in Parkinson's disease is to provide maximum relief of symptoms and maintain the patient's mobility and independence. No cure exists, and drug therapy is palliative, aimed at correcting or modifying neurotransmitter defects by inhibiting the dopamine-enhancing effects of acetylcholine.

Antiparkinsonian agents fall into two distinct categories: the anticholinergic agents, which block the effects of acetylcholine in the brain, and the dopaminergic agents, which directly and/or indirectly increase dopamine concentrations in the brain. Adjunctively, orphenadrine, a central-acting skeletal muscle relaxant, is used to relieve discomfort associated with Parkinson's disease.

Pharmacologic effects

● *Anticholinergic agents* (benztropine, biperiden, diphenhydramine, procyclidine, trihexyphenidyl) are centrally acting and especially useful as the disease progresses. Usually less effective than the dopaminergics in treating all forms of Parkinson's disease, anticholinergic agents reduce the incidence and severity of akinesia, rigidity, and tremor and secondary symptoms such as drooling. These agents may also inhibit the reuptake and storage of dopamine at central receptor sites, thus prolonging the action of dopamine.

● *Dopaminergic agents* (amantadine, bromocriptine, levodopa, levodopa-carbidopa, pergolide, selegiline) are the more effective agents, particularly against spasticity. Dopaminergic agents act primarily on the basal ganglia. Levodopa is the prototype of this group. As the immediate precursor of dopamine, levodopa is currently the most effective treatment, as dopaminergic deficiency appears to be central in the pathogenesis of Parkinson's disease. Unfortunately, it is useful for only 2 to 5 years, as patient response to it diminishes and eventually requires additional treatment with dopaminergic agonists.

● The *adjunctive agent* (orphenadrine) has anticholinergic actions; it produces symptomatic relief of tremor. It is used as an adjunct to physical therapy and with reduced doses of other more potent medications.

Mechanisms of action

● *Anticholinergic agents* may help to balance cholinergic and dopaminergic activity in the basal ganglia by partially blocking central cholinergic receptors.

● *Dopaminergic agents,* including levodopa, directly increase dopamine content in the brain. Current theory holds that a small amount of levodopa crosses the blood-brain barrier and is decarboxylated to dopamine, which then stimulates dopaminergic receptors in the basal ganglia, improving balance between cholinergic and dopaminergic activity. This improves modulation of voluntary nerve impulses transmitted to the motor cortex. Bromocriptine and pergolide directly stimulate dopamine receptors. Amantadine may increase dopamine release or block neuronal dopamine receptors. Selegiline increases dopaminergic activity through selective inhibition of MAO type B, which is found only in the brain. Other mechanisms, including interference with dopamine reuptake at the synapse, are also possible.

● The *adjunctive agent* (orphenadrine) has a mild anticholinergic action that produces its beneficial effect.

Pharmacokinetics

● *Absorption and distribution:* Anticholinergic agents are well-absorbed and widely distributed. Not much is known about their distribution other than they readily cross the blood-brain barrier.

COMPARING ANTIPARKINSONIAN DRUGS

CLASS AND DRUG	USUAL ADULT DOSAGE	SPECIAL CONSIDERATIONS
Anticholinergic agents		
benztropine biperiden procyclidine trihexyphenidyl	2 to 6 mg/day 6 to 30 mg/day 10 to 30 mg/day 6 to 15 mg/day	• Anticholinergic agents are useful in patients with autonomic symptoms (such as drooling or sweating). • May impair short term memory. • Titrate dosage slowly; observe for adverse effects.
Antihistamines		
diphenhydramine	50 to 150 mg/day	• Action may be related to drug's anticholinergic effects. • Monitor for excessive sedation.
Dopaminergic agents		
amantadine	200 mg/day	• Usually less effective than levodopa when used alone. • Commonly used with less than full doses of levodopa or with anticholinergic agents.
bromocriptine	2.5 to 7.5 mg/day	• Cardiovascular adverse reactions limit use. Watch for hypotension, especially at the start of therapy.
levodopa	1 to 2 g/day	• Cardiovascular side effects limit use. Watch for hypotension, nausea, vomiting, and arrhythmias, especially at the start of therapy.
levodopa-carbidopa	300 to 400 mg levodopa with 75 to 100 mg carbidopa daily	• Carbidopa suppresses peripheral metabolism of levodopa, reducing the amount of levodopa needed each day. • Daily dose of carbidopa should exceed 70 mg to inhibit peripheral levodopa metabolism.
pergolide	3 mg/day	• At start of therapy, drug may exacerbate dyskinesia, dizziness, or hallucinations. • Used with levodopa-carbidopa.
selegiline	10 mg/day	• Used with levodopa-carbidopa to reduce dosage and restore effectiveness of carbidopa.
Monoamine oxidase inhibitors		
selegiline	10 mg/day	• Higher than recommended doses may increase risk of toxicity. • Used with levodopa-carbidopa.

Levodopa is well-absorbed, but only about 1% actually crosses the blood-brain barrier and reaches the CNS because the drug is rapidly metabolized in the body.

• *Metabolism and excretion:* The metabolic fate of anticholinergics has not been studied in detail. Most are excreted in the urine as metabolites.

The small amount of levodopa that enters the CNS is rapidly converted by the L-aromatic amino acid decarboxylase to dopamine, which probably enters the normal pool of neurotransmitter available to the brain. Dopamine's action within the CNS is terminated by reuptake into dopaminergic nerve terminals, but small amounts may be metabolized to 3,4 dihydroxyphenylacetic acid (DOPAC) and homovanillic acid (HVA).

Most levodopa is metabolized in the stomach and intestines and during the first pass through the liver to dopamine by decarboxylase, an enzyme that is widely distributed. Carbidopa, a drug that inhibits this peripheral decarboxylation, may increase the availability of levodopa to the CNS.

Metabolites of levodopa include 3-*O*-methyldopa, dopamine, norepinephrine, and epinephrine. Dopamine may be converted to DOPAC and HVA, which are excreted in the urine.

Adverse reactions and toxicity

The anticholinergic agents and orphenadrine produce similar adverse reactions: dry mouth, dizziness, drowsiness, tachycardia, palpitations, nausea, vomiting, depression, confusion, blurred vision, increased intraocular pressure, urinary hesitancy, and urine retention.

Anticholinergic toxicity and overdose produce similar reactions that may include circulatory collapse, cardiac arrest, respiratory depression, foul-smelling breath, and dry, flushed hot skin.

Severe intoxication with orphenadrine develops rapidly; death can occur within 3 to 5 hours. Treatment of acute overdose is gastric lavage to prevent further absorption, followed by symptomatic and supportive treatment.

No overt adverse reactions or overdoses have been reported with carbidopa or bromocriptine. Any reactions reported have been associated with concurrent administration of levodopa, which produces adverse reactions in nearly every patient. Nausea, anorexia, flatulence, and dry mouth are most common; tolerance does develop. Abnormal involuntary movements, behavioral changes, easy sexual arousal, and olfactory hallucinations are also common.

Selegiline has been associated with reactions similar to those reported with the anticholinergic agents. Signs and symptoms of overdose may resemble those of nonselective MAO inhibitors; therefore, treatment should be modeled after MAO inhibitor poisoning. Pergolide most often causes dyskinesia, hallucination, somnolence, insomnia, nausea, and rhinitis. There is no clinical experience with massive overdose; however, 60-mg dosage produced vomiting, hypotension, and agitation. Treatment is symptomatic and supportive. Amantadine may cause hyperexcitability, tremor, anxiety, and slurred speech.

Clinical considerations

● Concurrent administration of amantadine and levodopa produces rapid therapeutic benefits.
● "On-off" phenomenon develops in 15% to 40% of patients taking levodopa.
● Diphenhydramine is useful initially in patients with minimal symptoms and is better tolerated by elderly patients.
● May be taken before or after meals as determined by patient response.
● Choreiform and other involuntary movements occur in 50% to 80% of patients, are usually dose-related, and may be minimized by combination therapy.
● Adverse reactions are more likely in elderly patients.
● Monitor blood cell counts, hepatic function, renal function, and blood pressure. Regular eye examinations are also recommended during therapy.
● Advise patients to avoid driving and other hazardous tasks that require alertness until drug's effects are known.
● Advise patients to use caution in hot weather because these drugs increase susceptibility to heat stroke.
● The anticholinergic agents useful in Parkinson's disease can suppress the extrapyramidal effects of the neuroleptic agents, but should not be used chronically as they mask the development of tardive dyskinesia.

---

amantadine hydrochloride
Symmetrel

● Pharmacologic classification: synthetic cyclic primary amine
● Therapeutic classification: antiparkinsonian agent
● Pregnancy risk category D

How supplied

Available by prescription only
Capsules: 100 mg
Syrup: 50 mg/5 ml

Indications, route, and dosage
Treatment of drug-induced extrapyramidal reactions
Adults: 100 mg P.O. b.i.d., up to 300 mg/day in divided doses. Patient may benefit from as much as 400 mg/day, but doses over 200 mg must be closely supervised.
Treatment of idiopathic parkinsonism, parkinsonian syndrome
Adults: 100 mg P.O. b.i.d.; in patients who are seriously ill or receiving other antiparkinsonian drugs, 100 mg daily for at least 1 week, then 100 mg b.i.d. p.r.n.

Patients with renal dysfunction require dosage reduction.

Dosage in renal failure

Base dosage on creatinine clearance value, as follows:

Creatinine clearance value (ml/minute/1.73 m²) determines maintenance dosage. Thus, if creatinine clearance is greater than 80 ml/minute, maintenance dosage is 100 mg b.i.d.; if 60 to 80 ml/minute, 200 mg or 100 mg on alternate days; 40 to 60 ml/minute, 100 mg once daily; 30 to 40 ml/minute, 200 mg twice weekly; 20 to 30 ml/minute, 100 mg three times weekly; 10 to 20 ml/minute, 200 mg or 100 mg alternating q 7 days.

Note: Patients on chronic hemodialysis should receive 200 mg or 100 mg alternating q 7 days.

Pharmacodynamics

Antiparkinsonian action: Amantadine is thought to cause the release of dopamine in the substantia nigra.

Pharmacokinetics

● *Absorption:* With oral administration, well absorbed from the GI tract. Peak serum levels occur in 1 to 8 hours; usual serum level is 0.2 to 0.9 mcg/ml. (Neurotoxicity may occur at levels exceeding 1.5 mcg/ml.)

● *Distribution:* Distributed widely throughout the body and crosses the blood-brain barrier.

● *Metabolism:* About 10% of dose is metabolized.

● *Excretion:* About 90% of dose is excreted unchanged in urine, primarily by tubular secretion. Portion of drug may be excreted in breast milk. Excretion rate depends on urine pH (acidic pH enhances excretion). In patients with normal renal function, elimination half-life is approximately 24 hours. In patients with renal dysfunction, elimination half-life may be prolonged to 10 days.

Contraindications and precautions

Amantadine is contraindicated in patients with known hypersensitivity to the drug.

Amantadine should be administered cautiously to patients with a history of hepatic disease, seizures, psychosis, renal disease, recurrent eczematoid dermatitis, CV disease (especially CHF), peripheral edema, or orthostatic hypotension because the drug may exacerbate these disorders. Do not administer to pregnant women or women of childbearing age without adequate contraceptive measures because animal studies have demonstrated embryotoxic and teratogenic potential.

Interactions

When used concomitantly, amantadine may potentiate anticholinergic adverse effects of trihexyphenidyl and benztropine (when these drugs are given in high doses), possibly causing confusion and hallucinations. Concomitant use with triamterene-hydrochlorothiazide may decrease urinary excretion of amantadine, resulting in increased serum amantadine levels and possible toxicity.

Concomitant use with CNS stimulants may cause additive stimulation. Concomitant use with alcohol may result in light-headedness, confusion, fainting, and hypotension.

Effects on diagnostic tests

None reported.

Adverse reactions

● CNS: depression, fatigue, confusion, dizziness, psychosis, hallucination, anxiety, irritability, ataxia, insomnia, weakness, headache, light-headedness, difficulty concentrating.

● CV: peripheral edema, orthostatic hypotension, CHF.

● DERM: livedo reticularis (with prolonged use).

● GI: anorexia, nausea, constipation, vomiting, dry mouth.

● GU: urine retention.

Note: Drug should be discontinued if patient develops hypersensitivity reaction.

Overdose and treatment

Clinical effects of overdose include nausea, vomiting, anorexia, hyperexcitability, tremor, slurred speech, blurred vision, lethargy, anticholinergic symptoms, seizures, and possible ventricular arrhythmias, including torsade de pointes and ventricular fibrillation.

Note: CNS effects result from increased levels of dopamine in the brain.

Treatment includes immediate gastric lavage or emesis induction along with supportive measures, forced fluids, and, if necessary, I.V. administration of fluids. Urine acidification may be used to increase drug excretion. Physostigmine may be given (1 to 2 mg by slow I.V. infusion at 1- to 2-hour intervals) to counteract CNS toxicity. Seizures or arrhythmias may be treated with conventional therapy. Patient should be monitored closely.

▶ Special considerations
- To prevent orthostatic hypotension, instruct patient to move slowly when changing position (especially when rising to standing position).
- If patient experiences insomnia, administer dose several hours before bedtime.

Information for the patient
- Warn patient that drug may impair mental alertness.
- Advise patient to take drug after meals to ensure best absorption.
- Caution patient to avoid abrupt position changes because these may cause light-headedness or dizziness.
- Warn patient who is taking drug to treat parkinsonism not to discontinue it abruptly, because that might precipitate a parkinsonian crisis.
- Warn patient to avoid alcohol while taking drug.
- Instruct patient to report adverse reactions promptly, especially dizziness, depression, anxiety, nausea, and urine retention.

Geriatric use
Elderly patients are more susceptible to adverse neurologic effects; dividing daily dosage into two doses may reduce this risk.

---

benztropine mesylate
Cogentin

- Pharmacologic classification: anticholinergic
- Therapeutic classification: antiparkinsonian agent
- Pregnancy risk category C

How supplied
Available by prescription only
Tablets: 0.5 mg, 1 mg, 2 mg
Injection: 1 mg/ml in 2-ml ampule

Indications, route, and dosage
Acute dystonic reaction
Adults: 2 mg I.V. or I.M. followed by 1 to 2 mg P.O. b.i.d. to prevent recurrence.
Parkinsonism
Adults: 0.5 to 6 mg P.O. daily. Initially, 0.5 to 1 mg, increased 0.5 mg q 5 to 6 days. Adjust dosage to meet individual requirements.

Pharmacodynamics
Antiparkinsonian action: Benztropine has both anticholinergic and antihistaminic activity. It probably acts by blocking central cholinergic receptors in the basal ganglia, restoring a normal balance of acetylcholine activity.

Pharmacokinetics
- *Absorption:* Absorbed from the GI tract.
- *Distribution:* Largely unknown; however, the drug crosses the blood-brain barrier and may cross the placenta.
- *Metabolism:* Unknown.
- *Excretion:* Like other muscarinics, excreted in the urine as unchanged drug and metabolites. After oral therapy, small amounts are probably excreted in feces as unabsorbed drug.

Contraindications and precautions
Benztropine is contraindicated in patients with narrow-angle glaucoma because drug-induced cycloplegia and mydriasis may increase intraocular pressure.

Administer benztropine cautiously to patients with prostatic hypertrophy because the drug may exacerbate urine retention; to patients with tachycardia because the drug may block vagal inhibition of the sinoatrial node pacemaker and exacerbate tachycardia; and to elderly patients because they may be more susceptible to the drug's effects.

Interactions
Concomitant use with amantadine may amplify such adverse anticholinergic effects as confusion and hallucinations. Benztropine dosage should be decreased before giving amantadine. Concomitant use with haloperidol and phenothiazines may decrease their effect, possibly reflecting direct CNS antagonism. Concomitant use with phenothiazines increases the risk of adverse anticholinergic effects.

Alcohol and other CNS depressants increase benztropine's sedative effects. Antacids and antidiarrheals may decrease benztropine absorption. Administer benztropine at least 1 hour before these agents.

Effects on diagnostic tests
None reported.

Adverse reactions
- CNS: disorientation, restlessness, agitation, confusion, excitement, memory loss, giddiness, psychoses, paranoia, delirium, delusions, euphoria, parasthesia, heaviness of extremities, hallucination, headache, depression, weakness.

- CV: palpitations, tachycardia, paradoxical bradycardia.
- DERM: urticaria, hypersensitivity rash, decreased sweating.
- EENT: dilated pupils, blurred vision, photophobia.
- GI: constipation, dry mouth, nausea, vomiting, epigastric distress, dysphagia.
- GU: dysuria, urinary hesitancy, urine retention.

Note: Drug should be discontinued if hypersensitivity, urine retention, confusion, hallucinations, dilated and nonreactive pupils, or hot, dry, flushed skin occurs.

Overdose and treatment
Clinical manifestations of overdose include central stimulation followed by depression and psychotic symptoms such as disorientation, confusion, hallucinations, delusions, anxiety, agitation, and restlessness. Peripheral effects may include dilated, nonreactive pupils; blurred vision; hot, flushed, dry skin; dryness of mucous membranes; dysphagia; decreased or absent bowel sounds; urine retention; hyperthermia; tachycardia; hypertension; and increased respiration.

Treatment is primarily symptomatic and supportive, as necessary. Maintain a patent airway. If patient is alert, induce emesis with ipecac syrup (or use gastric lavage) and follow with a saline cathartic and activated charcoal to prevent further absorption. In severe cases, physostigmine may be administered to block benztropine's antimuscarinic effects. Give fluids as needed to treat shock, diazepam to control psychotic symptoms, and pilocarpine (instilled into the eyes) to relieve mydriasis. If urine retention occurs, catheterization may be necessary.

▶ **Special considerations**
Besides those relevant to all *anticholinergics*, consider the following recommendations.
- To help prevent gastric irritation, administer drug after meals.
- Never discontinue drug abruptly.
- Monitor patient for intermittent constipation and abdominal distention and pain, which may indicate paralytic ileus.

Information for the patient
- Explain that drug's full effect may not occur for 2 to 3 days after therapy begins.
- Caution patient not to discontinue drug suddenly; dosage should be reduced gradually.

Geriatric use
Use cautiously in elderly patients because it can worsen memory impairment.

**biperiden hydrochloride,
biperiden lactate**
Akineton

- Pharmacologic classification: anticholinergic
- Therapeutic classification: antiparkinsonian agent
- Pregnancy risk category C

How supplied
Available by prescription only
Tablets: 2 mg
Injection: 5 mg/ml in 1-ml ampule

Indications, route, and dosage
Extrapyramidal disorders
Adults: 2 to 6 mg P.O. daily, b.i.d., or t.i.d., depending on severity. Usual dose is 2 mg daily, or 2 mg I.M. or I.V. q ½ hour, not to exceed four doses or 8 mg daily.
Parkinsonism
Adults: 2 mg P.O. t.i.d. to q.i.d.

Pharmacodynamics
Antiparkinsonian action: Biperiden blocks both the nicotinic and muscarinic actions of acetylcholine. It probably acts by blocking central cholinergic receptors in the basal ganglia, restoring a normal balance of acetylcholine activity.

Pharmacokinetics
- *Absorption:* Well absorbed from the GI tract.
- *Distribution:* Well distributed throughout the body.
- *Metabolism:* Exact metabolic fate is unknown.
- *Excretion:* Excreted in the urine as unchanged drug and metabolites. After oral therapy, small amounts are probably excreted as unabsorbed drug.

Contraindications and precautions
Administer biperiden cautiously to patients with prostatic hypertrophy because the drug may exacerbate urine retention; to patients with cardiac arrhythmias because it may block vagal inhibition of the sinoatrial node pacemaker; and to patients with narrow-angle glaucoma because drug-induced cycloplegia and mydriasis may increase intraocular pressure.

Interactions

Amantadine may amplify biperiden's anticholinergic adverse effects, such as confusion and hallucinations. Decrease biperiden dosage before amantadine administration.

Concomitant use with haloperidol or phenothiazines may decrease the antipsychotic effectiveness of these drugs, possibly by direct CNS antagonism. Concomitant use with phenothiazines increases risk of adverse anticholinergic effects.

Alcohol and other CNS depressants increase biperiden's sedative effects. Antacids and antidiarrheals may decrease biperiden absorption. Administer biperiden at least 1 hour before these drugs.

Effects on diagnostic tests

None reported.

Adverse reactions

● CNS: headache, disorientation, temporary euphoria, restlessness, drowsiness, confusion and excitement (in elderly), dizziness, transient psychosis, agitation, disturbed behavior.
● CV: transient postural hypotension.
● EENT: blurred vision.
● GI: constipation, dry mouth, nausea, vomiting, epigastric distress, abdominal distention.
● GU: urinary hesitancy, urine retention.

Note: Drug should be discontinued if hypersensitivity; urine retention; confusion; hallucinations; dilated, nonreactive pupils; or hot, dry, flushed skin occurs.

Overdose and treatment

Clinical effects of overdose include central stimulation followed by depression and psychotic symptoms such as disorientation, confusion, hallucination, delusions, anxiety, agitation, and restlessness. Peripheral effects may include dilated, nonreactive pupils; blurred vision; hot, dry, flushed skin; dry mucous membranes; dysphagia; decreased or absent bowel sounds; urine retention; hyperthermia; headache; tachycardia; hypertension; and increased respiration.

Treatment is primarily symptomatic and supportive, as necessary. Maintain patent airway. If the patient is alert, induce emesis (or use gastric lavage) and follow with a saline cathartic and activated charcoal to prevent further absorption of orally administered drug. In severe cases, physostigmine may be administered to block biperiden's antimuscarinic effects. Give fluids, as needed, to treat shock; diazepam to control psychotic symptoms; and pilocarpine (instilled into the eyes) to relieve mydriasis. If urine retention occurs, catheterization may be necessary.

▶ Special considerations

Besides those relevant to all *anticholinergics,* consider the following recommendations.
● When giving drug parenterally, keep patient supine; parenteral administration may cause transient postural hypotension and disturbed coordination.
● When giving biperiden I.V., inject the drug slowly.
● Because biperiden may cause dizziness, patient may need assistance when walking.
● In patients with severe parkinsonism, tremors may increase when drug is administered to relieve spasticity.

Information for the patient

Tell patient that, with chronic biperiden administration, tolerance to therapeutic effects and adverse reactions can occur.

Geriatric use

Use cautiously in elderly patients because it can worsen memory impairment. Lower doses are indicated.

Pediatric use

Biperiden is not recommended for children.

Breast-feeding

Biperiden may be excreted in breast milk, possibly resulting in infant toxicity. It may also decrease milk production. Breast-feeding women should avoid this drug.

---

bromocriptine mesylate
Parlodel

● Pharmacologic classification: dopamine receptor antagonist
● Therapeutic classification: antiparkinsonian agent
● Pregnancy risk category C

How supplied

Available by prescription only
Tablets: 2.5 mg
Capsules: 5 mg

Indications, route, and dosage
Parkinson's disease
Adults: Initial dose of 1.25 mg P.O. b.i.d. with meals. Dosage may be increased q 14 to 28 days, up to 100 mg daily or until a maximal therapeutic response is achieved. Safety in dosages over 100 mg daily has not been established.

Pharmacodynamics
Antiparkinsonian action: Bromocriptine activates dopaminergic receptors in the neostriatum of the CNS, which may produce its antiparkinsonian activity. Dysregulation of brain serotonin activity also may occur. The precise role of bromocriptine in treating parkinsonian syndrome requires further study of its safety and efficacy in long-term therapy.

Pharmacokinetics
• *Absorption:* Bromocriptine is 28% absorbed when given orally and reaches peak levels in about 1 to 3 hours. Plasma concentrations for therapeutic effects are unknown.
• *Distribution:* Bromocriptine is 90% to 96% bound to serum albumin.
• *Metabolism:* First-pass metabolism occurs with over 90% of the absorbed dose. Bromocriptine is metabolized completely in the liver, principally by hydrolysis, before excretion. The metabolites are not active or toxic.
• *Excretion:* The major route of bromocriptine excretion is through the bile. Only 2.5% to 5.5% of the dose is excreted in urine. Almost all (85%) of the dose is excreted in feces in 120 hours.

Contraindications and precautions
Bromocriptine is contraindicated in patients with a sensitivity to any ergot alkaloids and in those with severe ischemic heart disease or peripheral vascular disease because of the CV effects of the drug. Because bromocriptine prevents lactation, it should not be used by breast-feeding women.

Bromocriptine should be used cautiously in patients with Raynaud's disease, which may be exacerbated; in patients with hepatic and renal dysfunction or with a history of psychiatric disorders because the drug may worsen these disorders; and in patients with a history of MI with residual arrhythmias because drug may induce arrhythmias.

Interactions
Bromocriptine may potentiate antihypertensive agents, requiring a reduction of their dosage to prevent hypotension.

Alcohol intolerance may result when high doses of bromocriptine are administered; therefore, concomitant ingestion of alcohol should be limited.

Effects on diagnostic tests
Transient elevation of BUN, ALT (SGPT), AST (SGOT), CPK, alkaline phosphatase, and uric acid levels may occur.

Adverse reactions
Incidence of adverse reactions is high (68%); however, most are mild to moderate, and only 6% of patients discontinue the drug for this reason. Nausea is the most common adverse reaction, occurring in 51% of patients taking the drug. The potential for adverse reactions may be decreased by reducing dosage to one-half of a tablet one to three times daily initially, then gradually increasing it to the minimum effective dose.
• CNS: dizziness, headache, fatigue, mania, delusions, nervousness, insomnia, depression.
• CV: hypotension, postural hypotension, syncope.
• DERM: rash, mottling of the skin, urticaria.
• EENT: nasal congestion, tinnitus, blurred vision.
• GI: nausea, vomiting, abdominal cramps, constipation, diarrhea, metallic taste, dry mouth, dysphagia, anorexia.
• GU: urine retention, urinary frequency, incontinence, diuresis.
• Other: *pulmonary infiltrates* and *pleural effusions,* coolness and pallor of fingers and toes, facial pallor.

Overdose and treatment
Overdosage of bromocriptine may cause nausea, vomiting, and severe hypotension. Treatment includes emptying the stomach by aspiration and lavage and administering I.V. fluids to treat hypotension.

▶ Special considerations
• First-dose phenomenon occurs in 1% of patients. Sensitive patients may experience syncope for 15 to 60 minutes but can usually tolerate subsequent treatment without ill effects.
• Administer with meals, milk, or snacks to diminish GI distress.
• Alcohol intolerance may occur, especially when high doses of bromocriptine are administered; therefore, alcohol should be avoided.
• Bromocriptine is usually given with either levodopa alone or levodopa-carbidopa combination.

● Adverse reactions are more common when drug is given in high doses.

Information for the patient
● Tell patient to take first dose where and when he can lie down, because drowsiness is common at start of therapy.
● Instruct patient to report any visual problems, severe nausea and vomiting, or acute headaches.
● Warn patient to avoid hazardous tasks that require alertness and coordination until the drug's CNS effects are known.
● Advise patient to avoid alcohol during treatment.

Geriatric use
● Use with caution, particularly in patients receiving long-term, high-dose therapy. Regular physical assessment is recommended, with particular attention toward changes in pulmonary function.
● Safety not established for long-term use at the doses required to treat Parkinson's disease.

---

diphenhydramine hydrochloride
Beldin, Benadryl, Diahist, Diphen, Diphenadryl, Fenylhist, Fynex, Hydramine, Hydril

● Pharmacologic classification: ethanolamine-derivative antihistamine
● Therapeutic classification: antiparkinsonian (anticholinergic) agent
● Pregnancy risk category B

How supplied
Available with or without prescription
Tablets: 25 mg, 50 mg
Capsules: 25 mg, 50 mg
Elixir: 12.5 mg/5 ml (14% alcohol)
Syrup: 12.5 mg/5 ml, 13.3 mg/5 ml (5% alcohol)
Injection: 10 mg/ml, 50 mg/ml

Indications, route, and dosage
Symptomatic treatment of parkinsonian syndrome in elderly patients unable to tolerate levodopa therapy
Adults: Initially, 25 mg P.O. t.i.d. If necessary, gradually increase dosage to 50 mg P.O. q.i.d.
Control of dyskinetic movement
Adults: Initially, 25 mg t.i.d., increased to 50 mg q.i.d.; or 10 to 50 mg I.M. or I.V.

Pharmacodynamics
Antiparkinsonian action: Diphenhydramine blocks muscarinic receptors as well as histamine$_1$ receptors. Its central antimuscarinic effects help to balance cholinergic activity in the basal ganglia.

Pharmacokinetics
● *Absorption:* Diphenhydramine is well absorbed from the GI tract. Action begins within 15 to 30 minutes and peaks in 1 to 4 hours.
● *Distribution:* Diphenhydramine is distributed widely throughout the body, including the CNS; drug crosses the placenta. Diphenhydramine is approximately 82% protein-bound.
● *Metabolism:* About 50% to 60% of an oral dose of diphenhydramine is metabolized by the liver before reaching the systemic circulation (first-pass effect); virtually all available drug is metabolized by the liver within 24 to 48 hours.
● *Excretion:* Plasma elimination half-life of diphenhydramine is about 3½ hours; drug and metabolites are excreted primarily in urine. Drug is also excreted in breast milk.

Contraindications and precautions
Diphenhydramine is contraindicated in patients with known hypersensitivity to this drug or antihistamines with similar chemical structures (carbinoxamine and clemastine); during an acute asthma attack because diphenhydramine thickens bronchial secretions; and in patients who have taken MAO inhibitors within the past 2 weeks. (See "Interactions.")

Diphenhydramine should be used with caution in patients with narrow-angle glaucoma; in those with pyloroduodenal obstruction or urinary bladder obstruction from prostatic hypertrophy or narrowing of the bladder neck because of its marked anticholinergic effects; in patients with CV disease, hypertension, or hyperthyroidism because of the risk of palpitations and tachycardia; and in patients with renal disease, diabetes, bronchial asthma, urine retention, or stenosing peptic ulcers.

Diphenhydramine should not be used during pregnancy, especially in the third trimester, or during breast-feeding. Antihistamines have caused seizures and other severe reactions, especially in premature infants.

Benadryl 50 mg Kapseals, as well as some other formulations, contain bisulfites, which can cause severe reactions in individuals allergic to these chemicals.

Interactions

MAO inhibitors interfere with the detoxification of diphenhydramine and thus prolong its central depressant and anticholinergic effects; additive CNS depression may occur when diphenhydramine is given concomitantly with other CNS depressants, such as alcohol, barbiturates, tranquilizers, sleeping aids, and anxiolytics.

Diphenhydramine may diminish the effects of sulfonylureas, enhance the effects of epinephrine, and partially counteract the anticoagulant effects of heparin.

Effects on diagnostic tests

Discontinue diphenhydramine 4 days before diagnostic skin tests; antihistamines can prevent, reduce, or mask positive skin test response.

Adverse reactions

● CNS: drowsiness, sedation, dizziness, disturbed coordination, confusion, headache, insomnia, restlessness, vertigo; (in children) fever, ataxia, excitement, seizures, hallucination.
● CV: hypotension, palpitations, tachycardia, extrasystoles.
● DERM: photosensitivity, urticaria.
● EENT: blurred vision, diplopia, dry nose and throat.
● GI: dry mouth, nausea, vomiting, diarrhea, constipation, epigastric distress, anorexia.
● GU: urinary frequency, dysuria, urine retention.
● HEMA: leukopenia, agranulocytosis, hemolytic anemia.
● Respiratory: chest tightness, wheezing, thickened bronchial secretions, *anaphylaxis.*

Overdose and treatment

Drowsiness is the usual clinical manifestation of overdose. Seizures, coma, and respiratory depression may occur with profound overdose. Anticholinergic symptoms, such as dry mouth, flushed skin, fixed and dilated pupils, and GI symptoms, are common, especially in children.

Treat overdose by inducing emesis with ipecac syrup (in conscious patient), followed by activated charcoal to reduce further drug absorption. Use gastric lavage if patient is unconscious or ipecac syrup fails. Treat hypotension with vasopressors, and control seizures with diazepam or phenytoin. *Do not give stimulants.*

▶ Special considerations

Besides those relevant to all *antihistamines,* consider the following recommendations.
● Drowsiness is the most common adverse re-

action during initial therapy but usually disappears with continued use of the drug.
● Diphenhydramine injection is compatible with most I.V. solutions, but is *incompatible* with some drugs; check compatibility before mixing in the same I.V. line.
● When giving I.M., alternate injection sites to prevent sterile abscess. Administer deep I.M. into large muscle.
● Protect injection and elixir from light.

Geriatric use

Elderly patients are usually more sensitive to adverse effects of antihistamines and are especially likely to experience a greater degree of dizziness, sedation, hyperexcitability, dry mouth, and urine retention than younger patients. Symptoms usually respond to a decrease in medication dosage.

---

levodopa (L-dopa)
Dopar, Larodopa

● Pharmacologic classification: precursor of dopamine
● Therapeutic classification: antiparkinsonian agent
● Pregnancy risk category C

How supplied

Available by prescription only
Tablets: 100 mg, 250 mg, 500 mg
Capsules: 100 mg, 250 mg, 500 mg

Indications, route, and dosage
Parkinsonism

Levodopa is indicated in treating idiopathic, postencephalitic, arteriosclerotic parkinsonism and symptomatic parkinsonism that may follow injury to the nervous system by carbon monoxide intoxication and manganese intoxication.
Adults: Initially, 0.5 to 1 g P.O. daily, given b.i.d., t.i.d., or q.i.d. with food; increase by no more than 0.75 g daily q 3 to 7 days, as tolerated, until usual maximum of 8 g is reached. Do *not* exceed 8 g/daily, except for exceptional patients. A significant therapeutic response may not be obtained for 6 months. Larger dose requires close supervision.

Pharmacodynamics

Antiparkinsonian action: Precise mechanism has not been established. A small percentage of each dose crossing the blood-brain barrier

---

is decarboxylated. The dopamine then stimulates dopaminergic receptors in the basal ganglia to enhance the balance between cholinergic and dopaminergic activity, resulting in improved modulation of voluntary nerve impulses transmitted to the motor cortex.

Pharmacokinetics

● *Absorption:* Levodopa is absorbed rapidly from small intestine by an active amino acid transport system, with 30% to 50% reaching general circulation.

● *Distribution:* Levodopa is distributed widely to most body tissues, but not to the CNS, which receives less than 1% of dose because of extensive metabolism in the periphery.

● *Metabolism:* 95% of levodopa is converted to dopamine by L-aromatic amino acid decarboxylase in the lumen of the stomach and intestines and on the first pass through the liver.

● *Excretion:* Levodopa is excreted primarily in urine; 80% of dose is excreted within 24 hours as dopamine metabolites. The half-life is 1 to 3 hours.

Contraindications and precautions

Levodopa is contraindicated in patients with known hypersensitivity and in patients receiving MAO inhibitors. Because levodopa may activate a malignant melanoma, do not use in patients with suspicious undiagnosed skin lesions or history of melanoma.

Drug should be used cautiously in patients with CV, renal, hepatic, or endocrine disease; in patients with history of MI with residual arrhythmias, peptic ulcer, seizures, psychiatric disorders, chronic wide-angle glaucoma, diabetes, pulmonary diseases, or bronchial asthma; and in patients receiving antihypertensives.

Interactions

Anesthetics or hydrocarbon inhalation may cause cardiac arrhythmias because of increased endogenous dopamine concentration. (Levodopa should be discontinued 6 to 8 hours before administration of anesthetics such as halothane.)

Antacids containing calcium, magnesium, or sodium bicarbonate may increase absorption of levodopa.

Concurrent use of anticonvulsants (such as hydantoin), benzodiazepines, phenothiazines, haloperidol, papaverine, rauwolfia alkaloids, or thioxanthenes may decrease therapeutic effects of levodopa.

Antihypertensives used concurrently with levodopa may produce increased hypotensive effect.

Methyldopa may alter the antiparkinsonian effects of levodopa and may produce additive toxic CNS effects.

Combined use with MAO inhibitors may cause a hypertensive crisis. MAO inhibitors should be discontinued for 2 to 4 weeks before starting levodopa.

Pyridoxine in a small dose (10 mg) reverses the antiparkinsonian effects of levodopa.

Sympathomimetics may increase the risk of cardiac arrhythmias (dosage reduction of the sympathomimetic is recommended; the administration of carbidopa with levodopa reduces the tendency of sympathomimetics to cause dopamine-induced cardiac arrhythmias).

Anticholinergics used with levodopa may produce a mild synergy and increased efficacy (gradual reduction in anticholinergic dosage is necessary).

Tricyclic antidepressants may increase sympathetic activity, with sinus tachycardia and hypertension.

Effects on diagnostic tests

Coombs' test occasionally becomes positive during extended therapy. Colorimetric test for uric acid has shown false elevations. Copper-reduction method has shown false-positive results for urine glucose; glucose oxidase method has shown false-negative results. Levodopa also may interfere with tests for urine ketones.

Adverse reactions

● CNS: choreiform, dystonic, dyskinetic movements; involuntary grimacing, head movements, myoclonic body jerks, ataxia, tremor, muscle twitching; bradykinetic episodes; psychiatric disturbances, memory loss, nervousness, anxiety, disturbing dreams, euphoria, malaise, fatigue; severe depression, *suicidal tendencies,* dementia, delirium, hallucination (may necessitate reduction or withdrawal of drug).

● CV: orthostatic hypotension, irregular heartbeat, tachycardia, palpitations, hypertension, phlebitis, anemia, blood dyscrasias.

● DERM: diaphoresis, rash, alopecia, scleroderma-like skin changes.

● EENT: blepharospasm, diplopia, blurred vision, dilated pupils, rhinorrhea.

● GI: nausea, vomiting, anorexia, weight loss (at start of therapy), constipation, flatulence, dysphagia, diarrhea, epigastric pain, hiccups, sialorrhea, dry mouth, burning tongue, bitter taste, abdominal distress.

● GU: transiently increased levels of BUN, uri-

---

nary frequency, urine retention, incontinence, darkened urine, priapism, increased libido.

• HEMA: *hemolytic anemia;* leukopenia, possibly requiring temporary cessation of levodopa therapy.

• Hepatic: transiently elevated levels of bilirubin, AST (SGOT), ALT (SGPT), LDH, alkaline phosphatase; protein-bound iodine; hepatotoxicity.

• Other: decreased glucose tolerance, dark perspiration, hyperventilation.

Overdose and treatment

Clinical manifestations of overdose include spasm or closing of eyelids, irregular heartbeat, or palpitations. Treatment includes immediate gastric lavage, maintenance of an adequate airway, and judicious administration of I.V. fluids and may include antiarrhythmic drugs if necessary. Pyridoxine P.O. 10 to 25 mg has been reported to reverse toxic and therapeutic effects of levodopa. (Its usefulness has not been established in acute overdose.)

▶ Special considerations

• Drug should be taken between meals and with low-protein snack to maximize drug absorption. Foods high in protein appear to interfere with transport of the drug.

• Because this drug may cause orthostatic hypotension, check the patient's sitting and supine blood pressure after initial administration.

• Maximum effectiveness of medication may not occur for several weeks or months after therapy begins.

• Carefully monitor patients also receiving antihypertensive medication or hypoglycemic agents for possible drug interactions. Stop MAO inhibitors at least 2 weeks before levodopa therapy begins.

• Adjust dosage according to patient's response and tolerance. Observe and monitor vital signs, especially while adjusting dose.

• Monitor patient for muscle twitching and blepharospasm (twitching of eyelids), which may be an early sign of drug overdose.

• Patients on long-term therapy should be tested regularly for diabetes and acromegaly; check blood tests and liver and kidney function studies periodically for adverse effects. Leukopenia may require cessation of therapy.

• If restarting therapy after a long period of interruption, adjust drug dosage gradually to previous level.

• Patients who must undergo surgery should continue levodopa as long as oral intake is permitted, usually 6 to 24 hours before surgery.

Drug should be resumed as soon as patient is able to take oral medication.

• Monitor serum laboratory tests periodically for changes. Coombs' test occasionally becomes positive during extended use. Expect uric acid elevation with colorimetric method but not with uricase method.

• Alkaline phosphatase, AST (SGOT), ALT (SGPT), LDH, bilirubin, BUN, and protein-bound iodine levels show transient elevations in patients receiving levodopa; WBC count and hemoglobin and hematocrit levels show occasional reduction.

• Although controversial, a medically supervised period of drug discontinuance (drug holiday) may reestablish the effectiveness of a lower dose regimen.

• Combination of levodopa-carbidopa usually reduces amount of levodopa needed, thus reducing incidence of adverse reactions.

• Tablets may be crushed and mixed with applesauce or baby-food fruits for patients who have difficulty swallowing tablets.

• Protect from heat, light, and moisture. If preparation darkens, it has lost potency and should be discarded.

Information for the patient

• Warn patient and family not to increase drug dose without specific instruction. (They may be tempted to do this as disease symptoms of parkinsonism progress.)

• Explain that therapeutic response may not occur for up to 6 months.

• Advise patient and family that multivitamin preparations, fortified cereals, and certain OTC medications may contain pyridoxine (vitamin B_6), which can reverse the effects of levodopa.

• Warn patient of possible dizziness and orthostatic hypotension, especially at start of therapy. Tell patient to change position slowly and dangle legs before getting out of bed. Instruct patient in use of elastic stockings to control the adverse reaction if appropriate.

• Instruct patient about signs and symptoms of adverse reactions and therapeutic effects and the need to report any changes.

• Tell patient to take a missed dose as soon as possible and to skip dose if next scheduled dose is within 2 hours, but not to double up doses.

• Advise the patient not to take levodopa with food, but that eating something about 15 minutes after administration may help reduce GI upset.

Geriatric use
● Smaller doses may be required because of reduced tolerance to the effects of levodopa.
● Elderly patients, especially those with osteoporosis, should resume normal activity gradually, because increased mobility may increase the risk of fractures.
● Elderly patients are more likely to develop psychic adverse reactions such as anxiety, confusion, or nervousness; those with preexisting coronary disease are more susceptible to levodopa's cardiac effects.

---

levodopa-carbidopa
Sinemet

● Pharmacologic classification: decarboxylase inhibitor-dopamine precursor combination
● Therapeutic classification: antiparkinsonian agent
● Pregnancy risk category C

How supplied
Available by prescription only
Tablets: 10 mg carbidopa with 100 mg levodopa (Sinemet 10-100), 25 mg carbidopa with 100 mg levodopa (Sinemet 25-100), 25 mg carbidopa with 250 mg levodopa (Sinemet 25-250)

Indications, route, and dosage
Parkinsonism
Adults: 3 to 6 tablets of 25 mg carbidopa/250 mg levodopa daily in divided doses; do not exceed 8 tablets daily. Optimum daily dosage must be determined by careful titration for each patient.
    Most patients respond to a 25 mg/100 mg combination (1 tablet t.i.d.). Dose may be increased q 1 or 2 days. Maintenance therapy must be carefully adjusted according to individual tolerance and desired therapeutic response.
    The daily dose of carbidopa should be 70 mg or above to suppress the peripheral metabolism of levodopa.

Pharmacodynamics
Antiparkinsonian action: Carbidopa inhibits the peripheral decarboxylation of levodopa, thus slowing its conversion to dopamine in extracerebral tissues. This results in an increased availability of levodopa for transport to the brain, where it undergoes decarboxylation to dopamine.

Pharmacokinetics
● *Absorption:* 40% to 70% of the dose is absorbed after oral administration. Plasma levodopa concentrations are increased when carbidopa and levodopa are administered concomitantly because carbidopa inhibits the peripheral metabolism of levodopa.
● *Distribution:* Carbidopa is distributed widely in body tissues except the CNS. Levodopa is also distributed into breast milk.
● *Metabolism:* Carbidopa is not metabolized extensively. It inhibits metabolism of levodopa in the GI tract, thus increasing its absorption from the GI tract and its concentration in plasma.
● *Excretion:* 30% of dose is excreted unchanged in urine within 24 hours. When given with carbidopa, the amount of levodopa excreted unchanged in urine is increased by about 6%. The half-life is 1 to 2 hours.

Contraindications and precautions
Levodopa-carbidopa is contraindicated in patients known to be hypersensitive to either drug and in patients with bronchial asthma, emphysema, or other severe pulmonary disorders; severe CV disease; narrow-angle glaucoma; history of or suspected melanoma; or history of MI, because the drug may exacerbate symptoms of these disorders.

Interactions
Concomitant use with amantadine, benztropine, procyclidine, or trihexyphenidyl may increase the efficacy of levodopa. Bromocriptine may produce additive effects, allowing reduced levodopa dosage.
    Anesthetics or hydrocarbon inhalation may cause cardiac arrhythmias because of increased endogenous dopamine concentration. (Levodopa-carbidopa should be discontinued 6 to 8 hours before administration of anesthetics such as halothane.)
    Antacids containing calcium, magnesium, or sodium bicarbonate may increase absorption of levodopa.
    Concurrent use of anticonvulsants (hydantoins), benzodiazepines, droperidol, haloperidol, loxapine, metyrosine, papaverine, phenothiazines, rauwolfia alkaloids, and thioxanthenes may decrease therapeutic effects of levodopa.
    Concomitant use with antihypertensives may increase the hypotensive effect.
    Methyldopa may alter the antiparkinsonian effects of levodopa and may produce additive toxic CNS effects. Molindone may inhibit anti-

---

parkinsonian effects of levodopa by blocking dopamine receptors in the brain.

Concurrent use of MAO inhibitors may cause a hypertensive crisis. MAO inhibitors should be discontinued for 2 to 4 weeks before starting levodopa-carbidopa.

Sympathomimetics may increase the risk of cardiac arrhythmias (reduced dosage of the sympathomimetic is recommended; however, the administration of carbidopa with levodopa reduces the tendency of sympathomimetics to cause dopamine-induced cardiac arrhythmias).

Effects on diagnostic tests

Antiglobulin determinations (Coombs' test) are occasionally positive after long-term use. Levodopa-carbidopa therapy may elevate serum gonadotropin levels. Serum and urine uric acid determinations may show false elevations. Thyroid function determinations may inhibit thyroid-stimulating hormone response to protirelin.

Urine glucose determinations using copper reduction method may show false-positive results; with the glucose oxidase method, false-negative results. Urine ketone determination using dipstick method, urine norepinephrine determinations, and urine protein determinations using Lowery test may show false-positive results.

Systemic effects of this drug may elevate levels of BUN, ALT (SGPT), alkaline phosphatase, AST (SGOT), serum bilirubin, lactate dehydrogenase, and serum protein-bound iodine.

Adverse reactions

● CNS: choreiform, dystonic, dyskinetic movements; involuntary grimacing, head movements, myoclonic body jerks, ataxia, tremor, muscle twitching; bradykinetic episodes; psychiatric disturbances, confusion, memory loss, nervousness, anxiety, disturbing dreams, euphoria, malaise, weakness, fatigue; severe depression, *suicidal tendencies,* dementia, delirium, hallucination (may necessitate reduction or withdrawal of drug).

● CV: orthostatic hypotension, cardiac irregularities, flushing, hypertension, phlebitis.

● EENT: blepharospasm, blurred vision, diplopia, mydriasis or miosis, widening of palpebral fissures, activation of latent Horner's syndrome, oculogyric crises, nasal discharge.

● GI: nausea, vomiting, anorexia, weight loss may occur at start of therapy; constipation; flatulence; diarrhea; epigastric pain; hiccups; sialorrhea; dry mouth; bitter taste.

● GU: urinary frequency, urine retention, urinary incontinence, darkened urine, excessive and inappropriate sexual behavior, priapism.

● HEMA: *hemolytic anemia.*

● Hepatic: hepatotoxicity.

● Other: dark perspiration, hyperventilation.

Note: Drug should be discontinued if unusual and uncontrollable body movements, irregular heartbeat or palpitations, spasms or closing of eyelids, or severe and continuous nausea and vomiting occur.

Overdose and treatment

There have been no reports of overdosage with carbidopa. Clinical manifestations of levodopa overdose are irregular heartbeat and palpitations, severe continuous nausea and vomiting, and spasm or closing of eyelids.

Treatment of overdose includes immediate gastric lavage and antiarrhythmic medication if necessary. Pyridoxine is not effective in reversing the actions of levodopa-carbidopa combinations.

▶ Special considerations

● Because the drug may cause orthostatic hypotension, check the patient's sitting and supine blood pressure after initial administration.

● Carefully monitor patients also receiving antihypertensive or hypoglycemic agents. Discontinue MAO inhibitors at least 2 weeks before therapy begins.

● Dosage is adjusted according to patient's response and tolerance to the drug. Therapeutic effects and adverse reactions occur more rapidly with levodopa-carbidopa combination than with levodopa alone. Observe and monitor vital signs, especially while dosage is being adjusted; report significant changes.

● Muscle twitching and blepharospasm (twitching of eyelids) may be an early sign of overdose.

● Patients on long-term therapy should be tested regularly for diabetes and acromegaly; periodically repeat blood tests and liver and kidney function studies.

● If patient is being treated with levodopa, discontinue at least 8 hours before starting levodopa-carbidopa.

● The combination drug usually reduces the amount of levodopa needed by 75%, thereby reducing the incidence of adverse reactions.

● Pyridoxine (vitamin B_6) does not reverse the beneficial effects of levodopa-carbidopa. Multivitamins can be taken without fear of losing control of symptoms.

● If therapy is interrupted temporarily, the usual daily dosage may be given as soon as patient resumes oral medications.

● Maximum effectiveness of medication may not occur for several weeks or months after therapy begins.

Information for the patient
● Instruct patient to report adverse reactions and therapeutic effects.
● Warn patient of possible dizziness or orthostatic hypotension, especially at the start of therapy. Patient should change position slowly and dangle legs before getting out of bed. Elastic stockings may control this adverse reaction in some patients.
● Tell patient to take food shortly after taking medication to relieve gastric irritation.
● Tell patient medication may cause darkening of the urine or sweat.
● Tell patient to take a missed dose as soon as possible, to skip a missed dose if next scheduled dose is within 2 hours, and never to double-dose.

Geriatric use
● In elderly patients, smaller doses may be required because of reduced tolerance to the effects of carbidopa-levodopa. Elderly patients, especially those with osteoporosis, should resume normal activity gradually because increased mobility may increase the risk of fractures.
● Elderly patients are especially vulnerable to psychic adverse reactions, such as anxiety, confusion, or nervousness; those with preexisting coronary disease are more susceptible to cardiac effects.

---

orphenadrine citrate
Banflex, Flexoject, Flexon, Marflex, Myolin, Neocyten, Noradex, Norflex, Orflagen, Orphenate

● Pharmacologic classification: diphenhydramine analog
● Therapeutic classification: skeletal muscle relaxant
● Pregnancy risk category C

How supplied
Available by prescription only
Tablets: 50 mg, 100 mg
Tablets (extended-release): 100 mg
Injection: 30 mg/ml

Indications, route, and dosage
†*Symptomatic treatment of parkinsonian syndrome*
Adults: 50 mg P.O. t.i.d.
Relief of acute painful muscle spasticity
Adults: 60 mg I.M. or I.V. q 12 hours.

Pharmacodynamics
Antiparkinsonian action: Orphenadrine blocks muscarinic receptors as well as histamine₁ receptors. Its central antimuscarinic effects help to balance cholinergic activity in the ganglia.

Pharmacokinetics
● *Absorption:* Rapidly absorbed from the GI tract; its onset of action occurs within 1 hour, peaks within 2 hours, and persists for 4 to 6 hours.
● *Distribution:* Widely distributed throughout the body.
● *Metabolism:* Metabolic fate unknown, but drug is almost completely metabolized to at least eight metabolites.
● *Excretion:* Excreted in urine, mainly as metabolites. Small amounts are excreted unchanged. Its half-life is about 14 hours.

Contraindications and precautions
Orphenadrine is contraindicated in patients with known hypersensitivity to the drug and in patients in whom anticholinergic and antimuscarinic effects are undesirable: those with achalasia, bladder neck obstruction, glaucoma, myasthenia gravis, peptic ulcer, prostatic hypertrophy, or pyloric or duodenal obstruction.
    Administer cautiously to patients with cardiac, hepatic, or renal function impairment.

Interactions
Concomitant use with propoxyphene or CNS depressants, including alcohol, anxiolytics, tricyclic antidepressants, narcotics, and antipsychotics, may produce additive CNS effects; concurrent use requires reduction of both agents. Use with other anticholinergic agents may increase anticholinergic effects; with MAO inhibitors, may increase adverse CNS effects.

Effects on diagnostic tests
None reported.

Adverse reactions
● CNS: drowsiness, dizziness, weakness, headache, restlessness, irritability, confusion (especially in elderly patients), disorientation, hallucination, insomnia.

- CV: tachycardia, palpitations, transient syncope.
- DERM: rash, pruritus, urticaria.
- GI: nausea, dry mouth, constipation, paralytic ileus, epigastric distress, difficulty swallowing.
- GU: urine retention, urinary hesitancy.
- Other: blurred vision, allergic reactions, *anaphylaxis, aplastic anemia,* increased intraocular pressure, mydriasis.

Note: Drug should be discontinued if hypersensitivity or cardiac arrhythmias occur.

Overdose and treatment
Clinical manifestations of overdose include dry mouth, blurred vision, urine retention, tachycardia, confusion, paralytic ileus, deep coma, seizures, shock, respiratory arrest, cardiac arrhythmias, and death.

Treatment includes symptomatic and supportive measures. If ingestion is recent, induce emesis or gastric lavage followed by activated charcoal. Monitor vital signs and fluid and electrolyte balance.

▶ **Special considerations**
- Because this drug may cause orthostatic hypotension, check the patient's sitting and supine blood pressure after initial administration.
- Periodic blood, urine, and liver function tests are recommended in prolonged therapy.
- Monitor vital signs, especially intake and output, noting any urine retention.
- When giving orphenadrine I.V., inject slowly over 5 minutes. Keep patient supine during and 5 to 10 minutes after injection. Paradoxical initial bradycardia may occur when giving I.V.; usually disappears in 2 minutes.

Information for the patient
- Advise patient to relieve dry mouth with ice chips, sugarless gum, hard candy, or saliva substitutes.
- Orphenadrine may cause drowsiness. Tell patient to avoid hazardous activities that require alertness or physical coordination until CNS depressant effects can be determined.
- Warn patient to avoid alcoholic beverages and to use cough and cold preparations cautiously because some contain alcohol.
- Tell patient to store drug away from heat and light (not in bathroom medicine cabinet) and safely out of reach of children.
- Instruct patient to take missed dose if remembered within 1 hour. If beyond 1 hour, patient should skip that dose and return to regular schedule. Do not double dose.

Geriatric use
Elderly patients may be more sensitive to drug's effects.

---

pergolide mesylate
Permax

- Pharmacologic classification: dopaminergic agonist
- Therapeutic classification: antiparkinsonian agent
- Pregnancy risk category B

How supplied
Available by prescription only
Tablets: 0.05 mg, 0.25 mg, 1 mg

Indications, route, and dosage
Adjunct to levodopa-carbidopa in the management of Parkinson's disease
Adults: Initially, 0.05 mg P.O. daily for the first 2 days. Gradually increase dosage by 0.1 to 0.15 mg q third day over the next 12 days of therapy. Subsequent dosage can be increased by 0.25 mg q third day until optimum response occurs. The mean therapeutic daily dose is 3 mg.

The drug is usually administered in divided doses t.i.d. Gradual reductions in levodopa-carbidopa dosage may be made during dosage titration.

Pharmacodynamics
Antiparkinsonian action: Pergolide stimulates dopamine receptors at both D_1 and D_2 sites. It acts by directly stimulating postsynaptic receptors in the nigrostriatal system.

Pharmacokinetics
- *Absorption:* Well absorbed after oral administration.
- *Distribution:* Approximately 90% bound to plasma proteins.
- *Metabolism:* Metabolized to at least 10 different compounds, some of which retain some pharmacologic activity.
- *Excretion:* Primarily by the kidneys.

Contraindications and precautions
Pergolide is contraindicated in patients allergic to the drug or ergot alkaloids.

Symptomatic orthostatic or sustained hypotension may occur in some patients, especially at initial therapy.

Hallucinosis may occur in some patients. Tolerance to this adverse reaction was not seen in early clinical trials.

In premarketing trials, over 140 of approximately 2,300 patients died while taking pergolide. However, these deaths did not appear to be linked to use of the drug, since these patients were elderly and debilitated.

Interactions
Concomitant use of drugs that are dopamine antagonists, including phenothiazines, butyrophenones, thioxanthines, and metoclopramide, may antagonize the effects of pergolide.

Concomitant use with levodopa may cause or exacerbate preexisting dyskinesia; it may also initiate or worsen hallucinations.

Effects on diagnostic tests
None reported.

Adverse reactions
● CNS: headache, asthenia, dyskinesia, dizziness, hallucination, dystonia, confusion, somnolence, insomnia, anxiety, depression, tremor, abnormal dreams, personality disorder, psychosis, abnormal gait, akathisia, extrapyramidal syndrome, incoordination, paresthesia, akinesia, hypertonia, neuralgia, speech disorder.
● CV: postural hypotension, vasodilation, palpitation, hypotension, syncope, hypertension, arrhythmias, MI.
● DERM: rash, sweating.
● EENT: rhinitis, epistaxis, abnormal vision, diplopia, taste perversion, eye disorder.
● GI: abdominal pain, nausea, constipation, diarrhea, dyspepsia, anorexia, vomiting, dry mouth.
● GU: urinary frequency, urinary tract infection, hematuria.
● Other: accident or injury; flu syndrome; chills; infection; facial, peripheral, or generalized edema; weight gain; arthralgia; bursitis; myalgia; twitching; chest, neck, and back pain.
Note: The above adverse reactions, although not always attributable to the drug, occurred in less than 1% of the study population.

Overdose and treatment
One patient who intentionally ingested 60 mg of pergolide presented with hypotension and vomiting. Other cases of overdose revealed symptoms of hallucination, involuntary movements, palpitations, and arrhythmias.

Treatment should be supportive. Monitor cardiac function and protect the patient's airway. Antiarrhythmics and sympathomimetics may be necessary to support CV function. Adverse CNS effects may be treated with dopaminergic antagonists (such as phenothiazines). If indicated, gastric lavage or induced emesis may be used to empty the stomach of its contents. Orally administered activated charcoal may be useful in attenuating absorption.

▶ Special considerations
In early clinical trials, 27% of the patients who attempted pergolide therapy did not finish the trial because of adverse reactions (primarily hallucinations and confusion).

Information for the patient
● Because this drug may cause orthostatic hypotension, check the patient's sitting and supine blood pressure after initial administration.
● Inform patient of the potential for adverse reactions. Warn patient to avoid activities that could expose him to injury secondary to orthostatic hypotension and syncope.
● Caution the patient to rise slowly to avoid orthostatic hypotension, particularly at the beginning of therapy.

Geriatric use
Use cautiously in elderly patients. The drug may cause orthostatic hypotension.

---

procyclidine hydrochloride
Kemadrin

● Pharmacologic classification: anticholinergic
● Therapeutic classification: antiparkinsonian agent
● Pregnancy risk category C

How supplied
Available by prescription only
Tablets: 5 mg

Indications, route, and dosage
Parkinsonism, muscle rigidity
Adults: Initially, 2 to 2.5 mg P.O. t.i.d. after meals. Increase as needed to maximum 60 mg daily.

Procyclidine is also used to relieve extrapyramidal dysfunction that accompanies treatment with phenothiazines and rauwolfia derivatives; drug controls excessive salivation from neuroleptic medications.

Pharmacodynamics
Antiparkinsonian action: Procyclidine blocks central cholinergic receptors, helping to bal-

ance cholinergic activity in the basal ganglia. It may also prolong dopamine's effects by blocking dopamine reuptake and storage at central receptor sites.

Pharmacokinetics
- *Absorption:* Absorbed from the GI tract.
- *Distribution:* Crosses the blood-brain barrier; little else is known about its distribution.
- *Metabolism:* Exact metabolic fate is unknown.
- *Excretion:* Excreted in the urine as unchanged drug and metabolites.

Contraindications and precautions
Procyclidine is contraindicated in patients with narrow-angle glaucoma, because drug-induced cycloplegia and mydriasis may increase intraocular pressure.

Administer procyclidine cautiously to patients with tachycardia, because drug may block vagal inhibition of the sinoatrial node pacemaker, thus exacerbating tachycardia; and to patients with urine retention or prostatic hypertrophy, because drug may exacerbate these conditions.

Interactions
Procyclidine may reduce the antipsychotic effectiveness of haloperidol and phenothiazines, possibly by direct CNS antagonism; concomitant use with phenothiazines also increases the risk of adverse anticholinergic effects. Paralytic ileus may result from concomitant use with phenothiazines or TCAs. Concomitant use with alcohol and other CNS depressants increases procyclidine's sedative effects.

Antacids and antidiarrheals may decrease procyclidine's absorption, thus reducing its effectiveness.

Effects on diagnostic tests
None reported.

Adverse reactions
- CNS: light-headedness, giddiness, nervousness, headache, confusion, muscle weakness, parasthesia, disorientation, memory loss, agitation, delusions, delirium, paranoia, euphoria, excitement, psychoses, depression, heaviness of extremities.
- CV: tachycardia, palpitations.
- DERM: rash, flushing, decreased sweating.
- EENT: blurred vision, mydriasis.
- GI: constipation, dry mouth, nausea, vomiting, epigastric distress.
- GU: urinary hesitancy.
- Other: hypersensitivity.

Note: Drug should be discontinued if hypersensitivity or skin rash develops.

Overdose and treatment
Clinical effects of overdose include central stimulation followed by depression, and such psychotic symptoms as disorientation, confusion, hallucination, delusions, anxiety, agitation, and restlessness. Peripheral effects may include dilated, nonreactive pupils; blurred vision; flushed, hot, dry skin; dry mucous membranes; dysphagia; decreased or absent bowel sounds; urine retention; hyperthermia; tachycardia; hypertension; and increased respiration.

Treatment is primarily symptomatic and supportive, as needed. Maintain patent airway. If the patient is alert, induce emesis (or use gastric lavage) and follow with a saline cathartic and activated charcoal to prevent further drug absorption. In severe cases, physostigmine may be administered to block procyclidine's antimuscarinic effects. Give fluids, as needed, to treat shock; diazepam to control psychotic symptoms; and pilocarpine (instilled into the eyes) to relieve mydriasis. If urine retention develops, catheterization may be necessary.

▶ Special considerations
Besides those relevant to all *anticholinergics,* consider the following recommendations.
- Monitor the patient closely for confusion, disorientation, agitation, hallucination, and other psychotic symptoms, especially if patient is elderly.
- Give procyclidine with food to decrease adverse GI effects.
- In patients with severe parkinsonism, tremor may increase because drug relieves spasticity.

Geriatric use
Administer procyclidine cautiously to elderly patients because it can worsen memory impairment. Lower doses are indicated.

**selegiline hydrochloride
(L-deprenyl hydrochloride)**
Eldepryl

- Pharmacologic classification: MAO inhibitor
- Therapeutic classification: antiparkinsonian agent
- Pregnancy risk category C

How supplied
Available by prescription only
Tablets: 5 mg

Indications, route, and dosage
Adjunctive treatment in the management of the symptoms associated with Parkinson's disease in patients who exhibit diminished response to levodopa-carbidopa
Adults: 10 mg P.O. daily, taken as 5 mg at breakfast and 5 mg at lunch. After 2 or 3 days of therapy, begin gradual decrease of levodopa-carbidopa dosage.

Pharmacodynamics
Antiparkinsonian action: Probably acts by selectively inhibiting MAO type B (found mostly in the brain). At higher-than-recommended doses, it is a nonselective inhibitor of MAO, including MAO type A (found in the GI tract). It may also directly increase dopaminergic activity by decreasing the reuptake of dopamine into nerve cells. Its pharmacologically active metabolites (amphetamine and methamphetamine) may contribute to this effect.

Pharmacokinetics
- *Absorption:* Little is known about the absorption of selegiline.
- *Distribution:* After a single dose, plasma levels are below detectable levels (less than 10 ng/ml).
- *Metabolism:* Three metabolites have been detected in the serum and urine: N-desmethyl-deprenyl, amphetamine, and methamphetamine.
- *Excretion:* 45% of the drug appears as a metabolite in the urine after 48 hours.

Contraindications and precautions
Selegiline is contraindicated in patients hypersensitive to the drug.

Some patients may experience an exacerbation of levodopa-induced adverse reactions (including GI or CNS disturbances). Such effects may be ameliorated by reducing the dosage of levodopa-carbidopa.

Interactions
Concomitant use with adrenergic agents may increase pressor effects, particularly in patients who have taken an overdose of selegiline. MAO inhibitors have caused fatal interactions when used concomitantly with meperidine. Because the mechanism of this interaction is not known, do not use together. MAO inhibitors may prolong and intensify the anticholinergic effects of antihistamines.

Effects on diagnostic tests
None reported.

Adverse reactions
- CNS: dizziness, increased tremor, chorea, loss of balance, restlessness, blepharospasm, increased bradykinesia, facial grimace, stiff neck, dyskinesia, involuntary movements, increased apraxia, malaise, headache, taste disturbance.
- CV: orthostatic hypotension, hypertension, hypotension, arrhythmias, palpitations, new or increased anginal pain, tachycardia, peripheral edema, syncope, behavioral changes, tiredness.
- DERM: rash, hair loss, sweating.
- GI: nausea, vomiting, constipation, weight loss, anorexia or poor appetite, dysphagia, diarrhea, heartburn, dry mouth.
- GU: slow urination, transient nocturia, prostatic hypertrophy, urinary hesitancy or frequency, urine retention, sexual dysfunction.

Overdose and treatment
Limited experience with overdosage suggests that symptoms may include hypotension and psychomotor agitation. Because selegiline becomes a nonselective MAO inhibitor at high dosages, consider the possibility of symptoms of MAO inhibitor poisoning: drowsiness, dizziness, hyperactivity, agitation, seizures, coma, hypertension, hypotension, cardiac conduction disturbances, and CV collapse. These symptoms may not develop immediately after ingestion and may be delayed for 12 hours or longer.

Provide supportive treatment and closely monitor the patient for worsening of symptoms. Emesis or lavage may be helpful in the early stages of treatment. Avoid phenothiazine derivatives and CNS stimulants; adrenergic agents may provoke an exaggerated response. Diazepam may be useful in treating seizures.

▶ Special considerations

Besides those relevant to all *MAO inhibitors,* consider the following recommendations.

• In some patients who experience increased adverse reactions associated with levodopa (including muscle twitches), reduction of levodopa-carbidopa is necessary. Most of these patients require a dosage reduction of 10% to 30%.

• At dosages over 10 mg daily, selegiline loses specificity for MAO type B. At these higher doses, drug efficacy is not improved but there is a risk of hypertensive crisis unless the patient observes dietary restrictions recommended for nonspecific MAO inhibitors.

Information for the patient

• Advise patient not to take more than 10 mg daily. Higher dosage does not improve efficacy and may increase adverse reactions.

• Warn patient to move about cautiously at the start of therapy because he may experience dizziness, which can cause falls.

• Because the drug is an MAO inhibitor, tell patient about the possibility of an interaction with tyramine-containing foods such as red wines or aged cheese. Reportedly, however, this interaction does not occur at the recommended dosage; at 10 mg daily the drug inhibits only MAO type B. Therefore, dietary restrictions appear unnecessary, provided the patient does not exceed the recommended dose.

---

trihexyphenidyl hydrochloride

Aparkane∗, Apo-Trihex∗, Artane, Artane Sequels, Novohexidyl∗, Trihexane, Trihexidyl, Trihexy-2, Trihexy-5

• Pharmacologic classification: anticholinergic
• Therapeutic classification: antiparkinsonian agent
• Pregnancy risk category C

How supplied

Available by prescription only
Tablets: 2 mg, 5 mg
Capsules (sustained-release): 5 mg
Elixir: 2 mg/5 ml

Indications, route, and dosage
Drug-induced parkinsonism

Adults: 1 mg P.O. first day, 2 mg second day, then increase 2 mg q 3 to 5 days until total of 6 to 10 mg is given daily. Usually given t.i.d. with meals and, if needed, q.i.d. (last dose should be before bedtime). Postencephalitic parkinsonism may require 12 to 15 mg total daily dosage.

Pharmacodynamics

Antiparkinsonian action: Trihexyphenidyl blocks central cholinergic receptors, helping to balance cholinergic activity in the basal ganglia. It may also prolong dopamine's effects by blocking dopamine reuptake and storage at central receptor sites.

Pharmacokinetics

• *Absorption:* Rapidly absorbed after oral administration. Onset of action occurs within 1 hour.

• *Distribution:* Crosses the blood-brain barrier; little else is known about its distribution.

• *Metabolism:* Exact metabolic fate is unknown. Duration of effect is 6 to 12 hours.

• *Excretion:* Excreted in the urine as unchanged drug and metabolites.

Contraindications and precautions

Trihexyphenidyl is contraindicated in patients with a history of sensitivity to the drug. Administer trihexyphenidyl cautiously to patients with narrow-angle glaucoma, because drug-induced cycloplegia and mydriasis may increase intraocular pressure; to patients with cardiac disorders, arteriosclerosis, renal disorders, hepatic disorders, hypertension, obstructive GI or GU tract disease, or suspected prostatic hypertrophy, because the drug may exacerbate these conditions.

Interactions

Concomitant use with amantadine may amplify trihexyphenidyl's adverse anticholinergic effects, causing confusion and hallucinations. Concomitant use with haloperidol or phenothiazines may decrease the antipsychotic effectiveness of these drugs, possibly from direct CNS antagonism; concomitant phenothiazine use also increases the risk of adverse anticholinergic effects.

Concomitant use with CNS depressants, such as tranquilizers, sedative-hypnotics, and alcohol, increases trihexyphenidyl's sedative effects. When used with levodopa, dosage of both drugs may need adjustment because of synergistic anticholinergic effects and possible enhanced GI metabolism of levodopa from reduced gastric motility and delayed gastric emptying. Antacids and antidiarrheals may decrease trihexyphenidyl's absorption.

Effects on diagnostic tests
None reported.

Adverse reactions
● CNS: nervousness, dizziness, headache, restlessness, hallucination, insomnia, confusion and excitement (in elderly).
● CV: tachycardia, palpitations, orthostatic hypotension.
● EENT: blurred vision, mydriasis, increased intraocular pressure, photophobia.
● GI: constipation, dry mouth, nausea, vomiting, heartburn, dysphagia, abdominal distention.
● GU: urinary hesitancy, urine retention.
   Note: Drug should be discontinued if hypersensitivity, hallucinations, delusions, or urine retention occur.

Overdose and treatment
Clinical effects of overdose include central stimulation followed by depression, with such psychotic symptoms as disorientation, confusion, hallucination, delusions, anxiety, agitation, and restlessness. Peripheral effects may include dilated, nonreactive pupils; blurred vision; flushed, dry, hot skin; dry mucous membranes; dysphagia; decreased or absent bowel sounds; urine retention; hyperthermia; headache; tachycardia; hypertension; and increased respiration.

   Treatment is primarily symptomatic and supportive, as needed. Maintain patent airway. If the patient is alert, induce emesis (or use gastric lavage) and follow with saline cathartic and activated charcoal to prevent further drug absorption. In severe cases, physostigmine may be administered to block trihexyphenidyl's antimuscarinic effects. Give fluids, as needed, to treat shock; diazepam to control psychotic symptoms; and pilocarpine (instilled into the eyes) to relieve mydriasis. If urine retention occurs, catheterization may be necessary.

▶ Special considerations
Besides those relevant to all *anticholinergics,* consider the following recommendations.
● Because this drug may cause orthostatic hypotension, check the patient's sitting and supine blood pressure after initial administration.
● Store trihexyphenidyl in tight containers.
● Monitor patient for urinary hesitancy.
● Arrange for gonioscopic evaluation and close intraocular pressure monitoring, especially in patients over age 40.
● Patients may develop tolerance to this drug, necessitating higher doses.
● Advise patient to rise to standing position slowly to avoid orthostatic hypotension.

Geriatric use
Use caution when administering trihexyphenidyl to elderly patients because it can worsen memory impairment. Lower doses are indicated.

Breast-feeding
Trihexyphenidyl may be excreted in breast milk, possibly resulting in infant toxicity. Breast-feeding women should avoid this drug. Drug may also decrease milk production.

---

*Canada only   †Unlabeled clinical use   Italicized adverse reactions are life-threatening.

Antipsychotic agents

acetophenazine maleate
chlorpromazine hydrochloride
chlorprothixene
chlorprothixene hydrochloride
clozapine
droperidol
fluphenazine decanoate
fluphenazine enanthate
fluphenazine hydrochloride
haloperidol
haloperidol decanoate
haloperidol lactate
loxapine hydrochloride
loxapine succinate
mesoridazine besylate
molindone hydrochloride
perphenazine
pimozide
prochlorperazine
prochlorperazine edisylate
prochlorperazine maleate
promazine hydrochloride
thioridazine
thioridazine hydrochloride
thiothixene
thiothixene hydrochloride
trifluoperazine hydrochloride

Antipsychotic (neuroleptic) agents are most effectively used to treat schizophrenia, organic psychoses, the manic phase of manic-depressive illness, and other acute psychotic states. Such agents mainly include the phenothiazines, thioxanthenes, and butyrophenones, but also include dibenzodiazepines, dibenzoxazepines, rauwolfia alkaloids, and related amine-depleting agents. These agents' effectiveness in psychotic states is probably related to blockade of postsynaptic dopaminergic receptors in the mesolimbic area of the brain but may also involve other neurotransmitters. They have widespread beneficial use, but are often associated with severe adverse effects that can limit their usefulness.

At usual dosage levels, neuroleptic agents reduce affect and interest in the environment without causing cognitive impairment, dysarthria, ataxia, or incoordination. Typically, they cause psychotic patients to become less agitated, withdrawn, agressive, and impulsive and to become more communicative and responsive; they gradually relieve hallucinations, delusions, and disorganized thinking. Their additional neurologic effects, resembling those of Parkinson's disease, may include tremor, mild rigidity, and akathisia.

Pharmacologic effects
Phenothiazines (acetophenazine, chlorpromazine, fluphenazine, mesoridazine, perphenazine, prochlorperazine, promazine, thioridazine, trifluoperazine) and *thioxanthenes* (thiothixene, chlorprothixene) are potent and effective antipsychotic agents. Used primarily to alleviate acute psychotic illness, they also have other clinically useful properties, including antiemetic, antinausea, and antihistaminic effects and the ability to potentiate the effects of sedatives, analgesics, and anesthetics.
● *Butyrophenones* (droperidol, haloperidol), analogs of haloperidol, include some of the most potent antipsychotic agents known. Droperidol is used almost exclusively for anesthesia because of its potent sedative properties.
● *Miscellaneous agents* (clozapine, loxapine, pimozide, and molindone) are chemically unrelated to other antipsychotic agents.

Mechanism of action
Reportedly, neuroleptic agents act through antagonism of dopamine-mediated synaptic neurotransmission in the limbic, mesocortical, and hypothalamic systems. However, because some atypical antipsychotic agents (such as clozapine) lack antidopaminergic action, such action may not be required for effectiveness.

Pharmacokinetics
● *Absorption and distribution:* Antipsychotic agents tend to be absorbed erratically after oral administration, even of liquid preparations; I.M. administration greatly multiplies bioavailability. Highly lipophilic and membrane- or protein-bound, these agents accumulate in the brain, lungs, and other well-perfused tissues and readily enter fetal circulation.
● *Metabolism and excretion:* Usually, biological

ADVERSE REACTION POTENTIAL OF PHENOTHIAZINES

The chart below indicates the relative potential of phenothiazines and nonphenothiazines to produce specific adverse reactions.

DRUG	SEDATIVE EFFECTS	EXTRAPYRAMIDAL SYMPTOMS	HYPOTENSIVE EFFECTS	ANTICHOLINERGIC EFFECTS
Phenothiazines				
Aliphatic subgroup				
chlorpromazine	High	Moderate	High	High
promazine	Moderate	Moderate	Moderate	High
Piperazine subgroup				
acetophenazine	Moderate	Moderate	Low	Moderate
fluphenazine	Low	High	Low	Low
perphenazine	Moderate	Moderate	Low	Low
prochlorperazine	Moderate	High	Low	Moderate
trifluoperazine	Low	High	Low	Low
Piperidine subgroup				
mesoridazine	High	Low	Moderate	Moderate
thioridazine	High	Low	Moderate	Very high
Nonphenothiazines				
Butyrophenone subgroup				
droperidol	High	Low	Moderate	Moderate
haloperidol	Low	Very high	Low	Very low
Dibenzoxazepine subgroup				
loxapine	Low	Moderate	Low	Low
Dihydroindolone subgroup				
molindone	Moderate	Moderate	Low	Low
Thioxanthene subgroup				
chlorprothixene	High	Moderate	Moderate	Moderate
thiothixene	Low	Moderate	Moderate	Low
Diphenyl-butylpiperidine subgroup				
pimozide	Low	Very high	Low	Moderate
Tricyclic dibenzodiazepine group				
clozapine	High	Low	Low	Low

effects of a single dose persist for at least 24 hours; plasma half-life is typically 20 to 40 hours. However, elimination from plasma may be more rapid than from binding and lipid sites; metabolites of some agents have been detected several months after discontinuation of the drug. Metabolism occurs chiefly by oxidative processes mediated by hepatic microsomal and other drug-metabolizing enzymes. Metabolites are excreted mainly in the urine and, to a lesser extent, in the bile. Metabolism of antipsychotic agents is diminished in infants and fetuses and in elderly patients; it is more rapid in children.

Adverse reactions and toxicity

Aside from extension of pharmacologic effects, major adverse reactions affect the CNS, CV system, autonomic nervous system, and endocrine functions. Extrapyramidal effects include dystonia, akathisia, neuroleptic malignant syndrome, perioral tremor, and tardive dyskinesia.

Antipsychotic agents are relatively nontoxic. Fatal overdosage is rare. Adults have survived doses of chlorpromazine up to 10 g. Fatal overdose of haloperidol has not been reported.

Clinical considerations

• Selection of an antipsychotic drug is partially determined by the potential adverse effects, because these drugs affect autonomic, CV, and endocrine systems. A drug that has been used effectively for a patient in the past probably should be used for that patient again.

• Sedation is common after all of these agents but is most pronounced with high dosage of the less potent phenothiazines (including chlorpromazine, mesoridazine, and thioridazine). Sedation usually subsides during prolonged treatment, as many patients develop tolerance to it. However, to prevent daytime somnolence, administer these agents at bedtime.

• Antipsychotic agents cause alpha-adrenergic blockade, which can result in orthostatic hypotension, palpitations, and syncope. Hypotension is most likely after administration of phenothiazines with aliphatic side chains (such as chlorpromazine); it is less likely with piperazine derivatives and other nonphenothiazines.

• These agents' blockade of muscarinic cholinergic receptors can cause dry mouth, blurred vision, constipation, and, in males with prostatism, urine retention.

• Fatal overdosage with antipsychotic agents is rare, unless complicated by alcohol or other drugs.

• Neurologic adverse effects (such as extrapyramidal reactions) occur most frequently with high potency agents (tricyclic piperazines and butyrophenones). Acute extrapyramidal adverse effects are less likely with thioridazine and clozapine.

• Antipsychotic agents induce six characteristic neurologic syndromes: acute dystonia, akathisia, parkinsonism, neuroleptic malignant syndrome, perioral tremor, and tardive dyskinesia. Perioral tremor and tardive dyskinesia are delayed syndromes that occur after months or years of treatment.

• Acute dystonic reactions occur commonly in males under age 25 after parenteral therapy. These reactions usually respond to a centrally acting anticholinergic agent (such as benztropine) or an antihistamine (diphenhydramine).

acetophenazine maleate
Tindal

• Pharmacologic classification: phenothiazine (piperazine derivative)
• Therapeutic classification: antipsychotic
• Pregnancy risk category C

How supplied
Available by prescription only
Tablets: 20 mg

Indications, route, and dosage
Psychotic disorders
Adults: Initially, 20 mg P.O. t.i.d. or q.i.d. Daily dosage ranges from 40 to 80 mg in outpatients or 80 to 120 mg in hospitalized patients; however, in severe psychotic states, up to 600 mg daily has been administered safely. Smallest effective dose should be used at all times.

Pharmacodynamics
• *Antipsychotic action:* Acetophenazine is thought to exert its antipsychotic effects by postsynaptic blockade of CNS dopamine receptors, thereby inhibiting dopamine-mediated effects.

Acetophenazine has many other central and peripheral effects; it produces alpha and ganglionic blockade and counteracts histamine- and serotonin-mediated activity. Its most prominent adverse reactions are extrapyramidal.

Pharmacokinetics
• *Absorption:* Oral tablet absorption is erratic and variable, with onset of action ranging from ½ to 1 hour.
• *Distribution:* Acetophenazine is distributed widely into the body, including breast milk. CNS concentrations are higher than plasma concentrations. Drug is 91% to 99% protein-bound. Peak effect occurs at 2 to 4 hours; steady-state serum levels are achieved within 4 to 7 days.
• *Metabolism:* Acetophenazine is metabolized extensively by the liver, but no active metabolites are formed; duration of action is about 4 to 6 hours.
• *Excretion:* Most of the drug is excreted in urine as inactive metabolites; some is excreted in feces via the biliary tract.

Contraindications and precautions
Acetophenazine is contraindicated in patients with known hypersensitivity to phenothiazines

and related compounds, including allergic reactions involving hepatic function; in patients with blood dyscrasias and bone marrow depression because it may cause agranulocytosis; in patients in coma or with brain damage, CNS depression, circulatory collapse, or cerebrovascular disease because of its hypotensive effects; and in patients with adrenergic blocking agents or spinal or epidural anesthetics because of the potential for additive adrenergic blocking effects.

Acetophenazine should be used cautiously in patients with cardiac disease (arrhythmias, CHF, angina pectoris, valvular disease, or heart block), encephalitis, Reye's syndrome, head injury, respiratory disease, seizure disorders, glaucoma, prostatic hypertrophy, urine retention, hepatic or renal dysfunction, Parkinson's disease, pheochromocytoma, or hypocalcemia.

Interactions

Concomitant use of acetophenazine with sympathomimetics, including epinephrine, phenylephrine, phenylpropanolamine, and ephedrine (often found in nasal sprays), and appetite suppressants may decrease their stimulatory and pressor effects. Concomitant use of epinephrine as a pressor agent may cause epinephrine reversal because of its alpha-adrenergic blocking effects.

Acetophenazine may inhibit blood pressure response to centrally acting antihypertensive drugs, such as guanethidine, guanabenz, guanadrel, clonidine, methyldopa, and reserpine. Additive effects are likely after concomitant use of acetophenazine with CNS depressants (including alcohol, analgesics, barbiturates, narcotics, tranquilizers, and general, spinal, or epidural anesthetics) and parenteral magnesium sulfate (oversedation, respiratory depression, and hypotension); antiarrhythmic agents, including quinidine, disopyramide, or procainamide (increased incidence of cardiac arrhythmias and conduction defects); atropine and other anticholinergic drugs (including antidepressants, MAO inhibitors, phenothiazines, antihistamines, meperidine, and antiparkinsonian agents [oversedation, paralytic ileus, visual changes, and severe constipation]); nitrates (hypotension); or metrizamide (increased risk of seizures).

Beta blocking agents may inhibit acetophenazine metabolism, increasing plasma levels and toxicity.

Concomitant use with propylthiouracil increases risk of agranulocytosis; concomitant use with lithium may result in severe neurologic toxicity with an encephalitis-like syndrome and a decreased therapeutic response to acetophenazine.

Pharmacokinetic alterations and subsequent decreased therapeutic response to acetophenazine may follow concomitant use with phenobarbital (enhanced renal excretion), aluminum- and magnesium-containing antacids and antidiarrheals (decreased absorption), or caffeine and with heavy smoking (increased metabolism).

Acetophenazine may antagonize the therapeutic effects of bromocriptine on prolactin secretion; it may also decrease the vasoconstricting effects of high-dose dopamine and may decrease the effectiveness and increase toxicity of levodopa (by dopamine blockade). Acetophenazine may inhibit metabolism and increase toxicity of phenytoin.

Effects on diagnostic tests

Acetophenazine may cause false-positive test results for urinary porphyrins, urobilinogen, amylase, and 5-hydroxyindoleacetic acid because of darkening of urine by metabolites; it also causes false-positive results in urine pregnancy tests using human chorionic gonadotropin.

Acetophenazine elevates results of tests for liver function and protein-bound iodine and causes quinidine-like effects on the ECG.

Adverse reactions

● CNS: extrapyramidal symptoms, such as dystonia, akathisia, torticollis, and tardive dyskinesia (dose-related with long-term therapy); sedation (low incidence); pseudoparkinsonism, drowsiness (frequent); *neuroleptic malignant syndrome* (dose-related; fatal *respiratory failure* in over 10% of patients if untreated); dizziness, headache, insomnia, exacerbation of psychotic symptoms.
● CV: orthostatic hypotension, *asystole,* tachycardia, dizziness, fainting, arrhythmias, ECG changes, increased anginal pain (after I.M. injection).
● EENT: blurred vision, tinnitus, mydriasis, increased intraocular pressure, ocular changes (retinal pigmentary change with long-term use).
● GI: dry mouth, constipation, nausea, vomiting, anorexia, diarrhea.
● GU: urine retention, gynecomastia, hypermenorrhea, inhibited ejaculation.
● HEMA: transient leukopenia, *agranulocytosis,* thrombocytopenia, anemia (within 30 to 90 days).
● Local: contact dermatitis from concentrate or

injectable form, muscle necrosis from I.M. injection.
• Other: hyperprolactinemia, photosensitivity, increased appetite and weight gain, hypersensitivity (rash, urticaria, drug fever, edema, cholestatic jaundice [in 2% to 4% of patients within first 30 days]).

After abrupt withdrawal of long-term therapy, gastritis, nausea, vomiting, dizziness, tremor, feeling of heat or cold, sweating, tachycardia, headache, or insomnia may occur.

Note: Drug should be discontinued if the following reactions occur: hypersensitivity, jaundice, agranulocytosis, neuroleptic malignant syndrome (marked hyperthermia, extrapyramidal effects, autonomic dysfunction), and severe extrapyramidal symptoms that persist after dosage is lowered. Drug should be discontinued 48 hours before and 24 hours after myelography using metrizamide because of the risk of seizures. When feasible, drug should be withdrawn slowly and gradually; many drug effects persist after withdrawal.

Overdose and treatment
Acetophenazine overdose causes CNS depression characterized by deep, unarousable sleep and possible coma, hypotension or hypertension, extrapyramidal symptoms, dystonia, abnormal involuntary muscle movements, agitation, seizures, arrhythmias, ECG changes, hypothermia or hyperthermia, and autonomic nervous system dysfunction.

Treatment is symptomatic and supportive, including maintaining vital signs, airway, stable body temperature, and fluid and electrolyte balance.

Do not induce vomiting: drug inhibits cough reflex and aspiration may occur. Use gastric lavage and then activated charcoal and saline cathartics; drug is not dialyzable. Regulate body temperature as needed. Treat hypotension with I.V. fluids; *do not give epinephrine.* Treat seizures with parenteral diazepam or barbiturates; arrhythmias with parenteral phenytoin (1 mg/kg with rate titrated to blood pressure); extrapyramidal reactions with barbiturates, benztropine, or parenteral diphenhydramine at 2 mg/kg/minute.

▶ Special considerations
Besides those relevant to all *phenothiazines,* consider the following recommendations.
• Drug may cause a pink-brown discoloration of the patient's urine.
• Acetophenazine causes a high incidence of extrapyramidal effects and photosensitivity reactions. Patient should avoid exposure to sunlight or heat lamps.
• Drug may cause stomach upset; administer with food or fluid.
• Sugarless chewing gum or hard candy, or ice chips may help to alleviate dry mouth.
• Monitor blood pressure before and after oral administration.

Information for the patient
• Explain risks of dystonic reactions and tardive dyskinesia and tell patient to report abnormal body movements.
• Tell patient to avoid sun exposure and to use a sunscreen when going outdoors, to prevent photosensitivity reactions. (Note that heat lamps and tanning beds also may cause burning of the skin or skin discoloration.)
• Warn patient to avoid extremely hot or cold baths and exposure to temperature extremes, sunlamps, or tanning beds. Drug may cause thermoregulatory changes.
• Tell patient to take the drug exactly as prescribed, not to double dose for missed ones, and not to discontinue the drug suddenly.
• Explain that most adverse reactions can be relieved by a dosage reduction. Patient should promptly report persistent fever, difficulty urinating, sore throat, dizziness, or fainting.
• Tell patient that many drug interactions are possible. Patient should seek medical approval before taking *any* self-prescribed medications.
• Inform patient that he should become tolerant to the drug's sedative effects in several weeks.
• Tell patient to avoid hazardous activities that require alertness until the drug's effect is established.
• Tell patient to avoid alcohol and other medications that may cause excessive sedation.
• Suggest sugarless hard candy or chewing gum, or ice chips to relieve dry mouth.

Geriatric use
Elderly patients may require only 30% to 50% of regular adult dose. They are more likely to develop adverse reactions, especially tardive dyskinesia and other extrapyramidal effects.

Pediatric use
Drug is not recommended for pediatric use.

Breast-feeding
Because acetophenazine is distributed into the breast milk, this drug should be used with caution. The potential benefits to the mother should outweigh the potential harm to the breast-feeding infant.

---

chlorpromazine hydrochloride
Chlorpromanyl-5*, Chlorpromanyl-20*,
Chlorpromanyl-40*, Largactil*, Novo-
Chlorpromazine*, Ormazine, Promaz, Sonazine,
Thorazine, Thor-Prom

- Pharmacologic classification: phenothiazine
  (aliphatic derivative)
- Therapeutic classification: antipsychotic
- Pregnancy risk category C

How supplied
Available by prescription only
Tablets: 10 mg, 25 mg, 50 mg, 100 mg, 200 mg
Capsules (sustained-release): 30 mg, 75 mg, 150
mg, 200 mg, 300 mg
Injection: 25 mg/ml
Oral concentrate: 20 mg/ml*, 30 mg/ml*, 40 mg/
ml*
Syrup: 5 mg/ml, 10 mg/5ml
Suppositories: 25 mg, 100 mg

Indications, route, and dosage
Psychosis
Adults: 30 to 75 mg P.O. daily in two to four
divided doses. Dosage may be increased twice
weekly by 20 to 50 mg until symptoms are
controlled. Most patients respond to 200 mg
daily, but doses up to 800 mg may be necessary.
Children: 0.25 mg/kg P.O. q 4 to 6 hours; 0.25
mg/kg I.M. q 6 to 8 hours; or 0.5 mg/kg rectally
q 6 to 8 hours. Maximum dosage is 40 mg in
children under age 5 and 75 mg in children ages
5 to 12.
Acute management of psychosis in se-
verely agitated patients
Adults: 25 mg I.M.; may be repeated with 25 to
50 mg I.M. in 1 hour. May be gradually increased
over several days to a maximum of 400 mg q
4 to 6 hours.
Intractable hiccups
Adults: 25 to 50 mg P.O. or I.M. t.i.d. or q.i.d.
Mild alcohol withdrawal, acute intermit-
tent porphyria, and tetanus
Adults: 25 mg to 50 mg I.M. t.i.d. or q.i.d.

Pharmacodynamics
Antipsychotic action: Chlorpromazine is thought
to exert its antipsychotic effects by postsynaptic
blockade of CNS dopamine receptors, thereby
inhibiting dopamine-mediated effects; antiemetic effects are attributed to dopamine receptor blockade in the medullary chemoreceptor trigger zone. Chlorpromazine has many other
central and peripheral effects; it produces both
alpha and ganglionic blockade and counteracts
histamine- and serotonin-mediated activity. Its
most prominent adverse reactions are antimuscarinic and sedative; it causes fewer extrapyramidal effects than other antipsychotics.

Pharmacokinetics
- *Absorption:* Rate and extent of absorption
vary with route of administration. Oral tablet
absorption is erratic and variable, with onset
ranging from ½ to 1 hour; peak effects occur
at 2 to 4 hours and duration of action is 4 to 6
hours. Sustained-release preparations have similar absorption, but action lasts for 10 to 12
hours. Suppositories act in 60 minutes and last
3 to 4 hours. Oral concentrates and syrups are
much more predictable; I.M. drug is absorbed
rapidly.
- *Distribution:* Chlorpromazine is distributed
widely into the body, including breast milk; concentration is usually higher in CNS than plasma.
Steady-state serum level is achieved within 4
to 7 days. Drug is 91% to 99% protein-bound.
- *Metabolism:* Chlorpromazine is metabolized
extensively by the liver and forms 10 to 12 metabolites; some are pharmacologically active.
- *Excretion:* Most of drug is excreted as metabolites in urine; some is excreted in feces via the
biliary tract. It may undergo enterohepatic circulation.

Contraindications and precautions
Antipsychotics are contraindicated in patients
with known hypersensitivity to phenothiazines
and related compounds, including allergic reactions involving hepatic function; in patients
with blood dyscrasias and bone marrow depression because chlorpromazine may induce
agranulocytosis; in patients with disorders accompanied by coma, brain damage, or CNS depression because of additive CNS depressant
effects; in patients with circulatory collapse or
cerebrovascular disease because of the potential for hypotensive or adverse cardiac effects;
and for use with adrenergic blocking agents or
spinal or epidural anesthetics because of the
alpha blocking potential of chlorpromazine.
Chlorpromazine should be used cautiously in
patients with cardiac disease (arrhythmias,
CHF, angina pectoris, valvular disease, or heart
block), encephalitis, Reye's syndrome, head injury, respiratory disease, seizure disorders,
glaucoma, prostatic hypertrophy, urine retention, hepatic or renal dysfunction, Parkinson's
disease, pheochromocytoma, or hypocalcemia.

Interactions

Concomitant use of chlorpromazine with sympathomimetics, including epinephrine, phenylephrine, phenylpropanolamine, and ephedrine (often found in nasal sprays), and appetite suppressants may decrease their stimulatory and pressor effects. Chlorpromazine may cause epinephrine reversal: the beta-adrenergic agonist activity of epinephrine is evident while its alpha effects are blocked, leading to decreased diastolic and increased systolic pressures and tachycardia.

Chlorpromazine may inhibit blood pressure response to centrally acting antihypertensive drugs, such as guanethidine, guanabenz, guanadrel, clonidine, methyldopa, and reserpine. Additive effects are likely after concomitant use of chlorpromazine and CNS depressants (including alcohol, analgesics, barbiturates, narcotics, tranquilizers, and general, spinal, or epidural anesthetics), or parenteral magnesium sulfate (oversedation, respiratory depression, and hypotension); antiarrhythmic agents, including quinidine, disopyramide, and procainamide (increased incidence of cardiac arrhythmias and conduction defects); atropine and other anticholinergic drugs, including antidepressants, MAO inhibitors, phenothiazines, antihistamines, meperidine, and antiparkinsonian agents (oversedation, paralytic ileus, visual changes, and severe constipation); nitrates (hypotension); and metrizamide (increased risk of seizures).

Beta blocking agents may inhibit chlorpromazine metabolism, increasing plasma levels and toxicity.

Concomitant use with propylthiouracil increases risk of agranulocytosis; concomitant use with lithium may cause severe neurologic toxicity with an encephalitis-like syndrome, and a decreased therapeutic response to chlorpromazine.

Pharmacokinetic alterations and subsequent decreased therapeutic response to chlorpromazine may follow concomitant use with phenobarbital (enhanced renal excretion), aluminum- and magnesium-containing antacids and antidiarrheals (decreased absorption), caffeine, and heavy smoking (increased metabolism).

Chlorpromazine may antagonize therapeutic effect of bromocriptine on prolactin secretion; it also may decrease the vasoconstricting effects of high-dose dopamine and may decrease effectiveness and increase toxicity of levodopa (by dopamine blockade). Chlorpromazine may inhibit metabolism and increase toxicity of phenytoin.

Effects on diagnostic tests

Chlorpromazine causes false-positive test results for urinary porphyrins, urobilinogen, amylase, and 5-hydroxyindoleacetic acid because of darkening of urine by metabolites; it also causes false-positive results in urine pregnancy tests using human chorionic gonadotropin.

Chlorpromazine elevates tests for liver function and protein-bound iodine and causes quinidine-like ECG effects.

Adverse reactions

- CNS: extrapyramidal symptoms – dystonia, akathisia, torticollis, tardive dyskinesia; sedation, pseudoparkinsonism, drowsiness (frequent); *neuroleptic malignant syndrome* (fatal untreated); dizziness, headache, insomnia, exacerbation of psychotic symptoms.
- CV: *asystole,* orthostatic hypotension, tachycardia, dizziness, fainting, arrhythmias, ECG changes, increased anginal pain (after I.M. injection).
- EENT: blurred vision, tinnitus, mydriasis, increased intraocular pressure, ocular changes (retinal pigmentary change with long-term use).
- GI: dry mouth, constipation, nausea, vomiting, anorexia, diarrhea.
- GU: urine retention, gynecomastia, hypermenorrhea, inhibited ejaculation.
- HEMA: transient leukopenia, *agranulocytosis,* thrombocytopenia, anemia (within 30 to 90 days).
- Local: contact dermatitis from concentrate or injectable; muscle necrosis from I.M. injection.
- Other: hyperprolactinemia, photosensitivity, increased appetite or weight gain, hypersensitivity (rash, urticaria, drug fever, edema, cholestatic jaundice [in 2% to 4% of patients within first 30 days]).

After abrupt withdrawal of long-term therapy, gastritis, nausea, vomiting, dizziness, tremor, feeling of heat or cold, sweating, tachycardia, headache, or insomnia may occur.

Note: Drug should be discontinued immediately if the following reactions occur: hypersensitivity, jaundice, agranulocytosis; neuroleptic malignant syndrome (marked hyperthermia, extrapyramidal effects, autonomic dysfunction); and severe extrapyramidal symptoms even after dose is lowered. Chlorpromazine should be discontinued 48 hours before and 24 hours after myelography using metrizamide because of the risk of seizures. When feasible, withdraw drug

---

slowly and gradually; many drug effects persist after withdrawal.

Overdose and treatment

CNS depression is characterized by deep, un-arousable sleep and possible coma, hypotension or hypertension, extrapyramidal symptoms, abnormal involuntary muscle movements, agitation, seizures, arrhythmias, ECG changes, hypothermia or hyperthermia, and autonomic nervous system dysfunction.

Treatment is symptomatic and supportive, including maintaining vital signs, airway, stable body temperature, and fluid and electrolyte balance.

Do not induce vomiting: drug inhibits cough reflex and aspiration may occur. Use gastric lavage and then activated charcoal and saline cathartics; dialysis does not help. Regulate body temperature as needed. Treat hypotension with I.V. fluids; *do not give epinephrine.* Treat seizures with parenteral diazepam or barbiturates; arrhythmias with parenteral phenytoin (1 mg/kg with rate titrated to blood pressure); extrapyramidal reactions with barbiturates, benztropine, or parenteral diphenhydramine 2 mg/kg/minute.

▶ Special considerations

Besides those relevant to all *phenothiazines,* consider the following recommendations.
● A pink-brown discoloration of urine may be observed.
● Chlorpromazine has a high incidence of sedation, orthostatic hypotension, and photosensitivity reactions (3%). Patient should avoid exposure to sunlight or heat lamps.
● Sustained-release preparations should not be crushed or opened, but swallowed whole.
● Oral formulations may cause stomach upset and may be administered with food or fluid.
● Dilute the concentrate in 2 to 4 oz of liquid, preferably water, carbonated drinks, fruit juice, tomato juice, milk, puddings, or applesauce.
● Store the suppository form in a cool place.
● If tissue irritation occurs, chlorpromazine injection may be diluted with normal saline solution or 2% procaine.
● The I.V. form should be used only during surgery or for severe hiccups.
● Dilute the injection to 1 mg/ml with normal saline solution and administer at a rate of 1 mg/2 minutes for children and 1 mg/minute for adults.
● The I.M. injection should be given deep in the upper outer quadrant of the buttocks. Massaging the area after administration may prevent

abscess formation. Do not extravasate because skin necrosis can occur.
● The liquid and injectable formulations may cause a rash if skin contact occurs.
● Solution for injection may be slightly discolored. Do not use if drug is excessively discolored or if a precipitate is evident. Monitor blood pressure before and after parenteral administration.
● Shake the syrup before administration.

Information for the patient

● Explain the risks of dystonic reactions and tardive dyskinesia and tell the patient to report abnormal body movements.
● Tell patient to avoid sun exposure and to use a sunscreen when going outdoors, to prevent photosensitivity reactions. (Note that sunlamps and tanning beds also may cause burning of the skin or skin discoloration.)
● Warn patient to avoid extremely hot or cold baths or exposure to temperature extremes, sunlamps, or tanning beds. Drug may cause thermoregulatory changes.
● Tell patient not to spill the liquid preparation on the skin because rash and irritation may result.
● Tell patient to take the drug exactly as prescribed and not to double dose to compensate for missed ones.
● Explain that many drug interactions are possible. Patient should seek medical approval before taking *any* self-prescribed medications.
● Tell patient not to stop taking drug suddenly.
● Encourage patient to report persistent fever, difficulty urinating, sore throat, dizziness, or fainting.
● Tell patient to avoid hazardous activities that require alertness until the effect of the drug is established. Excessive sedative effects tend to subside after several weeks.
● Tell patient to avoid alcohol and medications that may cause excessive sedation.
● Explain what fluids are appropriate for diluting the concentrate and the dropper technique for measuring dose. Teach patient how to use the suppository form.
● Tell patient that sugarless hard candy or chewing gum, or ice chips can alleviate dry mouth.
● Tell patient to shake syrup before administration.

Geriatric use

Older patients tend to require lower doses, titrated individually. They also are more likely to develop adverse reactions, especially tardive dyskinesia and other extrapyramidal effects.

Pediatric use
Chlorpromazine is not recommended for patients under age 6 months. Sudden infant death syndrome has been reported to occur in children under age 1 receiving the drug.

Breast-feeding
Chlorpromazine enters into the breast milk. Potential benefits to the mother should outweigh the potential harm to the infant.

▬▬▬▬▬▬▬▬▬▬▬▬

chlorprothixene, chlorprothixene hydrochloride
Taractan, Tarasan*

- Pharmacologic classification: thioxanthene
- Therapeutic classification: antipsychotic
- Pregnancy risk category C

How supplied
Available by prescription only
chlorprothixene
Tablets: 10 mg, 25 mg, 50 mg, 100 mg
Oral concentrate: 100 mg/5 ml (fruit)
chlorprothixene hydrochloride
Injection: 12.5 mg/ml

Indications, route, and dosage
Psychotic disorders
Adults: Initially, 10 mg P.O. t.i.d. to q.i.d; increase gradually to maximum of 600 mg daily.
Children over age 6: 10 to 25 mg P.O. t.i.d. or q.i.d.
Agitation of severe neurosis, depression, schizophrenia
Adults: 25 to 50 mg P.O. or I.M. t.i.d. or q.i.d; increase as needed to maximum of 600 mg daily.

Pharmacodynamics
*Antipsychotic action:*Chlorprothixene is thought to exert its antipsychotic effects by postsynaptic blockade of CNS dopamine receptors, thereby inhibiting dopamine-mediated effects. Chlorprothixene has many other central and peripheral effects; it also acts as an alpha blocking agent. Its most prominent adverse reactions are extrapyramidal.

Pharmacokinetics
- *Absorption:* Oral absorption is rapid; I.M. onset of action is 10 to 30 minutes.
- *Distribution:* Chlorprothixene is distributed widely into the body. Peak effects occur at 1 to 3 hours; drug is 91% to 99% protein-bound.

- *Metabolism:* Metabolism of chlorprothixene is minimal; duration of action is 6 hours.
- *Excretion:* Most of drug is excreted as parent drug in feces via the biliary tract.

Contraindications and precautions
Chlorprothixene is contraindicated in patients with known hypersensitivity to thioxanthenes, phenothiazines, and related compounds, including that evidenced by jaundice and other allergic symptoms; in patients with blood dyscrasias and bone marrow depression because of its potential for agranulocytosis; in patients with disorders accompanied by coma, brain damage, or CNS depression because of additive CNS depressant effects; and in patients with circulatory collapse or cerebrovascular disease because of its potential for arrhythmogenic effects.

Chlorprothixene should be used cautiously in patients with cardiac disease (arrhythmias, CHF, angina pectoris, valvular disease, or heart block), encephalitis, Reye's syndrome, head injury, respiratory disease, seizure disorders, glaucoma, prostatic hypertrophy, urine retention, hepatic or renal dysfunction, Parkinson's disease, pheochromocytoma, or hypocalcemia.

Oral preparations of chlorprothixene may contain tartrazine; dye may cause allergic reaction in patients with aspirin allergy.

Interactions
Concomitant use of chlorprothixene with sympathomimetics, including epinephrine, phenylephrine, phenylpropanolamine, and ephedrine (often found in nasal sprays), or appetite suppressants may decrease their stimulatory and pressor effects.

Chlorprothixene may inhibit blood pressure response to centrally acting antihypertensive drugs, such as guanethidine, guanabenz, guanadrel, clonidine, methyldopa, and reserpine. Additive effects are likely after concomitant use of chlorprothixene with CNS depressants (including alcohol, analgesics, barbiturates, narcotics, tranquilizers, and general, spinal, or epidural anesthetics) or parenteral magnesium sulfate (oversedation, respiratory depression, and hypotension); antiarrhythmic agents, including quinidine, disopyramide, or procainamide (increased incidence of cardiac arrhythmias and conduction defects); atropine or other anticholinergic drugs, including antidepressants, MAO inhibitors, phenothiazines, antihistamines, meperidine, and antiparkinsonian agents (oversedation, paralytic ileus, visual changes, and

---

*Canada only   †Unlabeled clinical use   Italicized adverse reactions are life-threatening.

severe constipation); nitrates (hypotension); or metrizamide (increased risk of seizures.)

Beta blocking agents may inhibit chlorprothixene metabolism, increasing plasma levels and toxicity.

Concomitant use with propylthiouracil increases risk of agranulocytosis; concomitant use with lithium may result in severe neurologic toxicity with an encephalitis-like syndrome and a decreased therapeutic response to chlorprothixene.

Pharmacokinetic alterations and subsequent decreased therapeutic response to chlorprothixene may follow concomitant use with phenobarbital (enhanced renal excretion), aluminum- and magnesium-containing antacids and antidiarrheals (decreased absorption), or caffeine and with heavy smoking (increased metabolism).

Chlorprothixene may antagonize therapeutic effect of *bromocriptine* on prolactin secretion; it also may decrease the vasoconstricting effects of high-dose dopamine and may decrease effectiveness and increase toxicity of levodopa (by dopamine blockade). Chlorprothixene may inhibit metabolism and increase toxicity of phenytoin.

Effects on diagnostic tests

Chlorprothixene causes false-positive test results for urinary porphyrins, urobilinogen, amylase, and 5-hydroxyindoleacetic acid because of darkening of urine by metabolites; it also causes false-positive results in urine pregnancy tests using human chorionic gonadotropin.

Chlorprothixene elevates results of tests for liver enzymes and protein-bound iodine and causes quinidine-like ECG effects.

Adverse reactions

● CNS: extrapyramidal symptoms – dystonia, akathisia, torticollis, tardive dyskinesia, sedation, pseudoparkinsonism, drowsiness (frequent), *neuroleptic malignant syndrome* (if untreated, death follows *respiratory failure* in over 10% of patients), dizziness, headache, insomnia, exacerbation of psychotic symptoms.
● CV: *asystole*, orthostatic hypotension, tachycardia, dizziness or fainting, arrhythmias, ECG changes, increased anginal pain after I.M. injection.
● EENT: blurred vision, tinnitus, mydriasis, increased intraocular pressure, ocular changes (retinal pigmentary change with long-term use).
● GI: dry mouth, constipation, nausea, vomiting, anorexia, diarrhea.

● GU: urine retention, gynecomastia, hypermenorrhea, inhibited ejaculation.
● HEMA: transient leukopenia, *agranulocytosis,* thrombocytopenia, anemia (within 30 to 90 days).
● Local: contact dermatitis from concentrate or injectable form, muscle necrosis from I.M. injection.
● Other: hyperprolactinemia, photosensitivity, increased appetite or weight gain, hypersensitivity (rash, urticaria, drug fever, edema, cholestatic jaundice [in 2% to 4% of patients within first 30 days]).

After abrupt withdrawal of long-term therapy, gastritis, nausea, vomiting, dizziness, tremor, feeling of heat or cold, sweating, tachycardia, headache, or insomnia may occur.

Note: Drug should be discontinued immediately if the following reactions occur: hypersensitivity, jaundice, agranulocytosis; neuroleptic malignant syndrome (marked hyperthermia, extrapyramidal effects, autonomic dysfunction); and severe extrapyramidal symptoms even after dose is lowered. Chlorprothixene should be withdrawn 48 hours before and 24 hours after myelography using metrizamide because of the risk of seizures. When feasible, withdraw drug slowly and gradually; many drug effects persist after withdrawal.

Overdose and treatment

CNS depression is characterized by deep, unarousable sleep and possible coma, hypotension or hypertension, extrapyramidal symptoms, abnormal involuntary muscle movements, agitation, seizures, arrhythmias, ECG changes, hypothermia or hyperthermia, and autonomic nervous system dysfunction.

Treatment is symptomatic and supportive, including maintaining vital signs, airway, stable body temperature, and fluid and electrolyte balance.

Do not induce vomiting: drug inhibits cough reflex, and aspiration may occur. Use gastric lavage, then activated charcoal and saline cathartics; dialysis does not help. Regulate body temperature as needed. Treat hypotension with I.V. fluids; *do not give epinephrine.* Treat seizures with parenteral diazepam or barbiturates; arrhythmias, with parenteral phenytoin (1 mg/kg with rate titrated to blood pressure); extrapyramidal reactions, with barbiturates, benztropine, or parenteral diphenhydramine at 2 mg/kg/minute.

▶ **Special considerations**
Besides those relevant to all *phenothiazines*, consider the following recommendations.

● Chlorprothixene causes a high incidence of extrapyramidal effects and photosensitivity reactions.

● Oral formulations may cause stomach upset and may be administered with food or fluid.

● Concentrate must be diluted in 2 to 4 oz of liquid, preferably water, carbonated drinks, fruit juice, tomato juice, milk, or pudding.

● I.M. injection may cause skin necrosis; do not give I.V.

● The I.M. injection should be given deep in the upper outer quadrant of the buttocks. Massaging the area after administration may prevent the formation of abscesses.

● The liquid and injectable formulations may cause a rash if skin contact occurs.

● The injection solution may be slightly discolored. Do not use if drug is excessively discolored or if a precipitate is evident. Contact pharmacist.

● Protect the liquid formulation from light.

● The concentrate should be shaken and diluted before administration.

● Monitor blood pressure before and after parenteral administration.

● Drug is stable after reconstitution for 48 hours at room temperature.

● A dose of 65 mg is the therapeutic equivalent of 100 mg of chlorpramazine.

Information for the patient
● Explain the risks of dystonic reactions and tardive dyskinesia and tell patient to report abnormal body movements promptly.

● Tell patient to avoid sun exposure and to use a sunscreen when going outdoors, to prevent photosensitivity reactions. (Note that sunlamps and tanning beds also may cause burning of the skin or skin discoloration.)

● Warn patient to avoid extremely hot or cold baths or exposure to temperature extremes, sunlamps, or tanning beds because the drug may cause thermoregulatory changes.

● Tell patient not to spill the liquid preparation on the skin because rash and irritation may result.

● Tell patient to take the drug exactly as prescribed and not to double dose to compensate for missed ones.

● Tell patient that many drug interactions are possible. Patient should seek medical approval before taking *any* self-prescribed medication.

● Inform patient that he should become tolerant to the sedative effects of the drug in several weeks.

● Tell patient not to stop taking the drug suddenly.

● Encourage patient to report difficulty urinating, sore throat, dizziness, or fainting.

● Tell patient to avoid hazardous activities that require alertness until the effect of the drug is established.

● Tell patient to avoid alcohol and other medications that may cause excessive sedation.

● Suggest relieving dry mouth with sugarless hard candy or chewing gum, or ice chips.

● Tell patient to shake and dilute the concentrate before administration.

Geriatric use
Elderly patients tend to require lower doses, titrated to individual response. They also are more likely to develop adverse effects, especially tardive dyskinesia and other extrapyramidal effects.

Pediatric use
Drug is not recommended for patients under age 12.

clozapine
Clozaril

● Pharmacologic classification: tricyclic dibenzo-diazepine derivative
● Therapeutic classification: antipsychotic
● Pregnancy risk category B

How supplied
Available by prescription only
Tablets: 25 mg, 100 mg

Indications, route, and dosage
Treatment of schizophrenia in severely ill patients unresponsive to other therapies
Adults: Initially, 25 mg P.O. once or twice daily, titrated upward at 25 to 50 mg daily (if tolerated) to a daily dosage of 300 to 450 mg daily by the end of 2 weeks. Individual dosage is based on clinical response, patient tolerance, and adverse reactions. Subsequent increases of dosage should occur no more than once or twice weekly and should not exceed 100 mg. Many patients respond to doses of 300 to 600 mg daily, but some patients require as much as 900 mg daily. Do not exceed 900 mg/day.

Pharmacodynamics
Antipsychotic action: Clozapine binds to dopamine receptors (both D-1 and D-2) within the limbic system of the CNS. It also may interfere with adrenergic, cholinergic, histaminergic, and serotoninergic receptors.

Pharmacokinetics
● *Absorption:* Peak levels occur about 2.5 hours after oral administration. Food does not appear to interfere with bioavailability.
● *Distribution:* The drug is about 95% bound to serum proteins.
● *Metabolism:* Nearly complete; very little unchanged drug appears in the urine.
● *Excretion:* Approximately 50% of the drug appears in the urine and 30% in the feces, mostly as metabolites. Elimination half-life appears proportional to dose and may range from 8 to 12 hours.

Contraindications and precautions
Contraindicated in patients with a history of clozapine-induced agranulocytosis or severe granulocytopenia and in patients with severe CNS depression or coma. It is also contraindicated in patients currently taking other drugs that suppress bone marrow function and in patients with myelosuppressive disorders.

Because clozapine has potent anticholinergic effects, use cautiously in patients with prostatic hypertrophy or glaucoma.

Seizures may occur, especially in patients receiving high doses of the drug. Patients should avoid hazardous activities, such as driving, swimming, or climbing, while taking the drug.

Clozapine therapy carries a significant risk of agranulocytosis (early trials estimate the incidence at 1.3%). If possible, patients should receive at least two trials of a standard antipsychotic drug therapy before clozapine therapy is initiated. Baseline white blood cell (WBC) and differential counts are required before therapy; WBC counts must be monitored weekly and for at least 4 weeks after therapy is discontinued.

If WBC count drops below 3,500/mm³ after initiating therapy or drops substantially from baseline, monitor patient closely for signs of infection. If WBC count is 3,000/mm³ to 3,500/mm³ and granulocyte count is above 1,500/mm³, perform twice weekly WBC and differential counts. If WBC count drops below 3,000/mm³ and granulocyte count drops below 1,500/mm³, therapy should be interrupted and the patient monitored for signs of infection. Therapy may be cautiously restarted if WBC count returns above 3,000/mm³ and granulocyte count returns above 1,500/mm³, but twice weekly monitoring of WBC and differential counts should continue until the WBC count exceeds 3,500/mm³.

If the WBC count drops below 2,000/mm³ and granulocyte count drops below 1,000/mm³, the patient may require protective isolation. If the patient develops an infection, prepare cultures according to policy and administer antibiotics as appropriate. Some clinicians may perform bone marrow aspiration to assess bone marrow function. Subsequent clozapine therapy is contraindicated.

Interactions
Clozapine may potentiate the hypotensive effects of antihypertensives. Anticholinergics may potentiate the anticholinergic effects of clozapine. Administration of clozapine to a patient taking a benzodiazepine may pose a risk of respiratory failure. Avoid concomitant use.

Increased serum levels of warfarin, digoxin, and other highly protein-bound drugs may occur. Monitor closely for adverse reactions.

Potentially increased bone marrow toxicity may follow concomitant use with drugs that suppress bone marrow function.

Use together with other CNS-active drugs cautiously because of the potential for additive effects.

Effects on diagnostic tests
Toxic effects of the drug may be evidenced by depressed blood counts.

Adverse reactions
● CNS: drowsiness, sedation, *seizures,* dizziness, syncope, vertigo, headache, tremor, disturbed sleep or nightmares, restlessness, hypokinesia or akinesia, agitation, rigidity, akathisia, confusion, fatigue, insomnia, hyperkinesia, weakness, lethargy, ataxia, slurred speech, depression, myoclonia, anxiety.
● CV: tachycardia, hypotension, orthostatic hypotension, chest pain, ECG changes.
● DERM: rash.
● GI: constipation, nausea, vomiting, salivation, dry mouth.
● GU: urinary abnormalities, incontinence, abnormal ejaculation, urinary frequency or urgency, urine retention.
● HEMA: *leukopenia, granulocytopenia, agranulocytosis.*
● Other: fever, muscle pain or spasm, muscle weakness, weight gain.

Overdose and treatment
Fatalities have occurred at doses exceeding 2.5 g. Symptoms include drowsiness, delerium, coma, hypotension, hypersalivation, tachycardia, respiratory depression, and, rarely, seizures.

Treat symptomatically. Establish an airway and ensure adequate ventilation. Gastric lavage with activated charcoal and sorbitol may be effective. Monitor vital signs. Avoid epinephrine (and derivatives), quinidine, and procainamide when treating hypotension and cardiac arrhythmias.

▶ Special considerations
● Clozapine therapy should be given with a monitoring program that ensures weekly testing of WBC counts. Blood tests should be performed weekly, and no more than a 1-week supply of drug should be distributed.
● To discontinue clozapine therapy, withdraw drug gradually (over a 1- to 2-week period). However, changes in the patient's clinical status (including the development of leukopenia) may require abrupt discontinuation of the drug. If so, monitor closely for recurrence of psychotic symptoms.
● To reinstate therapy in patients withdrawn from the drug, follow usual guidelines for dosage buildup. However, reexposure of the patient may increase the risk and severity of adverse reactions. If therapy was terminated for WBC counts below 2,000/mm³ or granulocyte counts below 1,000/mm³, the drug should not be continued.
● Some patients experience transient fevers (temperature above 100.4° F. [38° C.]), especially in the first 3 weeks of therapy. Monitor patients closely.

Information for the patient
● Warn patient about the risk of developing agranulocytosis. He should know that the drug is available only with a special monitoring program that requires weekly blood tests to monitor for agranulocytosis. Advise patient to promptly report flulike symptoms, fever, sore throat, lethargy, malaise, or other signs of infection.
● Advise patient to check with physician before taking any OTC drugs or alcohol.
● Tell patient that ice chips or sugarless candy or gum may help to relieve dry mouth.
● Warn patient to rise slowly to upright position to avoid orthostatic hypotension.

Pediatric use
Safe use in children has not been established.

Breast-feeding
Animal studies have shown that the drug is excreted in breast milk. Women taking clozapine should not breast-feed.

███████████████

fluphenazine decanoate
Prolixin Decanoate

fluphenazine enanthate
Moditen Enanthate∗, Prolixin Enanthate

fluphenazine hydrochloride
Permitil Hydrochloride, Prolixin Hydrochloride

● Pharmacologic classification: phenothiazine (piperazine derivative)
● Therapeutic classification: antipsychotic
● Pregnancy risk category C

How supplied
Available by prescription only
fluphenazine hydrochloride
Tablets: 1 mg, 2.5 mg, 5 mg, 10 mg
Oral concentrate: 5 mg/ml (contains 14% alcohol)
Elixir: 2.5 mg/5 ml (with 14% alcohol)
I.M. injection: 2.5 mg/ml
fluphenazine enanthate
Depot injection: 25 mg/ml
fluphenazine decanoate
Depot injection: 25 mg/ml

Indications, route, and dosage
Psychotic disorders
Adults: Initially, 0.5 to 10 mg fluphenazine hydrochloride P.O. daily in divided doses q 6 to 8 hours; may increase cautiously to 20 mg. Maintenance dosage is 1 to 5 mg P.O. daily. I.M. doses are one-third to one-half that of oral doses. Lower doses for geriatric patients (1 to 2.5 mg daily).
Adults and children over age 12: 12.5 to 25 mg of long-acting esters (fluphenazine decanoate and enanthate) I.M. or S.C. q 1 to 6 weeks. Maintenance dosage is 25 to 100 mg p.r.n.
Children age 12 and under: 0.25 to 3.5 mg fluphenazine hydrochloride P.O. daily in divided doses q 4 to 6 hours; or one-third to one-half of oral dose I.M.; maximum dosage is 10 mg daily.

Pharmacodynamics
Antipsychotic action: Fluphenazine is thought to exert its antipsychotic effects by postsynaptic

blockade of CNS dopamine receptors, thereby inhibiting dopamine-mediated effects.

Fluphenazine has many other central and peripheral effects; it produces both alpha and ganglionic blockade and counteracts histamine- and serotonin-mediated activity. Its most prominent adverse reactions are extrapyramidal.

Pharmacokinetics

● *Absorption:* Rate and extent of absorption vary with route of administration; oral tablet absorption is erratic and variable. Oral and I.M. dosages have an onset of action within ½ to 1 hour. Long-acting decanoate and enanthate salts act within 24 to 72 hours.

● *Distribution:* Fluphenazine is distributed widely into the body, including breast milk. CNS concentrations are usually higher than those in plasma. Drug is 91% to 99% protein-bound. Peak effects of oral dose usually occur at 2 hours; steady-state serum levels are achieved within 4 to 7 days.

● *Metabolism:* Fluphenazine is metabolized extensively by the liver, but no active metabolites are formed; duration of action is about 6 to 8 hours after oral administration; 1 to 6 weeks (average, 2 weeks) after I.M. depot administration.

● *Excretion:* Most of drug is excreted in urine via the kidneys; some is excreted in feces via the biliary tract.

Contraindications and precautions

Fluphenazine is contraindicated in patients with known hypersensitivity to phenothiazines and related compounds, including allergic reactions involving hepatic function; in patients with blood dyscrasias and bone marrow depression because of possible agranulocytosis; in patients with disorders accompanied by coma, brain damage, or CNS depression because of additive CNS depression; in patients with circulatory collapse or cerebrovascular disease because of its hypotensive effect; and for use with adrenergic blocking agents or spinal or epidural anesthetics because of potential hypotension and alpha blockade.

Fluphenazine should be used cautiously in patients with cardiac disease (arrhythmias, CHF, angina pectoris, valvular disease, or heart block), encephalitis, Reye's syndrome, head injury, respiratory disease, seizure disorders, glaucoma, prostatic hypertrophy, urine retention, hepatic or renal dysfunction, Parkinson's disease, pheochromocytoma, or hypocalcemia. Some oral preparations of fluphenazine contain tartrazine; use of such products may cause allergic reaction in patients with aspirin allergy.

Interactions

Concomitant use of fluphenazine with sympathomimetics, including epinephrine, phenylephrine, phenylpropanolamine, and ephedrine (often found in nasal sprays), and appetite suppressants may decrease their stimulatory and pressor effects.

Fluphenazine may inhibit blood pressure response to centrally acting antihypertensive drugs, such as guanethidine, guanabenz, guanadrel, clonidine, methyldopa, and reserpine. Additive effects are likely after concomitant use of fluphenazine with CNS depressants, including alcohol, analgesics, barbiturates, narcotics, tranquilizers, and general, spinal, or epidural anesthetics, or parenteral magnesium sulfate (oversedation, respiratory depression, and hypotension); antiarrhythmic agents, including quinidine, disopyramide, and procainamide (increased incidence of cardiac arrhythmias and conduction defects); atropine or other anticholinergic drugs, including antidepressants, MAO inhibitors, phenothiazines, antihistamines, meperidine, and antiparkinsonian agents (oversedation, paralytic ileus, visual changes, and severe constipation); nitrates (hypotension); and metrizamide (increased risk of seizures).

Beta blocking agents may inhibit fluphenazine metabolism, increasing plasma levels and toxicity.

Concomitant use with propylthiouracil increases risk of agranulocytosis; concomitant use with lithium may result in severe neurologic toxicity with an encephalitis-like syndrome and a decreased therapeutic response to fluphenazine.

Pharmacokinetic alterations and subsequent decreased therapeutic response to fluphenazine may follow concomitant use with phenobarbital (enhanced renal excretion), aluminum- and magnesium-containing antacids and antidiarrheals (decreased absorption), or caffeine and with heavy smoking (increased metabolism).

Fluphenazine may antagonize therapeutic effect of bromocriptine on prolactin secretion; it also may decrease the vasoconstricting effects of high-dose dopamine and may decrease effectiveness and increase toxicity of levodopa (by dopamine blockade). Fluphenazine may inhibit metabolism and increase toxicity of phenytoin and tricyclic antidepressants.

Effects on diagnostic tests

Fluphenazine causes false-positive test results for urinary porphyrins, urobilinogen, amylase, and 5-hydroxyindoleacetic acid, because of darkening of urine by metabolites; it also causes false-positive urine pregnancy test results using human chorionic gonadotropin.

Fluphenazine elevates test results for liver enzymes and protein-bound iodine and causes quinidine-like ECG effects.

Adverse reactions

● CNS: extrapyramidal symptoms – dystonia, akathisia, torticollis, tardive dyskinesia, sedation (low incidence), pseudoparkinsonism, drowsiness (frequent), *neuroleptic malignant syndrome* (fatal *respiratory failure* in over 10% of patients if untreated), dizziness, headache, insomnia, exacerbation of psychotic symptoms.
● CV: *asystole*, orthostatic hypotension, tachycardia, dizziness and fainting, arrhythmias, ECG changes, increased anginal pain after I.M. injection.
● EENT: blurred vision, tinnitus, mydriasis, increased intraocular pressure, ocular changes (retinal pigmentary change with long-term use).
● GI: dry mouth, constipation, nausea, vomiting, anorexia, diarrhea.
● GU: urine retention, gynecomastia, hypermenorrhea, inhibited ejaculation.
● HEMA: transient leukopenia, *agranulocytosis*, thrombocytopenia, anemia (within 30 to 90 days).
● Local: contact dermatitis from concentrate or injectable form, muscle necrosis from I.M. injection.
● Other: hyperprolactinemia, photosensitivity, increased appetite or weight gain, hypersensitivity (rash, urticaria, drug fever, edema, cholestatic jaundice [in 2% to 4% of patients within first 30 days]).

After abrupt withdrawal of long-term therapy, patient may develop gastritis, nausea, vomiting, dizziness, tremor, feeling of heat or cold, sweating, tachycardia, headache, or insomnia.

Note: Drug should be discontinued immediately if any of the following occurs: hypersensitivity, jaundice, agranulocytosis or neuroleptic malignant syndrome (marked hyperthermia, extrapyramidal effects, autonomic dysfunction) or if severe extrapyramidal symptoms occur even after dosage is lowered. Drug should be discontinued 48 hours before and 24 hours after myelography using metrizamide because of the risk of seizures. When feasible, drug should be withdrawn slowly and gradually; many drug effects persist after withdrawal.

Overdose and treatment

CNS depression is characterized by deep, unarousable sleep and possible coma, hypotension or hypertension, extrapyramidal symptoms, dystonia, abnormal involuntary muscle movements, agitation, seizures, arrhythmias, ECG changes, hypothermia or hyperthermia, and autonomic nervous system dysfunction.

Treatment is symptomatic and supportive, including maintaining vital signs, airway, stable body temperature, and fluid and electrolyte balance.

Do not induce vomiting: drug inhibits cough reflex and aspiration may occur. Use gastric lavage and then activated charcoal and saline cathartics; dialysis does not help. Regulate body temperature as needed. Treat hypotension with I.V. fluids: *do not give epinephrine*. Treat seizures with parenteral diazepam or barbiturates; arrhythmias with parenteral phenytoin (1 mg/kg with rate titrated to blood pressure); extrapyramidal reactions with barbiturates, benztropine, or parenteral diphenhydramine at 2 mg/kg/minute.

▶ **Special considerations**

Besides those relevant to all *phenothiazines,* consider the following recommendations.
● Note that two parenteral forms are available: depot injection (25 mg/ml) and I.M. injection (2.5 mg/ml).
● The depot injection form is not recommended for patients who are not stabilized on a phenothiazine. This form has a prolonged elimination; its action could not be terminated in case of adverse reactions.

Information for the patient

● Explain risks of dystonic reactions and tardive dyskinesia and tell patient to report abnormal body movements.
● Tell patient to avoid sun exposure and to use a sunscreen when going outdoors, to prevent photosensitivity reactions. (Note that heat lamps and tanning beds also may cause burning of the skin or skin discoloration.)
● Warn patient to avoid extremely hot or cold baths and exposure to temperature extremes, sunlamps, or tanning beds. Drug may cause thermoregulatory changes.
● Tell patient to take the drug exactly as prescribed, not to double dose for missed ones, and not to discontinue the drug suddenly.
● Explain that most adverse reactions can be relieved by a dosage reduction. Patient should promptly report persistent fever, difficulty urinating, sore throat, dizziness, or fainting.

- Tell patient that many drug interactions are possible. Patient should seek medical approval before taking *any* OTC medications.
- Inform patient that he should become tolerant to the drug's sedative effects in several weeks.
- Tell patient to avoid hazardous activities that require alertness until the drug's effect is established.
- Tell patient to avoid alcohol and other medications that may cause excessive sedation.
- Suggest sugarless hard candy or chewing gum or ice chips to relieve dry mouth.

Pediatric use
Fluphenazine may be used in children over age 6.

Breast-feeding
Fluphenazine enters breast milk. Caution should be observed, and the potential benefits to the mother should outweigh the potential harm to the infant.

---

haloperidol
Apo-Haloperidol∗, Haldol, Novoperidol∗, Peridol∗

haloperidol decanoate
Haldol Decanoate, Haldol LA∗

haloperidol lactate
Haldol, Haldol Concentrate

- Pharmacologic classification: butyrophenone
- Therapeutic classification: antipsychotic
- Pregnancy risk category C

How supplied
Available by prescription only
haloperidol
Tablets: 0.5 mg, 1 mg, 2 mg, 5 mg, 10 mg, 20 mg
Injection: 5 mg/ml
haloperidol lactate
Oral concentrate: 2 mg/ml
Injection: 5 mg/ml
haloperidol decanoate
Injection: 50 mg/ml, 100 mg/ml

Indications, route, and dosage
Psychotic disorders
Adults: Dosage varies for each patient. Initial dosage range is 0.5 to 5 mg P.O. b.i.d. or t.i.d.; or 2 to 5 mg I.M. q 4 to 8 hours, increased rapidly if necessary for prompt control. Maximum dos-

age is 100 mg P.O. daily. Doses over 100 mg have been used for patients with severely resistant conditions. Reduce maintenance to lowest effective and tolerated level.
Chronic psychotic patients who require prolonged therapy
Adults: 50 to 100 mg I.M. of haloperidol decanoate q 4 weeks.
Control of tics, vocal utterances in Gilles de la Tourette's syndrome
Adults: 0.5 to 5 mg P.O. b.i.d. or t.i.d., increased p.r.n.
Children ages 3 to 12: 0.05 to 0.075 mg/kg/day given b.i.d. or t.i.d.

Pharmacodynamics
Antipsychotic action: Haloperidol is thought to exert its antipsychotic effects by strong postsynaptic blockade of CNS dopamine receptors, thereby inhibiting dopamine-mediated effects; its pharmacologic effects are most similar to those of piperazine antipsychotics. Its mechanism of action in Gilles de la Tourette's syndrome is unknown.
Haloperidol has many other central and peripheral effects; it has weak peripheral anticholinergic effects and antiemetic effects, produces both alpha and ganglionic blockade, and counteracts histamine- and serotonin-mediated activity. Its most prominent adverse reactions are extrapyramidal.

Pharmacokinetics
- *Absorption:* Rate and extent of absorption vary with route of administration: oral tablet absorption yields 60% to 70% bioavailability. I.M. dose is 70% absorbed within 30 minutes. Peak plasma levels after oral administration occur at 2 to 6 hours; after I.M. administration, 30 to 45 minutes; and after long-acting I.M. (decanoate) administration, 4 to 11 days.
- *Distribution:* Haloperidol is distributed widely into the body, with high concentrations in adipose tissue. Drug is 91% to 99% protein-bound.
- *Metabolism:* Haloperidol is metabolized extensively by the liver; there may be only one active metabolite that is less active than the parent drug.
- *Excretion:* About 40% of a given dose is excreted in urine within 5 days; about 15% is excreted in feces via the biliary tract.

Contraindications and precautions
Haloperidol is contraindicated in patients with known hypersensitivity to haloperidol, phenothiazines, and related compounds, including that expressed by jaundice because haloperidol may

impair liver function; in patients with blood dyscrasias and bone marrow depression because *agranulocytosis* can occur; in patients with disorders accompanied by coma, brain damage, or CNS depression because of additive CNS depression; and in circulatory collapse or cerebrovascular disease because of the drug's hypotensive and arrhythmogenic effects.

Use haloperidol cautiously in patients with cardiac disease (arrhythmias, CHF, angina pectoris, valvular disease, or heart block), encephalitis, Reye's syndrome, head injury, respiratory disease, seizure disorders, glaucoma, prostatic hypertrophy, urine retention, hepatic or renal dysfunction, Parkinson's disease, pheochromocytoma, or hypocalcemia.

Interactions

Concomitant use of haloperidol with sympathomimetics, including epinephrine, phenylephrine, phenylpropanolamine, and ephedrine (often found in nasal sprays), and appetite suppressants may decrease their stimulatory and pressor effects.

Haloperidol may inhibit blood pressure response to centrally acting antihypertensive drugs, such as guanethidine, guanabenz, guanadrel, clonidine, methyldopa, and reserpine. Additive effects are likely after concomitant use of haloperidol with CNS depressants, including alcohol, analgesics, barbiturates, narcotics, tranquilizers, and general, spinal, or epidural anesthetics, or with parenteral magnesium sulfate (oversedation, respiratory depression, and hypotension); antiarrhythmic agents, including quinidine, disopyramide, or procainamide (increased incidence of cardiac arrhythmias and conduction defects); atropine or other anticholinergic drugs, including antidepressants, MAO inhibitors, phenothiazines, antihistamines, meperidine, and antiparkinsonian agents (oversedation, paralytic ileus, visual changes, and severe constipation); nitrates (hypotension); and metrizamide (increased risk of seizures.)

Beta blocking agents may inhibit haloperidol metabolism, increasing plasma levels and toxicity.

Concomitant use with propylthiouracil increases risk of agranulocytosis; concomitant use with lithium may result in severe neurologic toxicity with an encephalitis-like syndrome and a decreased therapeutic response to haloperidol.

Pharmacokinetic alterations and subsequent decreased therapeutic response to haloperidol may follow concomitant use with phenobarbital (enhanced renal excretion); aluminum- and magnesium-containing antacids and antidiarrheals (decreased absorption); and heavy smoking (increased metabolism).

Haloperidol may antagonize therapeutic effect of bromocriptine on prolactin secretion; it also may decrease the vasoconstricting effects of high-dose dopamine and may decrease effectiveness and increase toxicity of levodopa (by dopamine blockade). Haloperidol may inhibit metabolism and increase toxicity of phenytoin.

Effects on diagnostic tests

Haloperidol causes quinidine-like effects on the ECG.

Adverse reactions

- CNS: extrapyramidal symptoms – dystonia, akathisia, torticollis, tardive dyskinesia, sedation, pseudoparkinsonism, drowsiness, *neuroleptic malignant syndrome* (fatal *respiratory failure* in over 10% of patients if untreated), dizziness, headache, insomnia, exacerbation of psychotic symptoms.
- CV: *asystole,* orthostatic hypotension, tachycardia, dizziness and fainting, arrhythmias, ECG changes, increased anginal pain (after I.M. injection).
- EENT: blurred vision, tinnitus, mydriasis, increased intraocular pressure, ocular changes (retinal pigmentary change with long-term use).
- GI: dry mouth, constipation, nausea, vomiting, anorexia, diarrhea.
- GU: urine retention, gynecomastia, hypermenorrhea, inhibited ejaculation.
- HEMA: transient leukopenia, *agranulocytosis,* thrombocytopenia, anemia (within 30 to 90 days).
- Local: contact dermatitis from concentrate or injectable form, muscle necrosis from I.M. injection more common with this drug.
- Other: hyperprolactinemia, photosensitivity, increased appetite or weight gain, hypersensitivity (rash, urticaria, drug fever, edema, cholestatic jaundice [in 2% to 4% of patients within first 30 days]).

Note: Drug should be discontinued immediately if any of the following occurs: hypersensitivity, jaundice, agranulocytosis; neuroleptic malignant syndrome (marked hyperthermia, extrapyramidal effects, autonomic dysfunction); or if severe extrapyramidal symptoms occur even after dosage is lowered; and 48 hours before and 24 hours after myelography using metrizamide because of the risk of seizures. When feasible, withdraw drug slowly and gradually; many drug effects persist after withdrawal.

Overdose and treatment
CNS depression is characterized by deep, unarousable sleep and possible coma, hypotension or hypertension, extrapyramidal symptoms, dystonia, abnormal involuntary muscle movements, agitation, seizures, arrhythmias, ECG changes (may show QT prolongation and torsades de pointes), hypothermia or hyperthermia, and autonomic nervous system dysfunction. Overdose with long-acting decanoate requires prolonged recovery time.

Treatment is symptomatic and supportive, including maintaining vital signs, airway, stable body temperature, and fluid and electrolyte balance. Ipecac syrup may be used to induce vomiting, with due regard for haloperidol's antiemetic properties and hazard of aspiration. Gastric lavage also may be used, followed by activated charcoal and saline cathartics; dialysis does not help.

Regulate body temperature as needed. Treat hypotension with I.V. fluids; *do not give epinephrine.* Treat seizures with parenteral diazepam or barbiturates; arrhythmias, with parenteral phenytoin (1 mg/kg with rate titrated to blood pressure); extrapyramidal reactions with barbiturates, benztropine, or parenteral diphenhydramine 2 mg/kg/minute.

▶ **Special considerations**
• Tardive dyskinesia may occur after prolonged use. It may not appear until months or years later and may disappear spontaneously or persist for life.
• Protect medication from light. Slight yellowing of injection or concentrate is common; does not affect potency. Discard markedly discolored solutions.
• Do not withdraw drug abruptly unless required by severe adverse reactions.
• A dose of 2 mg is the therapeutic equivalent of 100 mg chlorpromazine.
• When changing from tablets to decanoate injection, patient should receive 10 to 15 times the oral dose once a month (maximum 100 mg).
• Don't administer the decanoate form I.V.

Information for the patient
• Warn patient against activities that require alertness and good psychomotor coordination until CNS response to drug is determined. Drowsiness and dizziness usually subside after a few weeks.
• Explain the risks of dystonic reactions and tardive dyskinesia and tell the patient to report abnormal body movements.
• Tell patient to avoid sun exposure and to use a sunscreen when going outdoors, to prevent photosensitivity reactions. (Note that sunlamps and tanning beds also may cause burning of the skin or skin discoloration).
• Warn patient to avoid extremely hot or cold baths or exposure to temperature extremes, sunlamps, or tanning beds. Drug may cause thermoregulatory changes.
• Tell patient to take the drug exactly as prescribed and not to double dose to compensate for missed ones.
• Explain that many drug interactions are possible. Patient should seek medical approval before taking *any* self-prescribed medications.
• Tell patient not to stop taking drug suddenly.
• Encourage patient to report difficulty urinating, sore throat, persistent fever, dizziness, or fainting.
• Tell patient to avoid hazardous activities that require alertness until the effect of the drug is established. Excessive sedative effects tend to subside after several weeks.
• Tell patient to avoid alcohol and medications that may cause excessive sedation.
• Explain what fluids are appropriate for diluting the concentrate and the dropper technique for measuring dose.
• Tell patient that sugarless hard candy or chewing gum, or ice chips can alleviate dry mouth.
• Tell patient to shake concentrate before administration.

Geriatric use
• Especially useful for agitation associated with senile dementia.
• Elderly patients usually require lower initial doses and a more gradual dosage titration.

Pediatric use
Haloperidol is not recommended for children under age 3. Children are especially prone to extrapyramidal adverse reactions.

loxapine hydrochloride
Loxitane C, Loxitane IM

loxapine succinate
Loxapac*, Loxitane

- Pharmacologic classification: dibenzoxazepine
- Therapeutic classification: antipsychotic
- Pregnancy risk category C

How supplied
Available by prescription only
Capsules: 5 mg, 10 mg, 25 mg, 50 mg
Oral concentrate: 25 mg/ml
Injection: 50 mg/ml

Indications, route, and dosage
Psychotic disorders
Adults: 10 mg P.O. or I.M. b.i.d. to q.i.d., rapidly increasing to 60 to 100 mg P.O. daily for most patients; dose varies from patient to patient. Maximum daily dosage is 250 mg. Do not administer drug I.V.

Pharmacodynamics
Antipsychotic action: Loxapine is the only tricyclic antipsychotic; it is structurally similar to amoxapine. Loxapine is thought to exert its antipsychotic effects by postsynaptic blockade of CNS dopamine receptors, thus inhibiting dopamine-mediated effects. Loxapine has many central and peripheral effects; its most prominent adverse reactions are extrapyramidal.

Pharmacokinetics
- *Absorption:* Loxapine is absorbed rapidly and completely from the GI tract. Sedation occurs in 30 minutes.
- *Distribution:* Loxapine is distributed widely into the body, including breast milk. Peak effect occurs at 1½ to 3 hours; steady-state serum level is achieved within 3 to 4 days. Drug is 91% to 99% protein-bound.
- *Metabolism:* Drug is metabolized extensively by the liver, forming a few active metabolites; duration of action is 12 hours.
- *Excretion:* Most of drug is excreted as metabolites in urine; some is excreted in feces via the biliary tract. About 50% of drug is excreted in urine and feces within 24 hours.

Contraindications and precautions
Loxapine is contraindicated in patients with known hypersensitivity to loxapine and in patients with disorders accompanied by coma, CNS depression, brain damage, circulatory collapse, or cerebrovascular disease because of the potential hypotensive effects.

Loxapine should be used cautiously in patients with cardiac disease (arrhythmias, CHF, angina pectoris, valvular disease, or heart block), encephalitis, Reye's syndrome, head injury, respiratory disease, seizure disorders, glaucoma, prostatic hypertrophy, urine retention, hepatic or renal dysfunction, Parkinson's disease, pheochromocytoma, or hypocalcemia.

Interactions
Concomitant use of loxapine with sympathomimetics, including epinephrine, phenylephrine, phenylpropanolamine, and ephedrine (often found in nasal sprays), and with appetite suppressants may decrease their stimulatory and pressor effects. Loxapine may cause epinephrine reversal, an inhibition of epinephrine's vasopressor effect.

Loxapine may inhibit blood pressure response to centrally acting antihypertensive drugs, such as guanethidine, guanabenz, guanadrel, clonidine, methyldopa, and reserpine. Loxapine may antagonize therapeutic effect of bromocriptine on prolactin secretion; it may also decrease the vasoconstricting effects of high-dose dopamine and may decrease effectiveness and increase toxicity of levodopa (by dopamine blockade).

Additive effects are likely after concomitant use of loxapine and CNS depressants, including alcohol, analgesics, barbiturates, narcotics, tranquilizers, anesthetics (general, spinal, and epidural), and parenteral magnesium sulfate (oversedation, respiratory depression, and hypotension); antiarrhythmic agents, including quinidine, disopyramide, and procainamide (increased incidence of cardiac arrhythmias and conduction defects); atropine and other anticholinergic drugs, including antidepressants, MAO inhibitors, phenothiazines, antihistamines, meperidine, and antiparkinsonian agents (oversedation, paralytic ileus, visual changes, and severe constipation); and nitrates (hypotension).

Beta blocking agents may inhibit loxapine metabolism, increasing plasma levels and toxicity.

Concomitant use with lithium may result in severe neurologic toxicity with an encephalitis-like syndrome and in decreased therapeutic response to loxapine. Aluminum- and magnesium-containing antacids and antidiarrheals decrease loxapine absorption and, thus, its therapeutic effects.

Effects on diagnostic tests

Loxapine causes false-positive test results for urinary porphyrins, urobilinogen, amylase, and 5-hydroxyindoleacetic acid because of darkening of urine by metabolites; it also causes false-positive urine pregnancy test results using human chorionic gonadotropin.

Loxapine elevates test results for liver enzymes and protein-bound iodine and causes quinidine-like effects on the ECG.

Adverse reactions

● CNS: *extrapyramidal symptoms* – dystonia, akathisia, torticollis (more common with I.M. administration), tardive dyskinesia, sedation, pseudoparkinsonism, drowsiness (frequent), *neuroleptic malignant syndrome* (fatal *respiratory failure* in over 10% of patients if untreated), dizziness, headache, insomnia, exacerbation of psychotic symptoms.
● CV: *asystole,* orthostatic hypotension, tachycardia, dizziness and fainting, *arrhythmias,* ECG changes, increased anginal pain after I.M. injection.
● EENT: blurred vision, tinnitus, mydriasis, increased intraocular pressure, ocular changes (retinal pigmentary change on long-term use).
● GI: dry mouth, constipation, nausea, vomiting, anorexia, diarrhea.
● GU: urine retention, gynecomastia, hypermenorrhea, inhibited ejaculation.
● HEMA: transient leukopenia, *agranulocytosis,* thrombocytopenia, anemia (within 30 to 90 days).
● Local: contact dermatitis from concentrate or injectable, muscle necrosis from I.M. injection.
● Other: hyperprolactinemia, photosensitivity, increased appetite or weight gain, hypersensitivity (rash, urticaria, drug fever, edema, cholestatic jaundice [in 2% to 4% of patients within first 30 days]).

Note: Drug should be discontinued immediately if any of the following occur: hypersensitivity, jaundice, agranulocytosis, neuroleptic malignant syndrome (marked hyperthermia, extrapyramidal effects, autonomic dysfunction), or severe extrapyramidal symptoms that occur even after dose is lowered. Drug should be discontinued 48 hours before and 24 hours after myelography using metrizamide because of risk of seizures. When feasible, drug should be withdrawn slowly and gradually; many drug effects persist after withdrawal.

Overdose and treatment

CNS depression is characterized by deep, unarousable sleep and possible coma, hypotension or hypertension, extrapyramidal symptoms, abnormal involuntary muscle movements, agitation, seizures, arrhythmias, ECG changes, hypothermia or hyperthermia, and autonomic nervous system dysfunction.

Treatment is symptomatic and supportive, including maintaining vital signs, airway, stable body temperature, and fluid and electrolyte balance.

Do not induce vomiting: drug inhibits cough reflex and aspiration may occur. Use gastric lavage, then activated charcoal and saline cathartics; hemodialysis may be helpful. Regulate body temperature as needed. Treat hypotension with I.V. fluids; *do not give epinephrine.* Treat seizures with parenteral diazepam or barbiturates; arrhythmias with parenteral phenytoin (1 mg/kg with rate titrated to blood pressure); and extrapyramidal reactions with barbiturates, benztropine, or parenteral diphenhydramine 2 mg/kg/minute.

▶ Special considerations

● Tardive dyskinesia may occur after prolonged use. It may not appear until months or years after treatment and may disappear spontaneously or persist for life.
● Avoid combining with alcohol or other depressants.
● Obtain baseline blood pressure measurements before starting therapy and monitor regularly.
● Dilute liquid concentrate with orange or grapefruit juice just before giving.
● Periodic ophthalmic tests are recommended.
● A dose of 10 mg is the therapeutic equivalent of 100 mg chlorpromazine.
● Photosensitivity warnings may apply with loxapine.

Information for the patient

● Warn against activities that require alertness and good psychomotor coordination until CNS response to drug is determined. Drowsiness and dizziness usually subside after first few weeks.
● Tell patient that dry mouth may be relieved by sugarless gum, sugarless hard candy, or artificial saliva.
● Advise patient to get up slowly to avoid orthostatic hypotension.
● Tell patient to take the drug exactly as prescribed and not to double dose to compensate for missed ones.
● Explain that many drug interactions are pos-

sible. Patient should seek medical approval before taking *any* self-prescribed medications.
- Tell patient not to stop taking drug suddenly.
- Encourage patient to report difficulty urinating, sore throat, persistent fever, dizziness, or fainting.
- Explain the risks of dystonic reactions and tardive dyskinesia and tell the patient to report abnormal body movements.
- Tell patient to avoid sun exposure and to use a sunscreen when going outdoors, to prevent photosensitivity reactions. (Note that sunlamps and tanning beds also may cause burning of the skin or skin discoloration).
- Tell patient to avoid spilling oral concentrate on the skin because such contact can cause rash and irritation.

Geriatric use
Elderly patients are highly sensitive to the antimuscarinic, hypotensive, and sedative effects of loxapine and have a higher risk of developing extrapyramidal adverse reactions, such as parkinsonism and tardive dyskinesia. These patients develop higher plasma concentrations and therefore require lower initial dosage and more gradual titration.

Pediatric use
Loxapine is not recommended for children under age 16.

Breast-feeding
Excretion in breast milk is unknown. Use with caution.

---

mesoridazine besylate
Serentil

- Pharmacologic classification: phenothiazine (piperidine derivative)
- Therapeutic classification: antipsychotic
- Pregnancy risk category C

How supplied
Available by prescription only
Tablets: 10 mg, 25 mg, 50 mg, 100 mg
Oral concentrate: 25 mg/ml (0.6% alcohol)
Injection: 25 mg/ml

Indications, route, and dosage
Psychosis
Adults and children over age 12: 10 mg P.O. t.i.d. up to a maximum of 150 mg/day.

Schizophrenia
Adults and children over age 12: Initially, 50 mg P.O. t.i.d. to a maximum of 400 mg/day; or 25 mg I.M. repeated in 30 to 60 minutes p.r.n. not to exceed 200 mg I.M. daily.
Alcoholism
Adults and children over age 12: 25 mg P.O. b.i.d., up to a maximum of 200 mg/day.
Behavioral problems associated with chronic brain syndrome
Adults and children over age 12: 25 mg P.O. t.i.d., up to a maximum of 300 mg/day. I.M. dosage form is irritating.

Pharmacodynamics
Antipsychotic action: Mesoridazine is thought to exert its antipsychotic effects by postsynaptic blockade of CNS dopamine receptors, thereby inhibiting dopamine-mediated effects.

Mesoridazine has many other central and peripheral effects; it produces both alpha and ganglionic blockade and counteracts histamine- and serotonin-mediated activity. Its most prominent adverse reactions are antimuscarinic and sedative; it causes fewer extrapyramidal effects than other antipsychotics.

Pharmacokinetics
- *Absorption:* Rate and extent of absorption vary with route of administration. Oral tablet absorption is erratic and variable, with onset ranging from ½ to 1 hour. Oral liquids are much more predictable; I.M. dosage form is absorbed rapidly.
- *Distribution:* Mesoridazine is distributed widely into the body, including breast milk. Peak effects occur at 2 to 4 hours; steady-state serum level is achieved within 4 to 7 days. Drug is 91% to 99% protein-bound.
- *Metabolism:* Mesoridazine is metabolized extensively by the liver; no active metabolites are formed. Duration of action is 4 to 6 hours.
- *Excretion:* Most of drug is excreted as metabolites in urine; some drug is excreted in feces via the biliary tract.

Contraindications and precautions
Mesoridazine is contraindicated in patients with known hypersensitivity to phenothiazines and related compounds, including allergic reactions involving hepatic function, because it is potentially hepatotoxic; in patients with blood dyscrasias and bone marrow depression because it may induce agranulocytosis; in patients with disorders accompanied by coma, brain damage, or CNS depression because of additive CNS depression; in patients with circulatory collapse

or cerebrovascular disease because of its hypotensive effects; and for use with adrenergic blocking agents or spinal or epidural anesthetics because of its alpha blocking activity.

Mesoridazine should be used cautiously in patients with cardiac disease (arrhythmias, CHF, angina pectoris, valvular disease, or heart block), encephalitis, Reye's syndrome, head injury, respiratory disease, seizure disorders, glaucoma, prostatic hypertrophy, urine retention, hepatic or renal dysfunction, Parkinson's disease, pheochromocytoma, and hypocalcemia.

Oral dosage forms may contain tartrazine; dye may cause allergic reaction in aspirin-allergic patients.

Interactions

Concomitant use of mesoridazine with sympathomimetics, including epinephrine, phenylephrine, phenylpropanolamine, and ephedrine (often found in nasal sprays), or appetite suppressants may decrease their stimulatory and pressor effects. Phenothiazines can cause epinephrine reversal and produce hypotension when epinephrine is used as a pressor agent.

Mesoridazine may inhibit blood pressure response to centrally acting antihypertensive drugs, such as guanethidine, guanabenz, guanadrel, clonidine, methyldopa, and reserpine. Additive effects are likely after concomitant use of mesoridazine with CNS depressants, including alcohol, analgesics, barbiturates, narcotics, tranquilizers, and general, spinal, or epidural anesthetics, or parenteral magnesium sulfate (oversedation, respiratory depression, and hypotension); antiarrhythmic agents, including quinidine, disopyramide, or procainamide (increased incidence of cardiac arrhythmias and conduction defects); atropine and other anticholinergic drugs, including antidepressants, MAO inhibitors, phenothiazines, antihistamines, meperidine, and antiparkinsonian agents (oversedation, paralytic ileus, visual changes, and severe constipation); nitrates (hypotension); and metrizamide (increased risk of seizures).

Beta blocking agents may inhibit mesoridazine metabolism, increasing plasma levels and toxicity. Concomitant use with propylthiouracil increases risk of agranulocytosis; concomitant use with lithium may result in severe neurologic toxicity with an encephalitis-like syndrome and a decreased therapeutic response to mesoridazine.

Pharmacokinetic alterations and subsequent decreased therapeutic response to mesoridazine may follow concomitant use with phenobarbital (enhanced renal excretion); aluminum- and magnesium-containing antacids and antidiarrheals (decreased absorption); caffeine; or heavy smoking (increased metabolism).

Mesoridazine may antagonize therapeutic effect of bromocriptine on prolactin secretion; it also may decrease the vasoconstricting effects of high-dose dopamine and may decrease effectiveness and increase toxicity of levodopa (by dopamine blockade). Mesoridazine may inhibit metabolism and increase toxicity of phenytoin.

Effects on diagnostic tests

Mesoridazine causes false-positive test results for urinary porphyrins, urobilinogen, amylase, and 5-hydroxyindoleacetic acid because of darkening of urine by metabolites; it also causes false-positive urine pregnancy test results using human chorionic gonadotropin.

Mesoridazine elevates tests for liver function and protein-bound iodine and causes quinidine-like effects on the ECG.

Adverse reactions

● CNS: extrapyramidal symptoms—dystonia, akathisia, torticollis, tardive dyskinesia, sedation (high incidence), pseudoparkinsonism, drowsiness (frequent), *neuroleptic malignant syndrome* (fatal *respiratory failure* in over 10% of patients if untreated), dizziness, headache, insomnia, exacerbation of psychotic symptoms, changes in libido.

● CV: *asystole,* orthostatic hypotension (high incidence), tachycardia, dizziness/fainting, *arrhythmias,* ECG changes, increased anginal pain after I.M. injection.

● EENT: blurred vision, tinnitus, mydriasis, increased intraocular pressure, ocular changes (retinal pigmentary change with long-term use).

● GI: dry mouth, constipation, nausea, vomiting, anorexia, diarrhea.

● GU: urine retention, gynecomastia, hypermenorrhea, inhibited ejaculation.

● HEMA: transient leukopenia, *agranulocytosis,* thrombocytopenia, anemia (within 30 to 90 days).

● Local: contact dermatitis from concentrate or injectable form, muscle necrosis from I.M. injection.

● Other: hyperprolactinemia, photosensitivity, increased appetite/weight gain, hypersensitivity (rash, urticaria, drug fever, edema, cholestatic jaundice [in 2% to 4% of patients within first 30 days]).

After abrupt withdrawal of long-term therapy,

---

gastritis, nausea, vomiting, dizziness, tremor, feeling of heat or cold, sweating, tachycardia, headache, or insomnia may occur.

Note: Drug should be discontinued if hypersensitivity, jaundice, agranulocytosis, neuroleptic malignant syndrome (marked hyperthermia, extrapyramidal effects, autonomic dysfunction), or severe extrapyramidal symptoms occur even after dosage is lowered. Drug should be discontinued 48 hours before and 24 hours after myelography using metrizamide because of risk of seizures. When feasible, drug should be withdrawn slowly and gradually; many drug effects persist after withdrawal.

Overdose and treatment

CNS depression is characterized by deep, unarousable sleep and possible coma, hypotension or hypertension, extrapyramidal symptoms, abnormal involuntary muscle movements, agitation, seizures, arrhythmias, ECG changes, hypothermia or hyperthermia, and autonomic nervous system dysfunction.

Treatment is symptomatic and supportive, including maintaining vital signs, airway, stable body temperature, and fluid/electrolyte balance.

Do not induce vomiting: drug inhibits cough reflex and aspiration may occur. Use gastric lavage and then activated charcoal and saline cathartics; dialysis does not help. Regulate body temperature as needed. Treat hypotension with I.V. fluids; *do not give epinephrine.* Treat seizures with parenteral diazepam or barbiturates; arrhythmias, with parenteral phenytoin (1 mg/kg with rate titrated to blood pressure); extrapyramidal reactions, with barbiturates, benztropine, or parenteral diphenhydramine at 2 mg/kg/minute.

▶ **Special considerations**
A dose of 50 mg is the therapeutic equivalent of 100 mg of chlorpromazine.

Information for the patient

● Explain the risks of dystonic reactions and tardive dyskinesia and tell the patient to report abnormal body movements.
● Tell patient to avoid sun exposure and to use a sunscreen when going outdoors, to prevent photosensitivity reactions. (Note that sunlamps and tanning beds also may cause burning of the skin or skin discoloration).
● Tell patient to take the drug exactly as prescribed and not to double dose to compensate for missed ones.
● Explain that many drug interactions are possible. Patient should seek medical approval before taking *any* self-prescribed medications.
● Tell patient not to stop taking drug suddenly.
● Encourage patient to report difficulty urinating, sore throat, dizziness, or fainting.
● Tell patient to avoid hazardous activities that require alertness until the effect of the drug is established. Excessive sedative effects tend to subside after several weeks.
● Tell patient to avoid alcohol and medications that may cause excessive sedation.
● Tell patient that sugarless hard candy or chewing gum, or ice chips can alleviate dry mouth.

Pediatric use

Drug is not recommended in children under age 12.

███████████████

molindone hydrochloride
Moban

● Pharmacologic classification: dihydroindolone
● Therapeutic classification: antipsychotic
● Pregnancy risk category C

How supplied

Available by prescription only
Tablets: 5 mg, 10 mg, 25 mg, 50 mg, 100 mg
Oral solution: 20 mg/ml

Indications, route, and dosage
Psychotic disorders

Adults: 50 to 75 mg P.O. daily, increased to a maximum of 225 mg daily. Doses up to 400 mg may be required.

Pharmacodynamics

Antipsychotic action: Molindone is unrelated to all other antipsychotic drugs; it is thought to exert its antipsychotic effects by postsynaptic blockade of CNS dopamine receptors, thereby inhibiting dopamine-mediated effects.

Molindone has many other central and peripheral effects; it also produces alpha and ganglionic blockade. Its most prominent adverse reactions are extrapyramidal.

Pharmacokinetics

● *Absorption:* Data are limited, but absorption appears rapid; peak effects occur within 1½ hours.
● *Distribution:* Molindone is distributed widely into the body.

- *Metabolism:* Molindone is metabolized extensively; drug effects persist for 24 to 36 hours.
- *Excretion:* Most of drug is excreted as metabolites in urine; some is excreted in feces via the biliary tract. Overall, 90% of a given dose is excreted within 24 hours.

Contraindications and precautions
Molindone is contraindicated in patients with known hypersensitivity to molindone and in patients with disorders accompanied by coma, CNS depression, brain damage, circulatory collapse, or cerebrovascular disease because of additive CNS depression and adverse effects on blood pressure. Use molindone cautiously in patients with cardiac disease (arrhythmias, CHF, angina pectoris, valvular disease, or heart block); Reye's syndrome; encephalitits, head injury, or related conditions because drug may mask signs and symptoms; in patients with respiratory disease because molindone may worsen glaucoma; in patients with prostatic hypertrophy; in patients with urine retention; in patients with hepatic or renal dysfunction; in patients with Parkinson's disease; and in patients with pheochromocytoma, because drug may cause excessive buildup of transmitters, resulting in adverse CV effects.

Molindone lowers seizure threshold and may cause seizures in patients with seizure disorders.

Patients with hypocalcemia are more likely to develop extrapyramidal reactions. Administration of molindone may influence the CNS thermoregulatory center and predispose the patient to hyperthermia or hypothermia.

In patients with hepatic or renal dysfunction, decreased metabolsim and excretion may cause the drug to accumulate in plasma.

Sulfite preservatives in oral solution could induce acute asthmatic attack in asthma patients.

Interactions
Concomitant use with sympathomimetics, including epinephrine, phenylephrine, phenylpropanolamine, and ephedrine (often found in nasal sprays), or appetite suppressants may decrease their stimulatory and pressor effects. Because of its alpha blocking potential, molindone may cause epinephrine reversal – a hypotensive response to epinephrine.

Molindone may inhibit blood pressure response to centrally acting antihypertensive drugs, such as guanethidine, guanabenz, guanadrel, clonidine, methyldopa, and reserpine. Additive effects are likely after concomitant use of molindone with CNS depressants, including alcohol, analgesics, barbiturates, narcotics, tranquilizers, and general, spinal, or epidural anesthetics, or parenteral magnesium sulfate (oversedation, respiratory depression, and hypotension); antiarrhythmic agents, including quinidine, disopyramide, or procainamide (increased incidence of cardiac arrhythmias and conduction defects); atropine or other anticholinergic drugs, including antidepressants, MAO inhibitors, phenothiazines, antihistamines, meperidine, and antiparkinsonian agents (oversedation, paralytic ileus, visual changes, and severe constipation); nitrates (hypotension); and metrizamide (increased risk of seizures).

Beta blocking agents may inhibit molindone metabolism, increasing plasma levels and toxicity.

Concomitant use with propylthiouracil increases risk of agranulocytosis; concomitant use with lithium may result in severe neurologic toxicity with an encephalitis-like syndrome and a decreased therapeutic response to molindone.

Decreased therapeutic response to molindone may follow concomitant use with calcium-containing drugs, such as phenytoin and tetracyclines, aluminum- and magnesium-containing antacids, or antidiarrheals (decreased absorption); or caffeine (increased metabolism).

Molindone may antagonize therapeutic effect of bromocriptine on prolactin secretion; it may also decrease the vasoconstricting effects of high-dose dopamine and may decrease effectiveness and increase toxicity of levodopa (by dopamine blockade). Calcium sulfate in molindone tablets may inhibit the absorption of phenytoin or tetracyclines.

Effects on diagnostic tests
Molindone causes false-positive results in urine pregnancy tests using human chorionic gonadotropin and additive potential for causing seizures with metrizamide myelography.

Molindone elevates levels of liver enzymes (AST [SGOT] and ALT [SGPT]), free fatty acids, and BUN; drug may alter white blood cell (WBC) counts and may increase or decrease serum glucose levels.

Adverse reactions
- CNS: extrapyramidal symptoms – dystonia, akathisia, torticollis, tardive dyskinesia, sedation (high incidence), pseudoparkinsonism, drowsiness (frequent), *neuroleptic malignant syndrome* (fatal *respiratory failure* in over 10% of patients if untreated), dizziness, headache,

insomnia (early awakening), exacerbation of psychotic symptoms.

• CV: *asystole*, orthostatic hypotension, tachycardia, dizziness/fainting, arrhythmias, ECG changes, increased anginal pain after I.M. injection.

• EENT: blurred vision, tinnitus, mydriasis, increased intraocular pressure, ocular changes (retinal pigmentary change with long-term use).

• GI: dry mouth, constipation, nausea, vomiting, anorexia, diarrhea.

• GU: urine retention, gynecomastia, hypermenorrhea, inhibited ejaculation.

• HEMA: transient leukopenia, *agranulocytosis*, thrombocytopenia, anemia (within 30 to 90 days).

• Hepatic: cholestatic jaundice in 2% to 4% of patients (within 30 days).

• Local: contact dermatitis from concentrate or injectable form, muscle necrosis from I.M. injection.

• Other: hyperprolactinemia, photosensitivity, increased appetite or weight gain, neuroleptic malignant syndrome, hypersensitivity (rash, urticaria, drug fever, edema, cholestatic jaundice [in 2% to 4% of patients within first 30 days]).

Note: Drug should be discontinued if hypersensitivity, jaundice, agranulocytosis, or neuroleptic malignant syndrome (marked hyperthermia, extrapyramidal effects, autonomic dysfunction) occurs; if WBC count falls below 4,000; or if severe extrapyramidal symptoms occur even after dosage is lowered. Drug should be discontinued 48 hours before and 24 hours after myelography using metrizamide because of the additive risk of seizures. When feasible, withdraw drug slowly and gradually; many drug effects persist after withdrawal.

Overdose and treatment

CNS depression is characterized by deep, unarousable sleep and possible coma, hypotension or hypertension, extrapyramidal symptoms, abnormal involuntary muscle movements, agitation, seizures, arrhythmias, ECG changes, hypothermia or hyperthermia, and autonomic nervous system dysfunction.

Treatment is symptomatic and supportive, including maintaining vital signs, airway, stable body temperature, and fluid and electrolyte balance.

Do not induce vomiting: drug inhibits cough reflex and aspiration may occur. Use gastric lavage, then activated charcoal and saline cathartics; dialysis does not help. Regulate body temperature as needed. Treat hypotension with I.V. fluids; *do not give epinephrine.* Treat seizures with parenteral diazepam or barbiturates; arrhythmias, with parenteral phenytoin (1 mg/kg with rate titrated to blood pressure); extrapyramidal reactions, with barbiturates, benztropine, or parenteral diphenhydramine at 2 mg/kg/minute.

▶ **Special considerations**

• Drug may cause GI distress and should be administered with food or fluids.

• Dilute concentrate in 2 to 4 oz of liquid, preferably soup, water, juice, carbonated drinks, milk, or puddings.

• Drug may cause pink to brown discoloration of urine.

• Protect liquid forms from light.

• A dose of 10 mg is the therapeutic equivalent of 100 mg of chlorpromazine.

Information for the patient

• Explain the risks of dystonic reaction and tardive dyskinesia and advise patient to report abnormal body movements.

• Warn patient to avoid spilling liquid preparations on the skin; rash and irritation may result.

• Advise the patient to avoid temperature extremes (hot or cold baths, sunlamps, or tanning beds) because drug may cause thermoregulatory changes.

• Suggest sugarless chewing gum or candy, or ice chips to relieve dry mouth.

• Warn patient not to take drug with antacids or antidiarrheals; not to drink alcoholic beverages or take other drugs that cause sedation; not to stop taking the drug or take *any* other drug except as instructed; and to take drug exactly as prescribed, without doubling after missing a dose.

• Warn patient about sedative effect. Tell patient to report difficult urination, sore throat, dizziness, or fainting.

Geriatric use

Lower doses are recommended; 30% to 50% of usual dose may be effective. Elderly patients are at greater risk for tardive dyskinesia and other extrapyramidal effects.

Pediatric use

Drug is not recommended for children under age 12.

perphenazine
Apo-Perphenazine∗, Phenazine∗, Trilafon

- Pharmacologic classification: phenothiazine (piperazine derivative)
- Therapeutic classification: antipsychotic
- Pregnancy risk category C

How supplied
Available by prescription only
Tablets: 2 mg, 4 mg, 8 mg, 16 mg
Repetabs (sustained-release): 8 mg
Oral concentrate: 16 mg/5ml
Injection: 5 mg/ml

Indications, route, and dosage
Psychosis
Adults: Initially, 8 to 16 mg P.O. b.i.d., t.i.d., or q.i.d., increasing to 64 mg daily.
Children over age 12: 6 to 12 mg P.O. daily in divided doses.
Mental disturbances, acute alcoholism
Adults and children over age 12: 5 to 10 mg I.M. p.r.n. Maximum dosage is 15 mg daily in ambulatory patients, 30 mg daily in hospitalized patients.

Perphenazine may be given slowly by I.V. drip at a rate of 1 mg/2 minutes with continuous blood pressure monitoring (rarely used). Extended-release preparation may be given 8 to 16 mg P.O. b.i.d. for outpatients; 8 to 32 mg P.O. b.i.d. for inpatients.

Pharmacodynamics
Antipsychotic action: Perphenazine is thought to exert its antipsychotic effects by postsynaptic blockade of CNS dopamine receptors, thus inhibiting dopamine-mediated effects; antiemetic effects are attributed to dopamine receptor blockade in the medullary chemoreceptor trigger zone. Perphenazine has many other central and peripheral effects: it produces both alpha and ganglionic blockade and counteracts histamine- and serotonin-mediated activity. Its most serious adverse reactions are extrapyramidal.

Pharmacokinetics
- *Absorption:* Rate and extent of absorption vary with administration route: oral tablet absorption is erratic and variable, with onset of action ranging from ½ to 1 hour; oral concentrate absorption is much more predictable. I.M. drug is absorbed rapidly.

- *Distribution:* Perphenazine is distributed widely into the body, including breast milk. Drug is 91% to 99% protein-bound. After oral tablet administration, peak effect occurs at 2 to 4 hours; steady-state serum levels are achieved within 4 to 7 days.
- *Metabolism:* Perphenazine is metabolized extensively by the liver but no active metabolites are formed.
- *Excretion:* Most of drug is excreted in urine via the kidneys; some is excreted in feces via the biliary tract.

Contraindications and precautions
Perphenazine is contraindicated in patients with known hypersensitivity to phenothiazines and related compounds, including allergic reactions involving hepatic function because perphenazine may be hepatotoxic; in patients with blood dyscrasias and bone marrow depression because drug may have adverse effects on bone marrow and blood cell lines; in disorders accompanied by coma, brain damage, or CNS depression because of additive CNS and respiratory depression; in patients with circulatory collapse or cerebrovascular disease because drug may adversely affect blood pressure through its alpha blocking effects; and with adrenergic blocking agents or spinal or epidural anesthetics because of the potential for alpha blockade.

Perphenazine should be used cautiously in patients with cardiac disease (arrhythmias, CHF, angina pectoris, valvular disease, or heart block); encephalitis; Reye's syndrome; head injury; respiratory disease; seizure disorders (drug may lower seizure threshold); glaucoma (drug may raise intraocular pressure); prostatic hypertrophy, Parkinson's disease, urine retention (drug may worsen these conditions); hepatic or renal dysfunction (impaired metabolism and excretion may cause drug accumulation); pheochromocytoma; or hypocalcemia (increased risk of extrapyramidal reactions). Exposure to temperature extremes may predispose the patient to hyperthermia or hypothermia.

Interactions
Concomitant use of perphenazine with sympathomimetics, including epinephrine, phenylephrine, phenylpropanolamine, and ephedrine (often found in nasal sprays), and with appetite suppressants may decrease their stimulatory and pressor effects. Phenothiazines can cause epinephrine reversal and a hypotensive response when epinephrine is used for its pressor effects.

Perphenazine may inhibit blood pressure response to centrally acting antihypertensive drugs, such as guanethidine, guanabenz, guanadrel, clonidine, methyldopa, and reserpine. Additive effects are likely after concomitant use of perphenazine with CNS depressants, including alcohol, analgesics, barbiturates, narcotics, tranquilizers, and general, spinal, or epidural anesthetics, or parenteral magnesium sulfate (oversedation, respiratory depression, and hypotension); antiarrhythmic agents, including quinidine, disopyramide, and procainamide (increased incidence of cardiac arrhythmias and conduction defects); atropine or other anticholinergic drugs, including antidepressants, MAO inhibitors, phenothiazines, antihistamines, meperidine, and antiparkinsonian agents (oversedation, paralytic ileus, visual changes, and severe constipation); nitrates (hypotension); and metrizamide (increased risk of seizures).

Beta blocking agents may inhibit perphenazine metabolism, increasing plasma levels and toxicity.

Concomitant use with propylthiouracil increases risk of agranulocytosis; concomitant use with lithium may result in severe neurologic toxicity with an encephalitis-like syndrome and a decreased therapeutic response to perphenazine.

Pharmacokinetic alterations and subsequent decreased therapeutic response to perphenazine may follow concomitant use with phenobarbital (enhanced renal excretion), aluminum and magnesium-containing antacids and antidiarrheals (decreased absorption), caffeine, or heavy smoking (increased metabolism).

Perphenazine may antagonize therapeutic effect of bromocriptine on prolactin secretion; it may also decrease vasoconstricting effects of high-dose dopamine and may decrease effectiveness and increase toxicity of levodopa (by dopamine blockade). Perphenazine may inhibit metabolism and increase toxicity of phenytoin.

Effects on diagnostic tests

Perphenazine causes false-positive test results for urinary porphyrins, urobilinogen, amylase, and 5-hydroxyindoleacetic acid because of darkening of urine by metabolites; it also causes false-positive urine pregnancy test results using human chorionic gonadotropin.

Perphenazine elevates test results for liver enzymes and protein-bound iodine and causes quinidine-like effects on the ECG.

Adverse reactions

● CNS: extrapyramidal symptoms—dystonia, akathisia, torticollis, tardive dyskinesia, sedation (low incidence), pseudoparkinsonism, drowsiness (frequent), *neuroleptic malignant syndrome* (fatal *respiratory failure* in over 10% of patients if untreated), dizziness, fainting, headache, insomnia, exacerbation of psychotic symptoms, decreased libido.
● CV: *asystole*, orthostatic hypotension, tachycardia, arrhythmias, ECG changes, increased anginal pain after I.M. injection.
● EENT: blurred vision, tinnitus, mydriasis, increased intraocular pressure, ocular changes (retinal pigmentary change on long-term use).
● GI: dry mouth, constipation, nausea, vomiting, anorexia, diarrhea.
● GU: urine retention, gynecomastia, hypermenorrhea, inhibited ejaculation.
● HEMA: transient leukopenia, *agranulocytosis,* thrombocytopenia, anemia (within 30 to 90 days).
● Local: contact dermatitis from concentrate or injectable form, muscle necrosis from I.M. injection.
● Other: hyperprolactinemia, photosensitivity, increased appetite or weight gain, hypersensitivity (rash, urticaria, drug fever, edema, cholestatic jaundice [in 2% to 4% of patients within first 30 days]).

After abrupt withdrawal of long-term therapy, gastritis, nausea, vomiting, dizziness, tremor, feeling of heat or cold, sweating, tachycardia, headache, or insomnia may occur.

Note: Drug should be discontinued if hypersensitivity, jaundice, agranulocytosis, or neuroleptic malignant syndrome (marked hyperthermia, extrapyramidal effects, autonomic dysfunction) occurs or if severe extrapyramidal symptoms occur even after dose is lowered. Drug should be discontinued 48 hours before and 24 hours after myelography using metrizamide because of the risk of seizures. When feasible, drug should be withdrawn slowly and gradually; many drug effects persist after withdrawal.

Overdose and treatment

CNS depression is characterized by deep, unarousable sleep and possible coma, hypotension or hypertension, extrapyramidal symptoms, dystonia, abnormal involuntary muscle movements, agitation, seizures, arrhythmias, ECG changes, hypothermia or hyperthermia, and autonomic nervous system dysfunction.

Treatment is symptomatic and supportive, including maintaining vital signs, airway, stable body temperature, and fluid and electrolyte balance.

Do not induce vomiting: drug inhibits cough

reflex and aspiration may occur. Use gastric lavage, then activated charcoal and saline cathartics; dialysis is usually ineffective. Regulate body temperature as needed. Treat hypotension with I.V. fluids; *do not give epinephrine.* Treat seizures with parenteral diazepam or barbiturates; arrhythmias with parenteral phenytoin (1 mg/kg with rate titrated to blood pressure); and extrapyramidal reactions with barbiturates, benztropine, or parenteral diphenhydramine 2 mg/kg/minute.

▶ **Special considerations**
Besides those relevant to all *phenothiazines,* consider the following recommendations.
● Oral formulations may cause stomach upset; administer with food or fluid.
● Dilute the concentrate in 2 to 4 oz of liquid (water, carbonated drinks, fruit juice, tomato juice, milk, or puddings). Dilute every 5 ml of concentrate with 60 ml of suitable fluid.
● Liquid formulation may cause rash upon contact with skin.
● I.M. injection may cause skin necrosis; avoid extravasation.
● Administer I.M. injection deep into upper outer quadrant of buttocks. Massaging the injection site may prevent formation of abscesses.
● Do not administer drug for injection if it is excessively discolored or contains precipitate.
● Monitor blood pressure before and after parenteral administration.
● Shake oral concentrate before administration.
● A dose of 10 mg is the therapeutic equivalent of 100 mg of chlorpromazine.

Information for the patient
● Explain the risks of dystonic reactions and tardive dyskinesia and tell patient to report abnormal body movements.
● Tell patient to avoid sun exposure and to use a sunscreen when going outdoors, to prevent photosensitivity reactions. (Note that using heat lamps and tanning beds may cause burning of the skin or skin discoloration.)
● Tell patient to avoid spilling the liquid; contact with skin may cause rash and irritation.
● Warn patient not to take extremely hot or cold baths and to avoid exposure to temperature extremes, sun lamp, or tanning beds; the drug may cause thermoregulatory changes.
● Advise patient to take drug exactly as prescribed and not to double doses for missed doses.
● Tell patient that interactions with many other drugs are possible. Advise patient to seek medical approval before taking any self-prescribed medication.
● Tell patient not to stop taking the drug suddenly; any adverse reactions may be alleviated by a dosage reduction. Patient should promptly report difficulty urinating, sore throat, dizziness, or fainting.
● Tell patient to avoid hazardous activities that require alertness until the drug's effect is established. Reassure patient that sedative effects of the drug should become tolerable in several weeks.
● Tell patient not to drink alcohol or take other medications that may cause excessive sedation.
● Explain which fluids are appropriate for diluting the concentrate (not apple juice or caffeine-containing drinks); explain dropper technique of measuring dose.
● Suggest sugarless hard candy or chewing gum, or ice chips to relieve dry mouth.
● Tell patient not to crush or chew sustained-release form.

Geriatric use
Elderly patients tend to require lower doses. Dose must be titrated to effects; 30% to 50% of the usual dose may be effective. Elderly patients are at greater risk for adverse reactions, especially tardive dyskinesia and other extrapyramidal effects.

Pediatric use
Drug is not recommended for children under age 12.

Breast-feeding
Perphenazine may enter breast milk. Use with caution. Potential benefits to the mother should outweigh the potential harm to the infant.

---

pimozide
Orap

● Pharmacologic classification: diphenylbutylpiperidine
● Therapeutic classification: antipsychotic
● Pregnancy risk category C

How supplied
Available by prescription only
Tablets: 2 mg

Indications, route, and dosage
Suppression of severe motor and phonic tics in patients with Gilles de la Tourette's syndrome
Adults and children over age 12: Initially, 1 to 2 mg/day in divided doses. Then, increase dosage as needed every other day.
Maintenance dose: From 7 to 16 mg/day. Maximum dosage is 20 mg/day.

Pharmacodynamics
Antipsychotic action: Pimozide's mechanism of action in Gilles de la Tourette's syndrome is unknown: it is thought to exert its effects by postsynaptic and/or presynaptic blockade of CNS dopamine receptors, thus inhibiting dopamine-mediated effects. Pimozide also has anticholinergic, antiemetic, and anxiolytic effects and produces alpha blockade.

Pharmacokinetics
• *Absorption:* Pimozide is absorbed slowly and incompletely from the GI tract; bioavailability is about 50%. Peak plasma levels may occur from 4 to 12 hours (usually in 6 to 8 hours).
• *Distribution:* Pimozide is distributed widely into the body.
• *Metabolism:* Pimozide is metabolized by the liver; a significant first-pass effect exists.
• *Excretion:* About 40% of a given dose is excreted in urine as parent drug and metabolites in 3 to 4 days; about 15% is excreted in feces via the biliary tract within 3 to 6 days.

Contraindications and precautions
Pimozide is contraindicated in patients with known hypersensitivity to phenothiazines, thioxanthenes, haloperidol, and molindone; in patients with any form of mild or severe tic, including those induced by pemoline, methylphenidate, or amphetamines; in patients with arrhythmias because drug may cause ventricular arrhythmias or aggravate existing arrhythmias; in patients with congenital long QT syndrome because drug may cause conduction defects and sudden death; and in comatose states and CNS depression because of the risk of additive effects.

Pimozide should be used with extreme caution in patients taking antiarrhythmic drugs, tricyclic antidepressants, or other antipsychotic agents because additive effect may further depress cardiac conduction and prolong QT interval and may induce arrhythmias. Use pimozide cautiously in patients with other cardiac disease (CHF, angina pectoris, valvular disease, or heart block), encephalitis, Reye's syndrome, hematologic disorders, seizure disorders, glaucoma, prostatic hypertrophy, urine retention, hepatic or renal dysfunction, and Parkinson's disease because drug may worsen these conditions.

Interactions
Concomitant use of pimozide with quinidine, procainamide, disopyramide and other antiarrhythmics, phenothiazines, other antipsychotics, and antidepressants may further depress cardiac conduction and prolong QT interval, resulting in serious arrhythmias.

Concomitant use with anticonvulsants (phenytoin, carbamazepine, or phenobarbital) may induce seizures, even in patients previously stabilized on anticonvulsants; an anticonvulsant dosage increase may be required.

Concomitant use with amphetamines, methylphenidate, or pemoline may induce Tourette-like tic and may exacerbate existing tics.

Concomitant use with CNS depressants, including alcohol, analgesics, barbiturates, narcotics, anxiolytics, parenteral magnesium sulfate, tranquilizers, and general, spinal, or epidural anesthetics may cause oversedation and respiratory depression because of additive CNS depressant effects.

Effects on diagnostic tests
Pimozide causes quinidine-like ECG effects (including prolongation of QT interval and flattened T waves).

Adverse reactions
• CNS: parkinsonian symptoms, other extrapyramidal symptoms (dystonia, akathisia, hyperreflexia, opisthotonos, oculogyric crisis), tardive dyskinesia, sedation, headache, *neuroleptic malignant syndrome* (fatal *respiratory failure* in over 10% of patients if untreated), *hyperpyrexia. Seizures and sudden death* have occurred with doses above 20 mg/day.
• CV: *ventricular arrhythmias* (rare), ECG changes (prolonged QT interval, hypotension).
• EENT: visual disturbances, photophobia.
• GI: dry mouth, constipation, nausea, vomiting, taste changes.
• GU: impotence.
• Other: muscle tightness.

Note: Drug should be discontinued immediately if hypersensitivity or neuroleptic malignant syndrome (marked hyperthermia, extrapyramidal effects, autonomic dysfunction) occurs; if severe extrapyramidal symptoms occur even after dose is lowered; if ventricular arrhythmias occur; or if QT interval is prolonged

---

*Canada only   †Unlabeled clinical use   Italicized adverse reactions are life-threatening.

as follows: beyond 0.52 second in adults, beyond 0.47 second in children, or over 25% of patient's original baseline.

When feasible, drug should be withdrawn slowly and gradually; many drug effects persist after withdrawal.

Overdose and treatment
Clinical signs of overdose include severe extrapyramidal reactions, hypotension, respiratory depression, coma, and ECG abnormalities, including prolongation of QT interval, inversion or flattening of T waves, and/or new appearance of U waves.

Treat with gastric lavage to remove unabsorbed drug. Maintain blood pressure with I.V. fluids, plasma expanders, or norepinephrine. *Do not use epinephrine.*

Do not induce vomiting because of the potential for aspiration.

Treat extrapyramidal symptoms with parenteral diphenhydramine. Monitor for adverse reactions for at least 4 days because of prolonged half-life (55 hours) of drug.

▶ **Special considerations**
● Elderly patients may be at greater risk for adverse CV effects.
● All patients should have have baseline ECGs before therapy begins and periodic ECGs thereafter to monitor CV effects.
● Patient's serum potassium level should be maintained within normal range at all times; decreased potassium concentrations increase risk of arrhythmias. Monitor potassium level in patients with diarrhea and those who are taking diuretics.
● Extrapyramidal reactions develop in approximately 10% to 15% of patients at normal doses. They are especially likely to occur during early days of therapy.
● If excessive restlessness and agitation occur, therapy with a beta blocker, such as propranolol or metoprolol, may be helpful.
● A dose of 0.5 mg is the therapeutic equivalent of 100 mg of chlorpromazine.

Information for the patient
● Inform patient of the risks, signs, and symptoms of dystonic reactions and tardive dyskinesia.
● Advise patient to take pimozide exactly as prescribed, not to double doses for missed doses, not to share drug with others, and not to stop taking it suddenly.
● Explain that pimozide's therapeutic effect may not be apparent for several weeks.

● Urge patient to promptly report unusual effects, such as fever and abnormal muscle movement.
● Tell patient not to take pimozide with alcohol, sleeping medications, or any other drugs that may cause drowsiness without medical approval.
● Suggest using sugarless hard candy or chewing gum to relieve dry mouth.
● To prevent dizziness at start of therapy, patient should lie down for 30 minutes after taking each dose and should avoid sudden changes in posture, especially when rising to upright position.
● To minimize daytime sedation, suggest taking entire daily dose at bedtime.
● Warn patient to avoid hazardous activities that require alertness until the drug's effects are known.

Geriatric use
Elderly patients are more likely to develop cardiac toxicity and tardive dyskinesia even at normal doses.

Pediatric use
Use and efficacy in children under age 12 are limited. Dosage should be kept at the lowest possible level. Use of the drug in children for any disorder other than Gilles de la Tourette's syndrome is not recommended.

---

prochlorperazine
Compazine, Stemetil∗

prochlorperazine edisylate
Compazine

prochlorperazine maleate
Compazine, Compazine Spansule, Stemetil∗

● Pharmacologic classification: phenothiazine (piperazine derivative)
● Therapeutic classification: antipsychotic, anxiolytic
● Pregnancy risk category C

How supplied
Available by prescription only
prochlorperazine maleate
Tablets: 5 mg, 10 mg, 25 mg
prochlorperazine edisylate
Spansules (sustained-release): 10 mg, 15 mg, 30 mg

Syrup: 1 mg/ml
Injection: 5 mg/ml
Suppositories: 2.5 mg, 5 mg, 25 mg

Indications, route, and dosage
Nonpsychotic anxiety
Adults: 5 mg P.O. t.i.d. or q.i.d. or 10 mg sustained-release capsule P.O. b.i.d. Some patients respond well to 15 mg sustained-release capsule once daily in the morning.
Psychotic disorders
Adults: For mild conditions, 5 to 10 mg P.O. t.i.d. or q.i.d. In moderate to severe conditions, usual starting dosage is 10 mg P.O. t.i.d. or q.i.d. Increase dosage gradually (every 2 or 3 days). Some patients respond to 50 to 75 mg daily. In severe disturbances, optimum dosage is 100 to 150 mg daily in divided doses. For severely agitated patients requiring immediate control, give 10 to 20 mg I.M. deeply into the upper outer quadrant of the buttock. Repeat as needed q 1 to 4 hours; substitute oral dosage as soon as feasible.
Children ages 2 to 12: 2.5 mg P.O. or rectally b.i.d. or t.i.d., not to exceed 10 mg on the first day. Increase dosage based on age and response. For ages 2 to 5 years, total daily dosage usually does not exceed 20 mg. For ages 6 to 12 years, total daily dosage usually does not exceed 25 mg.

Pharmacodynamics
• *Antipsychotic action:* Prochlorperazine is thought to exert its antipsychotic effects by postsynaptic blockade of CNS dopamine receptors, thus inhibiting dopamine-mediated effects.
  Prochlorperazine has many other central and peripheral effects: it produces alpha and ganglionic blockade and counteracts histamine- and serotonin-mediated activity. Its most prevalent adverse reactions are extrapyramidal. It is used primarily as an antiemetic; it is ineffective against motion sickness.

Pharmacokinetics
• *Absorption:* Rate and extent of absorption vary with administration route: oral tablet absorption is erratic and variable, with onset of action ranging from ½ to 1 hour; oral concentrate absorption is more predictable. I.M. drug is absorbed rapidly.
• *Distribution:* Prochlorperazine is distributed widely into the body, including breast milk. Drug is 91% to 99% protein-bound. Peak effect occurs at 2 to 4 hours; steady-state serum levels are achieved within 4 to 7 days.
• *Metabolism:* Prochlorperazine is metabolized

extensively by the liver, but no active metabolites are formed; duration of action is about 4 to 6 hours.
• *Excretion:* Most of drug is excreted in urine via the kidneys; some is excreted in feces via the biliary tract.

Contraindications and precautions
Prochlorperazine is contraindicated in patients with known hypersensitivity to phenothiazines and related compounds, including allergic reactions involving hepatic function; in patients with blood dyscrasias and bone marrow depression; and in patients with disorders accompanied by coma, brain damage, CNS depression, circulatory collapse, or cerebrovascular disease, because of adverse effects on blood pressure and possible additive CNS depression. It also is contraindicated for use with adrenergic blocking agents or spinal or epidural anesthetics.
  Prochlorperazine should be used cautiously in patients with cardiac disease (arrhythmias, CHF, angina pectoris, valvular disease, or heart block) because of additive arrhythmic effects; encephalitis; Reye's syndrome, head injury, or respiratory disease because of additive CNS and respiratory depression; seizure disorders because of lowered seizure threshold; glaucoma because of increased intraocular pressure; prostatic hypertrophy; urine retention; hepatic or renal dysfunction; Parkinson's disease; pheochromocytoma because excessive buildup of neurotransmitters may have adverse CV effects; and hypocalcemia, which increases the risk of extrapyramidal symptoms.

Interactions
Concomitant use of prochlorperazine with sympathomimetics, including epinephrine, phenylephrine, phenylpropanolamine, and ephedrine (often found in nasal sprays), and with appetite suppressants may decrease their stimulatory and pressor effects and may cause epinephrine reversal (hypotensive response to epinephrine).
  Prochlorperazine may inhibit blood pressure response to centrally acting antihypertensive drugs, such as guanethidine, guanabenz, guanadrel, clonidine, methyldopa, and reserpine. Additive effects are likely after concomitant use of prochlorperazine with CNS depressants, including alcohol, analgesics, barbiturates, narcotics, tranquilizers, and anesthetics (general, spinal, or epidural), and parenteral magnesium sulfate (oversedation, respiratory depression, and hypotension); antiarrhythmic agents, including quinidine, disopyramide, and procain-

amide (increased incidence of cardiac arrhythmias and conduction defects); atropine and other anticholinergic drugs, including antidepressants, MAO inhibitors, phenothiazines, antihistamines, meperidine, and antiparkinsonian agents (oversedation, paralytic ileus, visual changes, and severe constipation); nitrates (hypotension); and metrizamide (increased risk of seizures).

Beta blocking agents may inhibit prochlorperazine metabolism, increasing plasma levels and toxicity.

Concomitant use with propylthiouracil increases risk of agranulocytosis; concomitant use with lithium may result in severe neurologic toxicity with an encephalitis-like syndrome and in decreased therapeutic response to prochlorperazine.

Pharmacokinetic alterations and subsequent decreased therapeutic response to prochlorperazine may follow concomitant use with phenobarbital (enhanced renal excretion); aluminum- and magnesium-containing antacids and antidiarrheals (decreased absorption); caffeine; or heavy smoking (increased metabolism).

Prochlorperazine may antagonize therapeutic effect of bromocriptine on prolactin secretion; it also may decrease the vasoconstricting effects of high-dose dopamine and may decrease effectiveness and increase toxicity of levodopa (by dopamine blockade). Prochlorperazine may inhibit metabolism and increase toxicity of phenytoin.

Effects on diagnostic tests

Prochlorperazine causes false-positive test results for urinary porphyrins, urobilinogen, amylase, and 5-hydroxyindoleacetic acid because of darkening of urine by metabolites; it also causes false-positive urine pregnancy results in tests using human chorionic gonadotropin as the indicator.

Prochlorperazine elevates test results for liver enzymes and protein-bound iodine and causes quinidine-like ECG effects.

Adverse reactions

● CNS: extrapyramidal symptoms – dystonia, akathisia, torticollis, tardive dyskinesia, pseudoparkinsonism, *neuroleptic malignant syndrome* (fatal *respiratory failure* in over 10% of patients if untreated), dizziness, drowsiness, sedation, headache, exacerbation of psychotic symptoms.
● CV: *asystole*, orthostatic hypotension, tachycardia, dizziness or fainting, arrhythmias, ECG changes, increased anginal pain after I.M. injection.
● EENT: blurred vision, tinnitus, mydriasis, increased intraocular pressure, ocular changes (retinal pigmentary change with long-term use).
● GI: dry mouth, constipation, nausea, vomiting, anorexia, diarrhea.
● GU: urine retention, gynecomastia, hypermenorrhea, inhibited ejaculation.
● HEMA: transient leukopenia, *agranulocytosis,* thrombocytopenia, anemia (within 30 to 90 days).
● Local: contact dermatitis from concentrate or injectable form, muscle necrosis from I.M. injection.
● Other: hyperprolactinemia, photosensitivity, increased appetite (weight gain), hypersensitivity (rash, urticaria, drug fever, edema, cholestatic jaundice [in 2% to 4% of patients within first 30 days]).

After abrupt withdrawal of long-term therapy, gastritis, nausea, vomiting, dizziness, tremor, feeling of heat or cold, sweating, tachycardia, headache, or insomnia may occur.

Note: Drug should be discontinued if hypersensitivity, jaundice, agranulocytosis, or neuroleptic malignant syndrome (marked hyperthermia, extrapyramidal effects, autonomic dysfunction) occur or if severe extrapyramidal symptoms occur even after dose is lowered. Drug should be discontinued 48 hours before and 24 hours after myelography using metrizamide because of the risk of seizures. When feasible, drug should be withdrawn slowly and gradually; many drug effects persist after withdrawal.

Overdose and treatment

CNS depression is characterized by deep, unarousable sleep and possible coma, hypotension or hypertension, extrapyramidal symptoms, dystonia, abnormal involuntary muscle movements, agitation, seizures, arrhythmias, ECG changes, hypothermia or hyperthermia, and autonomic nervous system dysfunction.

Treatment is symptomatic and supportive and includes maintaining vital signs, airway, stable body temperature, and fluid and electrolyte balance.

Do not induce vomiting: drug inhibits cough reflex and aspiration may occur. Use gastric lavage and then activated charcoal and saline cathartics; dialysis does not help. Regulate body temperature as needed. Treat hypotension with I.V. fluids; *do not give epinephrine.* Treat seizures with parenteral diazepam or barbiturates; arrhythmias with parenteral phenytoin (1 mg/

---

kg with rate titrated to blood pressure); and extrapyramidal reactions with barbiturates, benztropine, or parenteral diphenhydramine 2 mg/kg/minute.

▶ **Special considerations**
Besides those relevant to all *phenothiazines*, consider the following recommendations.
● The liquid and injectable formulations may cause a rash after contact with skin.
● Drug may cause a pink to brown discoloration of urine.
● Prochlorperazine is associated with a high incidence of extrapyramidal effects and in institutionalized mental patients, photosensitivity reactions; patient should avoid exposure to sunlight or heat lamps.
● Oral formulations may cause stomach upset. Administer with food or fluid.
● Dilute the concentrate in 2 to 4 oz of water. The suppository form should be stored in a cool place.
● Give I.V. dose slowly (5 mg/minute). I.M. injection may cause skin necrosis; take care to prevent extravasation. Do not administer subcutaneously.
● Administer I.M. injection deep into the upper outer quadrant of the buttock. Massaging the area after administration may prevent formation of abscesses.
● Solution for injection may be slightly discolored. Do not use if excessively discolored or if a precipitate is evident. Contact pharmacist.
● Monitor patient's blood pressure before and after parenteral administration.
● The sustained-release form should not be given to children.
● Prochlorperazine is ineffective in treating motion sickness.
● Chewing gum, hard candy, or ice chips may help relieve dry mouth.
● Protect the liquid formulation from light.

Information for the patient
● Explain the risks of dystonic reactions and tardive dyskinesia. Tell patient to report abnormal body movements promptly.
● Tell patient to avoid sun exposure and to use a sunscreen when going outdoors, to prevent photosensitivity reactions. (Note that heat lamps and tanning beds also may cause burning of the skin or skin discoloration.)
● Tell patient to avoid spilling the liquid form. Contact with skin may cause rash and irritation.
● Warn patient to avoid extremely hot or cold baths and exposure to temperature extremes, sunlamps, or tanning beds; drug may cause thermoregulatory changes.
● Advise patient to take the drug exactly as prescribed, not to double doses after missing one, and not to share drug with others.
● Tell patient not to drink alcohol or take other medications that may cause excessive sedation.
● Tell patient to dilute the concentrate in water; explain the dropper technique of measuring dose; teach correct use of suppository.
● Tell patient that sugarless hard candy or chewing gum, or ice chips can alleviate dry mouth.
● Urge patient to store this drug safely away from children.
● Tell patient that interactions are possible with many drugs. Warn him to seek medical approval before taking *any* self-prescribed medication.
● Warn patient not to stop taking the drug suddenly and to promptly report persistent fever, difficulty urinating, sore throat, dizziness, or fainting. Reassure patient that most reactions can be relieved by reducing dose.
● Warn patient to avoid hazardous activities that require alertness until the drug's effect is established. Reassure patient that sedative effects subside and become tolerable in several weeks.

Geriatric use
Elderly patients tend to require lower doses, titrated to individual effects. These patients are at greater risk for adverse reactions, especially tardive dyskinesia, other extrapyramidal effects, and hypotension.

Pediatric use
Prochlorperazine is not recommended for patients under age 2 or weighing less than 9 kg.

Breast-feeding
Prochlorperazine may enter breast milk and should be used with caution. Potential benefits to the mother should outweigh potential harm to the infant.

promazine hydrochloride
Prozine-50, Sparine

- Pharmacologic classification: phenothiazine (aliphatic derivative)
- Therapeutic classification: antipsychotic
- Pregnancy risk category C

How supplied
Available by prescription only
Tablets: 25 mg, 50 mg, 100 mg
Syrup: 10 mg/5 ml
Injection: 25 mg, 50 mg/ml

Indications, route, and dosage
Psychosis
Adults: 10 to 200 mg P.O. or I.M. q 4 to 6 hours, up to 1 g daily; in acutely agitated patients, the initial I.M. or I.V. dose is 50 to 150 mg. Dose may be repeated within 5 to 10 minutes if necessary. Give I.V. dose in concentrations no greater than 25 mg/ml.
Children over age 12: 10 to 25 mg P.O. or I.M. q 4 to 6 hours.

Use of doses over 1,000 mg/day has not increased therapeutic effect.

Pharmacodynamics
Antipsychotic action: Promazine is thought to exert its antipsychotic effects by postsynaptic blockade of CNS dopamine receptors, thus inhibiting dopamine-mediated effects; antiemetic effects are attributed to dopamine receptor blockade in the medullary chemoreceptor trigger zone. Promazine has many other central and peripheral effects: it produces both alpha and ganglionic blockade and counteracts histamine- and serotonin-mediated activity. Its most prevalent adverse reactions are antimuscarinic and sedative; it causes fewer extrapyramidal effects than other drugs in this class.

Pharmacokinetics
- *Absorption:* Promazine usually is absorbed well from the GI tract. Liquid forms have the most predictable effect, whereas tablets have erratic and variable absorption. Onset of effect ranges from ½ to 1 hour. I.M. drug is absorbed rapidly.
- *Distribution:* Promazine is distributed widely into the body, including breast milk. Peak effect occurs at 2 to 4 hours; steady-state serum level is achieved within 4 to 7 days. Drug is 91% to 99% protein-bound.

- *Metabolism:* Promazine is metabolized extensively by the liver, but no active metabolites are formed.
- *Excretion:* Most of drug is excreted as metabolites in urine; some is excreted in feces via the biliary tract.

Contraindications and precautions
Promazine is contraindicated in patients with known hypersensitivity to phenothiazines and related compounds, including allergic reactions involving hepatic function; in patients with blood dyscrasias and bone marrow depression because of adverse hematologic effects; in patients with disorders accompanied by coma or CNS depression or in patients with brain damage because of additive CNS depression; in patients with circulatory collapse or cerebrovascular disease because of adverse effects on blood pressure; and in patients who are receiving adrenergic blocking agents or spinal or epidural anesthetics because of potential for excessive hypotensive response.

Promazine should be used cautiously in patients with cardiac disease (arrhythmias, CHF, angina pectoris, valvular disease, or heart block), encephalitis, Reye's syndrome, head injury, respiratory disease, seizure disorders, glaucoma, prostatic hypertrophy, urine retention, hepatic or renal dysfunction, Parkinson's disease, pheochromocytoma, or hypocalcemia. Some oral preparations of promazine contain tartrazine; dyes may cause allergic reaction in aspirin-allergic patients.

Interactions
Concomitant use of promazine with sympathomimetics, including epinephrine, phenylephrine, phenylpropanolamine, and ephedrine (often found in nasal sprays), and with appetite suppressants may decrease their stimulatory and pressor effects.

Promazine may inhibit blood pressure response to centrally acting antihypertensive drugs, such as guanethidine, guanabenz, guanadrel, clonidine, methyldopa, and reserpine. Additive effects are likely after concomitant use of promazine with CNS depressants, including alcohol, analgesics, barbiturates, narcotics, tranquilizers, anesthetics (general, spinal or epidural), and parenteral magnesium sulfate (oversedation, respiratory depression, and hypotension); antiarrhythmic agents, including quinidine, disopyramide, and procainamide (increased incidence of cardiac arrhythmias and conduction defects); atropine and other anticholinergic drugs, including antidepressants,

MAO inhibitors, phenothiazines, antihistamines, meperidine, and antiparkinsonian agents (oversedation, paralytic ileus, visual changes, and severe constipation); nitrates (hypotension); and metrizamide (increased risk of seizures).

Beta blocking agents may inhibit promazine metabolism, increasing plasma levels and toxicity.

Concomitant use with propylthiouracil increases risk of agranulocytosis; concomitant use with lithium may result in severe neurologic toxicity with an encephalitis-like syndrome and in decreased therapeutic response to promazine.

Pharmacokinetic alterations and subsequent decreased therapeutic response to promazine may follow concomitant use with phenobarbital (enhanced renal excretion); aluminum- and magnesium-containing antacids and antidiarrheals (decreased absorption); caffeine; or heavy smoking (increased metabolism).

Promazine may antagonize the therapeutic effect of bromocriptine on prolactin secretion; it also may decrease the vasoconstricting effects of high-dose dopamine and may decrease effectiveness and increase toxicity of levodopa (by dopamine blockade). Promazine may inhibit metabolism and increase toxicity of phenytoin.

Effects on diagnostic tests

Promazine causes false-positive test results for urinary porphyrins, urobilinogen, amylase, and 5-hydroxyindoleacetic acid because of darkening of urine by metabolites; it also causes false-positive urine pregnancy results in tests using human chorionic gonadotropin as the indicator.

Promazine elevates test results for liver enzymes and protein-bound iodine and causes quinidine-like effects on the ECG.

Adverse reactions

● CNS: extrapyramidal symptoms – dystonia, akathisia, torticollis, tardive dyskinesia, sedation, pseudoparkinsonism, drowsiness (frequent), *neuroleptic malignant syndrome* (fatal *respiratory failure* in over 10% of patients if untreated), dizziness, headache, insomnia, exacerbation of psychotic symptoms.
● CV: *asystole,* orthostatic hypotension, tachycardia, dizziness or fainting, arrhythmias, ECG changes, increased anginal pain after I.M. injection.
● EENT: blurred vision, tinnitus, mydriasis, increased intraocular pressure, ocular changes (retinal pigmentary change with long-term use).

● GI: dry mouth, constipation, nausea, vomiting, anorexia, diarrhea.
● GU: urine retention, gynecomastia, hypermenorrhea, inhibited ejaculation.
● HEMA: transient leukopenia, *agranulocytosis,* thrombocytopenia, anemia (within 30 to 90 days).
● Local: contact dermatitis from concentrate or injectable form, muscle necrosis from I.M. injection.
● Other: hyperprolactinemia, photosensitivity (high incidence), increased appetite or weight gain, hypersensitivity (rash, urticaria, drug fever, edema, cholestatic jaundice [in 2% to 4% of patients within first 30 days]).

After abrupt withdrawal of long-term therapy, gastritis, nausea, vomiting, dizziness, tremor, feeling of heat or cold, sweating, tachycardia, headache, or insomnia may occur.

Note: Drug should be discontinued immediately if any of the following occurs: hypersensitivity, jaundice, agranulocytosis, neuroleptic malignant syndrome (marked hyperthermia, extrapyramidal effects, autonomic dysfunction), or severe extrapyramidal symptoms even after dosage is lowered. Drug should be discontinued 48 hours before and 24 hours after myelography using metrizamide because of the risk of seizures. When feasible, drug should be withdrawn slowly and gradually; many drug effects persist after withdrawal.

Overdose and treatment

CNS depression is characterized by deep, unarousable sleep and possible coma, hypotension or hypertension, extrapyramidal symptoms, abnormal involuntary muscle movements, agitation, seizures, arrhythmias, ECG changes, hypothermia or hyperthermia, and autonomic nervous system dysfunction.

Treatment is symptomatic and supportive and includes maintaining vital signs, airway, stable body temperature, and fluid and electrolyte balance.

Do not induce vomiting: drug inhibits cough reflex and aspiration may occur. Use gastric lavage and then activated charcoal and saline cathartics; dialysis does not help. Regulate body temperature as needed. Treat hypotension with I.V. fluids; *do not give epinephrine.* Treat seizures with parenteral diazepam or barbiturates; arrhythmias with parenteral phenytoin (1 mg/kg with rate titrated to blood pressure); and extrapyramidal reactions with barbiturates, benztropine, or parenteral diphenhydramine 2 mg/kg/minute.

▶ **Special considerations**

Besides those relevant to all *phenothiazines*, consider the following recommendations.

● Liquid and injectable formulations may cause a rash after contact with skin.

● Drug may cause a pink to brown discoloration of the urine.

● Promazine is associated with a high incidence of sedation and orthostatic hypotension.

● Oral formulations may cause stomach upset. Administer with food or fluid.

● Dilute the concentrate in 2 to 4 oz of liquid, preferably water, carbonated drinks, fruit juice, tomato juice, milk, or pudding. Recommended dilution is 10 ml of liquid per 25 mg of drug.

● I.V. use is not recommended; however, if it is necessary, drug should be diluted to not more than 25 mg/ml, given slowly with special care to prevent extravasation. I.V. route should be used during surgery or for severe hiccups.

● To prevent photosensitivity reactions, patient should avoid exposure to sunlight or heat lamps.

● Administer I.M. injection deep into the upper outer quadrant of the buttock. Massaging the area after administration may prevent the formation of abscesses. I.M. injection may cause skin necrosis; take care to avoid extravasation. Monitor blood pressure before and after parenteral administration.

● Shake syrup before administration.

● Sugarless chewing gum, hard candy, or ice chips may help relieve dry mouth.

● The injection may be slightly discolored. Do not use if excessively discolored or if a precipitate is evident. Contact pharmacist.

● Protect the liquid formulation from light.

Information for the patient

● Explain the risks of dystonic reactions and tardive dyskinesia and tell patient to report abnormal body movements promptly.

● Tell patient to avoid sun exposure and to use a sunscreen when going outdoors, to prevent photosensitivity reactions. (Note that heat lamps and tanning beds also may cause burning of the skin or skin discoloration.)

● Tell patient to avoid spilling the liquid form. Contact with skin may cause rash and irritation.

● Warn patient to avoid extremely hot or cold baths or exposure to temperature extremes, sunlamps, or tanning beds; drug may cause thermoregulatory changes.

● Urge patient to take drug exactly as prescribed; not to double doses for missed doses; not to share drug with others; and not to stop taking the drug suddenly.

● Reassure patient that most adverse reactions can be alleviated by dosage reduction, but tell patient to call promptly if difficulty urinating, sore throat, dizziness, or fainting develops.

● Warn patient to avoid hazardous activities that require alertness until the drug's effect is established. Reassure patient that excessive sedative effects usually subside after several weeks.

● Tell patient to avoid alcohol and other medications that may cause excessive sedation.

● Explain which fluids are appropriate for diluting the concentrate. Explain the dropper technique of measuring dose. Tell patient to shake syrup form before administration.

● Suggest sugarless hard candy or chewing gum, or ice chips to relieve dry mouth.

● Store drug safely away from children.

● Tell patient that many drug interactions are possible. Patient should seek medical approval before taking *any* self-prescribed medication.

Geriatric use

Elderly patients tend to require lower dosages, titrated to individual response. Such patients are more likely to develop adverse reactions, especially tardive dyskinesia and other extrapyramidal effects.

Pediatric use

Promazine is not recommended for children under age 12.

Breast-feeding

Promazine enters into breast milk. Potential benefits to the mother should outweigh the potential harm to the infant.

thioridazine
Mellaril-S

thioridazine hydrochloride
Apo-Thioridazine∗, Mellaril, , Novo-Ridazine∗, PMS Thioridazine∗

● Pharmacologic classification: phenothiazine (piperidine derivative)
● Therapeutic classification: antipsychotic
● Pregnancy risk category C

How supplied
Available by prescription only
Tablets: 10 mg, 15 mg, 25 mg, 50 mg, 100 mg, 200 mg
Syrup: 10 mg/5 ml

Oral concentrate: 30 mg/ml, 100 mg/ml (3% to 4.2% alcohol)
Suspension: 25 mg/5 ml, 100 mg/5 ml

Indications, route, and dosage
Psychosis
Adults: Initially, 50 to 100 mg P.O. t.i.d., with gradual increments up to 800 mg daily in divided doses, if needed. Dosage varies.
Adults over age 65: Initial dose is 25 mg t.i.d.
Dysthymic disorder (neurotic depression), alcohol withdrawal, dementia in geriatric patients, behavioral problems in children
Adults: Initially, 25 mg P.O. t.i.d. Maintenance dosage is 20 to 200 mg daily.
Children over age 2: Usually, 1 mg/kg/day P.O. in divided doses.

Pharmacodynamics
Antipsychotic action: Thioridazine is thought to exert its antipsychotic effects by postsynaptic blockade of CNS dopamine receptors, thereby inhibiting dopamine-mediated effects.

Thioridazine has many other central and peripheral effects: it produces both alpha and ganglionic blockade and counteracts histamine- and serotonin-mediated activity. Its most prevalent adverse reactions are antimuscarinic and sedative; it causes fewer extrapyramidal effects than other antipsychotics.

Pharmacokinetics
• *Absorption:* Rate and extent of absorption vary with administration route: oral tablet absorption is erratic and variable, with onset ranging from ½ to 1 hour. Oral concentrates and syrups are much more predictable.
• *Distribution:* Thioridazine is distributed widely into the body, including breast milk. Peak effects occur at 2 to 4 hours; steady-state serum level is achieved within 4 to 7 days. Drug is 91% to 99% protein-bound.
• *Metabolism:* Thioridazine is metabolized extensively by the liver and forms the active metabolite mesoridazine; duration of action is 4 to 6 hours.
• *Excretion:* Most of drug is excreted as metabolites in urine; some is excreted in feces via the biliary tract.

Contraindications and precautions
Thioridazine is contraindicated in patients with known hypersensitivity to phenothiazines and related compounds, including allergic reactions involving hepatic function; in patients with blood dyscrasias or bone marrow depression (adverse hematologic effects); in patients with disorders accompanied by coma, brain damage, CNS depression, circulatory collapse, or cerebrovascular disease (additive CNS depression and adverse effects on blood pressure); and in patients receiving adrenergic blocking agents or spinal or epidural anesthetics (excessive respiratory, cardiac, and CNS depression).

Thioridazine should be used cautiously in patients with cardiac disease (arrhythmias, CHF, angina pectoris, valvular disease, or heart block), encephalitis, Reye's syndrome, head injury, respiratory disease, seizure disorders, glaucoma, prostatic hypertrophy, urine retention, Parkinson's disease, and pheochromocytoma because drug may exacerbate these conditions and in hypocalcemia because it increases the risk of extrapyramidal reactions.

Interactions
Concomitant use of thioridazine with sympathomimetics, including epinephrine, phenylephrine, phenylpropanolamine, and ephedrine (often found in nasal sprays), and with appetite suppressants may decrease their stimulatory and pressor effects. Thioridazine may cause epinephrine reversal.

Thioridazine may inhibit blood pressure response to centrally acting antihypertensive drugs, such as guanethidine, guanabenz, guanadrel, clonidine, methyldopa, and reserpine. Additive effects are likely after concomitant use of thioridazine with CNS depressants, including alcohol, analgesics, barbiturates, narcotics, tranquilizers, anesthetics (general, spinal, or epidural), and parenteral magnesium sulfate (oversedation, respiratory depression, and hypotension); antiarrhythmic agents, including quinidine, disopyramide, and procainamide (increased incidence of cardiac arrhythmias and conduction defects); atropine and other anticholinergic drugs, including antidepressants, MAO inhibitors, phenothiazines, antihistamines, meperidine, and antiparkinsonian agents (oversedation, paralytic ileus, visual changes, and severe constipation); nitrates (hypotension); and metrizamide (increased risk of seizures).

Beta blocking agents may inhibit thioridazine metabolism, increasing plasma levels and toxicity.

Concomitant use with propylthiouracil increases risk of agranulocytosis; concomitant use with lithium may result in severe neurologic toxicity with an encephalitis-like syndrome and in decreased therapeutic response to thioridazine.

Pharmacokinetic alterations and subsequent decreased therapeutic response to thioridazine may follow concomitant use with phenobarbital (enhanced renal excretion); aluminum- and magnesium-containing antacids and antidiarrheals (decreased absorption); caffeine; or heavy smoking (increased metabolism).

Thioridazine may antagonize therapeutic effect of bromocriptine on prolactin secretion; it also may decrease the vasoconstricting effects of high-dose dopamine and may decrease effectiveness and increase toxicity of levodopa (by dopamine blockade). Thioridazine may inhibit metabolism and increase toxicity of phenytoin.

Effects on diagnostic tests

Thioridazine causes false-positive test results for urinary porphyrins, urobilinogen, amylase, and 5-hydroxyindoleacetic acid, because of darkening of urine by metabolites; it also causes false-positive urine pregnancy results in tests using human chorionic gonadotropin as the indicator.

Thioridazine elevates test results for liver enzymes and protein-bound iodine and causes quinidine-like effects on the ECG.

Adverse reactions

● CNS: extrapyramidal symptoms – dystonia, akathisia, torticollis, tardive dyskinesia, sedation (high incidence), pseudoparkinsonism, drowsiness (frequent), *neuroleptic malignant syndrome* (fatal *respiratory failure* in over 20% of patients if untreated), dizziness, headache, insomnia, exacerbation of psychotic symptoms.
● CV: *asystole,* orthostatic hypotension (high incidence), tachycardia, dizziness or fainting, *arrhythmias,* ECG changes.
● EENT: blurred vision, tinnitus, mydriasis, increased intraocular pressure, ocular changes (retinal pigmentary change with long-term use), especially when dosage exceeds 800 mg/day).
● GI: dry mouth, constipation, nausea, vomiting, anorexia, diarrhea.
● GU: urine retention, gynecomastia, hypermenorrhea, inhibited ejaculation.
● HEMA: transient leukopenia, *agranulocytosis,* thrombocytopenia, anemia (within 30 to 90 days).
● Local: contact dermatitis from concentrate or injectable form, muscle necrosis from I.M. injection.
● Other: hyperprolactinemia, photosensitivity (high incidence), increased appetite or weight gain, hypersensitivity (rash, urticaria, drug fe-

ver, edema, cholestatic jaundice [in 2% to 4% of patients within first 30 days]).

After abrupt withdrawal of long-term therapy, gastritis, nausea, vomiting, dizziness, tremor, feeling of heat or cold, sweating, tachycardia, headache, or insomnia may occur.

Note: Drug should be discontinued if any of the following occur: hypersensitivity, jaundice, agranulocytosis, neuroleptic malignant syndrome (marked hyperthermia, extrapyramidal effects, autonomic dysfunction), or severe extrapyramidal symptoms even after dose is lowered. Drug should be discontinued 48 hours before and 24 hours after myelography using metrizamide because of the risk of seizures. When feasible, drug should be withdrawn slowly and gradually; many drug effects persist after withdrawal.

Overdose and treatment

CNS depression is characterized by deep, unarousable sleep and possible coma, hypotension or hypertension, extrapyramidal symptoms, abnormal involuntary muscle movements, agitation, seizures, arrhythmias, ECG changes, hypothermia or hyperthermia, and autonomic nervous system dysfunction.

Treatment is symptomatic and supportive and includes maintaining vital signs, airway, stable body temperature, and fluid and electrolyte balance.

Do not induce vomiting: drug inhibits cough reflex and aspiration may occur. Use gastric lavage and then activated charcoal and saline cathartics; dialysis does not help. Regulate body temperature as needed. Treat hypotension with I.V. fluids; *do not give epinephrine.* Treat seizures with parenteral diazepam or barbiturates; arrhythmias with parenteral phenytoin (1 mg/kg with rate titrated to blood pressure); and extrapyramidal reactions with barbiturates, benztropine, or parenteral diphenhydramine 2 mg/kg/minute.

▶ Special considerations

Besides those relevant to all *phenothiazines,* consider the following recommendations.
● Doses greater than 300 mg/day are usually reserved for adults with severe psychosis. Dosage should not exceed 800 mg/day.
● Liquid and injectable formulations may cause a rash if skin contact occurs.
● Drug causes pink to brown discoloration of patient's urine.
● Thioridazine is associated with a high incidence of sedation, anticholinergic effects, or-

---

thostatic hypotension, and photosensitivity reactions.

• Oral formulations may cause stomach upset. Administer with food or fluid.

• Check patient regularly for abnormal body movements (at least once every 6 months).

• Concentrate must be diluted in 2 to 4 oz of liquid, preferably water, carbonated drinks, fruit juice, tomato juice, milk, or pudding.

• Sugarless chewing gum or hard candy, or ice chips may help alleviate dry mouth.

• Protect liquid formulation from light.

• A 100-mg dose is about equivalent to 100 mg of chlorpromazine.

Information for the patient

• Explain the risks of dystonic reactions and tardive dyskinesia and tell patient to report any abnormal body movements.

• Tell patient to avoid sun exposure and to use a sunscreen when going outdoors, to prevent photosensitivity reactions. (Note that heat lamps and tanning beds also may cause burning of the skin or skin discoloration.)

• Warn patient not to spill the liquid on the skin; rash and irritation may result.

• Warn patient to avoid extremely hot or cold baths or exposure to temperature extremes, sunlamps, or tanning beds; drug may cause thermoregulatory changes.

• Advise patient to take the drug exactly as prescribed and not to double doses for missed doses.

• Explain that many drug interactions are possible. Patient should seek medical approval before taking any self-prescribed medication.

• Tell patient not to stop taking the drug suddenly; most adverse reactions may be relieved by dosage reduction. However, patient should call promptly if persistent fever, difficulty urinating, sore throat, dizziness or fainting, or any visual changes develop.

• Warn patient to avoid hazardous activities that require alertness until the drug's effect is established. Reassure patient that excessive sedation usually subsides after several weeks.

• Tell patient not to drink alcohol or take other medications that may cause excessive sedation.

• Explain which fluids are appropriate for diluting the concentrate and the dropper technique of measuring dose.

• Suggest hard candy, chewing gum, or ice chips to relieve dry mouth.

• Store drug safely away from children.

Geriatric use

Elderly patients tend to require lower dosages, titrated to individual response. Such patients also are more likely to develop adverse reactions, especially tardive dyskinesia and other extrapyramidal effects.

Pediatric use

Thioridazine is not recommended for patients under age 2. For patients over age 2, dosage is 1 mg/kg/day in divided doses.

Breast-feeding

Thioridazine may enter breast milk. Potential benefits to the mother should outweigh the potential harm to the infant.

---

thiothixene, thiothixene hydrochloride
Navane

• Pharmacologic classification: thioxanthene
• Therapeutic classification: antipsychotic
• Pregnancy risk category C

How supplied
Available by prescription only
Capsules: 1 mg, 2 mg, 5 mg, 10 mg, 20 mg
Solution: 2.5 mg/ml
Oral concentrate: 5 mg/ml (7% alcohol)
Injection: 2 mg, 5 mg/ml

Indications, route, and dosage
Acute agitation
Adults: 4 mg I.M. b.i.d. to q.i.d.; maximum dosage is 30 mg I.M. daily. Change to P.O. form as soon as possible; I.M. dosage form is irritating.
Mild to moderate psychosis
Adults: Initially, 2 mg P.O. t.i.d.; may increase gradually to 15 mg daily.
Severe psychosis
Adults: Initially, 5 mg P.O. b.i.d.; may increase gradually to 15 to 30 mg daily. Maximum recommended daily dosage is 60 mg.

Pharmacodynamics
Antipsychotic action: Thiothixene is thought to exert its antipsychotic effects by postsynaptic blockade of CNS dopamine receptors, thereby inhibiting dopamine-mediated effects.

Thiothixene has many other central and peripheral effects: it also acts as an alpha blocking agent. Its most prominent adverse reactions are extrapyramidal.

Pharmacokinetics

● *Absorption:* Absorption is rapid; I.M. onset of action is 10 to 30 minutes.

● *Distribution:* Thiothixene is distributed widely into the body. Peak effects occur at 1 to 6 hours after I.M. administration; drug is 91% to 99% protein-bound.

● *Metabolism:* Metabolism of thiothixene is minimal.

● *Excretion:* Most of drug is excreted as parent drug in feces via the biliary tract.

Contraindications and precautions

Thiothixene is contraindicated in patients with known hypersensitivity to thioxanthenes, phenothiazines, and related compounds, including that evidenced by jaundice and other allergic symptoms; in patients with blood dyscrasias and bone marrow depression (adverse hematologic effects); and in patients with disorders accompanied by coma, brain damage, CNS depression, circulatory collapse, or cerebrovascular disease (additive CNS depression and adverse effects on blood pressure).

Thiothixene should be used cautiously in patients with cardiac disease (arrhythmias, CHF, angina pectoris, valvular disease, or heart block), encephalitis, Reye's syndrome, head injury, respiratory disease, seizure disorders, glaucoma, prostatic hypertrophy, urine retention, Parkinson's disease, or pheochromocytoma because it may exacerbate these conditions; in patients with hypocalcemia because it increases the risk of extrapyramidal reactions; and in patients with hepatic or renal impairment because diminished metabolism and excretion cause drug to accumulate.

Interactions

Concomitant use of thiothixene with sympathomimetics, including epinephrine, phenylephrine, phenylpropanolamine, and ephedrine (often found in nasal sprays), and with appetite suppressants may decrease their stimulatory and pressor effects. Thiothixene may cause epinephrine reversal; patients taking thiothixene may experience a decrease in blood pressure when epinephrine is used as a pressor agent.

Thiothixene may inhibit blood pressure response to centrally acting antihypertensive drugs, such as guanethidine, guanabenz, guanadrel, clonidine, methyldopa, and reserpine. Additive effects are likely after concomitant use of thiothixene with CNS depressants, including alcohol, analgesics, barbiturates, narcotics, tranquilizers, anesthetics (general, spinal, or epidural) and parenteral magnesium sulfate (over-

sedation, respiratory depression, and hypotension); antiarrhythmic agents, including quinidine, disopyramide, and procainamide (increased incidence of cardiac arrhythmias and conduction defects); atropine and other anticholinergic drugs, including antidepressants, MAO inhibitors, phenothiazines, antihistamines, meperidine, and antiparkinsonian agents (oversedation, paralytic ileus, visual changes, and severe constipation); nitrates (hypotension); and metrizamide (increased risk of seizures).

Beta blocking agents may inhibit thiothixene metabolism, increasing plasma levels and toxicity.

Concomitant use with propylthiouracil increases risk of agranulocytosis; concomitant use with lithium may result in severe neurologic toxicity with an encephalitis-like syndrome and in decreased therapeutic response to thiothixene.

Pharmacokinetic alterations and subsequent decreased therapeutic response to thiothixene may follow concomitant use with phenobarbital (enhanced renal excretion); aluminum- and magnesium-containing antacids and antidiarrheals (decreased absorption); caffeine; or heavy smoking (increased metabolism).

Thiothixene may antagonize therapeutic effect of bromocriptine on prolactin secretion; it may also decrease the vasoconstricting effects of high-dose dopamine and may decrease effectiveness and increase toxicity of levodopa (by dopamine blockade). Thiothixene may inhibit metabolism and increase toxicity of phenytoin.

Effects on diagnostic tests

Thiothixene causes false-positive test results for urinary porphyrins, urobilinogen, amylase, and 5-hydroxyindoleacetic acid because of darkening of urine by metabolites; it also causes false-positive urine pregnancy results in tests using human chorionic gonadotropin as the indicator.

Thiothixene elevates test results for liver enzymes and protein-bound iodine and causes quinidine-like effects on the ECG.

Adverse reactions

● CNS: extrapyramidal symptoms—dystonia, akathisia, torticollis, tardive dyskinesia, sedation, pseudoparkinsonism, drowsiness (frequent), *neuroleptic malignant syndrome* (fatal *respiratory failure* in over 10% of patients if untreated), dizziness, headache, insomnia, exacerbation of psychotic symptoms.

- CV: *asystole,* orthostatic hypotension, tachycardia, dizziness or fainting, *arrhythmias,* ECG changes, increased anginal pain after I.M. injection.
- EENT: blurred vision, tinnitus, mydriasis, increased intraocular pressure, ocular changes (retinal pigmentary change with long-term use).
- GI: dry mouth, constipation, nausea, vomiting, anorexia, diarrhea.
- GU: urine retention, gynecomastia, hypermenorrhea, inhibited ejaculation.
- HEMA: transient leukopenia, *agranulocytosis,* thrombocytopenia, anemia (within 30 to 90 days).
- Local: contact dermatitis from concentrate or injectable form, muscle necrosis from I.M. injection.
- Other: hyperprolactinemia, photosensitivity, increased appetite or weight gain, hypersensitivity (rash, urticaria, drug fever, edema, cholestatic jaundice [in 2% to 4% of patients within first 30 days]).

After abrupt withdrawal of long-term therapy, gastritis, nausea, vomiting, dizziness, tremor, feeling of heat or cold, sweating, tachycardia, headache, or insomnia may occur.

Note: Drug should be discontinued if any of the following occur: hypersensitivity, jaundice, agranulocytosis, neuroleptic malignant syndrome (marked hyperthermia, extrapyramidal effects, autonomic dysfunction), or severe extrapyramidal symptoms even after dose is lowered. Drug should be discontinued 48 hours before and 24 hours after myelography using metrizamide because of risk of seizures. When feasible, drug should be withdrawn slowly and gradually; many drug effects persist after withdrawal.

Overdose and treatment

CNS depression is characterized by deep, unarousable sleep and possible coma, hypotension or hypertension, extrapyramidal symptoms, abnormal involuntary muscle movements, agitation, seizures, arrhythmias, ECG changes, hypothermia or hyperthermia, and autonomic nervous system dysfunction.

Treatment is symptomatic and supportive and includes maintaining vital signs, airway, stable body temperature, and fluid and electrolyte balance.

Do not induce vomiting: drug inhibits cough reflex and aspiration may occur. Use gastric lavage and then activated charcoal and saline cathartics; dialysis does not help. Regulate body temperature as needed. Treat hypotension with I.V. fluids; *do not give epinephrine.* Seizures may

be treated with parenteral diazepam or barbiturates; arrhythmias with parenteral phenytoin (1 mg/kg with rate titrated to blood pressure); and extrapyramidal reactions with barbiturates, benztropine, or parenteral diphenhydramine 2 mg/kg/minute.

▶ Special considerations

- Liquid and injectable formulations may cause a rash if skin contact occurs.
- Thiothixene is associated with a high incidence of extrapyramidal effects.
- Oral formulations may cause stomach upset. Administer with food or fluid.
- Check patient regularly for abnormal body movements (at last once every 6 months).
- Dilute the concentrate in 2 to 4 oz of liquid, preferably water, carbonated drinks, fruit juice, tomato juice, milk, or pudding.
- Photosensitivity reactions may occur; patient should avoid exposure to sunlight or heat lamps.
- Administer I.M. injection deep into upper outer quadrant of the buttock. Massaging the area after administration may prevent formation of abscesses. I.M. injection may cause skin necrosis; do not extravasate or give I.V.
- Solution for injection may be slightly discolored. Do not use if excessively discolored or if a precipitate is evident. Contact pharmacist.
- Monitor blood pressure before and after parenteral administration.
- Shake concentrate before administration.
- Sugarless chewing gum or hard candy as well as ice chips may help relieve dry mouth.
- Drug is stable after reconstitution for 48 hours at room temperature.
- Protect liquid formulation from light.
- A 5-mg dose is the therapeutic equivalent of 100 mg chlorpromazine.

Information for the patient

- Explain the risks of dystonic reactions and tardive dyskinesia and tell patient to report any abnormal body movements.
- Tell patient to avoid sun exposure and to use a sunscreen when going outdoors, to prevent photosensitivity reactions. (Note that heat lamps and tanning beds also may cause burning of the skin or skin discoloration.)
- Tell patient not to spill the liquid. Contact with skin may cause rash and irritation.
- Warn patient to avoid extremely hot or cold baths or exposure to temperature extremes, sunlamps, or tanning beds; drug may cause thermoregulatory changes.
- Tell patient to take drug exactly as prescribed,

not to double dose for missed doses, and not to share drug with others.

● Explain that many drug interactions are possible. Patient should seek medical approval before taking *any* self-prescribed medication.

● Patient should become tolerant to the drug's sedative effects in several weeks.

● Tell patient not to stop taking the drug suddenly; most adverse reactions may be relieved by reducing the dosage. However, patient should call if difficulty urinating, sore throat, dizziness, or fainting develops.

● Warn patient against hazardous activities that require alertness until the drug's effect is established. Reassure patient that sedation usually subsides after several weeks.

● Tell patient not to drink alcohol or take other medications that may cause excessive sedation.

● Explain which fluids are appropriate for diluting the concentrate and the dropper technique of measuring dose.

● Tell patient that sugarless hard candy or chewing gum, or ice chips can alleviate dry mouth.

● Tell patient to shake concentrate before administration.

● Store drug safely away from children.

Geriatric use
Elderly patients tend to require lower dosages, titrated to individual response. Such patients also are more likely to develop adverse reactions, especially tardive dyskinesia and other extrapyramidal effects.

Pediatric use
Drug is not recommended for children under age 12.

---

trifluoperazine hydrochloride
Apo-Trifluoperazine∗, Novo-Flurazine∗, Solazine∗, Stelazine, Suprazine, Terfluzine∗

● Pharmacologic classification: phenothiazine (piperazine derivative)
● Therapeutic classification: antipsychotic
● Pregnancy risk category C

How supplied
Available by prescription only
Tablets (regular and film-coated): 1 mg, 2 mg, 5 mg, 10 mg
Oral concentrate: 10 mg/ml
Injection: 2 mg/ml

Indications, route, and dosage
Anxiety states
Adults: 1 to 2 mg P.O. b.i.d.
Schizophrenia and other psychotic disorders
Adults: For outpatients, 1 to 2 mg P.O. b.i.d., increased as needed. For hospitalized patients, 2 to 5 mg P.O. b.i.d.; may increase gradually to 40 mg daily. For I.M. injection, 1 to 2 mg q 4 to 6 hours p.r.n.
Children ages 6 to 12 (hospitalized or under close supervision): 1 mg P.O. daily or b.i.d.; may increase gradually to 15 mg daily.

Pharmacodynamics
Antipsychotic action: Trifluoperazine is thought to exert its antipsychotic effects by postsynaptic blockade of CNS dopamine receptors, thereby inhibiting dopamine-mediated effects; antiemetic effects are attributed to dopamine receptor blockade in the medullary chemoreceptor trigger zone. Trifluoperazine has many other central and peripheral effects; it produces alpha and ganglionic blockade and counteracts histamine- and serotonin-mediated activity. Its most prevalent adverse reactions are extrapyramidal; it has less sedative and autonomic activity than aliphatic phenothiazines.

Pharmacokinetics
● *Absorption:* Rate and extent of absorption vary with route of administration—oral tablet absorption is erratic and variable, with onset of action ranging from ½ to 1 hour; oral concentrate absorption is much more predictable. I.M. drug is absorbed rapidly.
● *Distribution:* Trifluoperazine is distributed widely in the body, including breast milk. Drug is 91% to 99% protein-bound. Peak effect occurs in 2 to 4 hours; steady-state serum levels are achieved within 4 to 7 days.
● *Metabolism:* Trifluoperazine is metabolized extensively by the liver, but no active metabolites are formed; duration of action is about 4 to 6 hours.
● *Excretion:* Most of drug is excreted in urine via the kidneys; some is excreted in feces via the biliary tract.

Contraindications and precautions
Trifluoperazine is contraindicated in patients with known hypersensitivity to phenothiazines and related compounds, including allergic reactions involving hepatic function; in patients with blood dyscrasias and bone marrow depression (adverse hematologic effects); in patients with disorders accompanied by coma,

---

∗Canada only   †Unlabeled clinical use   Italicized adverse reactions are life-threatening.

brain damage, CNS depression, circulatory collapse, or cerebrovascular disease (additive CNS depression and adverse blood pressure effects); and in patients taking adrenergic blocking agents or spinal or epidural anesthetics (excessive respiratory, cardiac, and CNS depression).

Trifluoperazine should be used with caution in patients with cardiac disease (arrhythmias, CHF, angina pectoris, valvular disease, or heart block), encephalitis, Reye's syndrome, head injury, respiratory disease, seizure disorders, glaucoma, prostatic hypertrophy, urine retention, Parkinson's disease, and pheochromocytoma because it may exacerbate these conditions; in patients with hypocalcemia because it increases the risk of extrapyramidal reactions; and in patients with hepatic or renal dysfunction (diminished metabolism and excretion cause the drug to accumulate).

Interactions

Concomitant use of trifluoperazine with sympathomimetics, including epinephrine, phenylephrine, phenylpropanolamine, and ephedrine (often found in nasal sprays), and appetite suppressants may decrease their stimulatory and pressor effects. Using epinephrine as a pressor agent in patients taking trifluoperazine may result in epinephrine reversal or further lowering of blood pressure.

Trifluoperazine may inhibit blood pressure response to centrally acting antihypertensive drugs, such as guanethidine, guanabenz, guanadrel, clonidine, methyldopa, and reserpine. Additive effects are likely after concomitant use of trifluoperazine with CNS depressants, including alcohol, analgesics, barbiturates, narcotics, tranquilizers, anesthetics (general, spinal, epidural), and parenteral magnesium sulfate (oversedation, respiratory depression, and hypotension); antiarrhythmic agents, including quinidine, disopyramide, and procainamide (increased incidence of cardiac arrhythmias and conduction defects); atropine and other anticholinergic drugs, including antidepressants, MAO inhibitors, phenothiazines, antihistamines, meperidine, and antiparkinsonian agents (oversedation, paralytic ileus, visual changes, and severe constipation); nitrates (hypotension); and metrizamide (increased risk of seizures).

Beta blocking agents may inhibit trifluoperazine metabolism, increasing plasma levels and toxicity.

Concomitant use of trifluoperazine with propylthiouracil increases risk of agranulocytosis;

concomitant use with lithium may result in severe neurologic toxicity with an encephalitis-like syndrome and in decreased therapeutic response to trifluoperazine.

Pharmacokinetic alterations and subsequent decreased therapeutic response to trifluoperazine may follow concomitant use with phenobarbital (enhanced renal excretion), aluminum and magnesium-containing antacids and antidiarrheals (decreased absorption), caffeine, and heavy smoking (increased metabolism).

Trifluoperazine may antagonize therapeutic effect of bromocriptine on prolactin secretion; it also may decrease the vasoconstricting effects of high-dose dopamine and may decrease effectiveness and increase toxicity of levodopa (by dopamine blockade). Trifluoperazine may inhibit metabolism and increase toxicity of phenytoin.

Effects on diagnostic tests

Trifluoperazine causes false-positive test results for urine porphyrins, urobilinogen, amylase, and 5-hydroxyindoleacetic acid levels from darkening of urine by metabolites; it also causes false-positive urine pregnancy results in tests using human chorionic gonadotropin as the indicator.

Trifluoperazine elevates tests for liver function and protein-bound iodine and causes quinidine-like effects on the ECG.

Adverse reactions

● CNS: extrapyramidal symptoms—dystonia, akathisia, torticollis, tardive dyskinesia, sedation (low incidence), pseudoparkinsonism, drowsiness (frequent), *neuroleptic malignant syndrome* (fatal *respiratory failure* in over 10% of patients if untreated), dizziness, headache, insomnia, exacerbation of psychotic symptoms.
● CV: *asystole,* orthostatic hypotension, tachycardia, dizziness or fainting, *arrhythmias,* ECG changes, increased anginal pain after I.M. injection.
● EENT: blurred vision, tinnitus, mydriasis, increased intraocular pressure, ocular changes (retinal pigmentary change with long-term use).
● GI: dry mouth, constipation, nausea, vomiting, anorexia, diarrhea.
● GU: urine retention, gynecomastia, hypermenorrhea, inhibited ejaculation.
● HEMA: transient leukopenia, *agranulocytosis,* thrombocytopenia, anemia (within 30 to 90 days).
● Local: contact dermatitis from concentrate or injection, muscle necrosis from I.M. injection.
● Other: hyperprolactinemia, photosensitivity,

increased appetite or weight gain, hypersensitivity (rash, urticaria, drug fever, edema, cholestatic jaundice [2% to 4% in first 30 days]).

After abrupt withdrawal of long-term therapy, gastritis, nausea, vomiting, dizziness, tremor, feeling of heat or cold, sweating, tachycardia, headache, or insomnia may occur.

Note: Drug should be discontinued immediately if any of the following occur: hypersensitivity, jaundice, agranulocytosis, neuroleptic malignant syndrome (marked hyperthermia, extrapyramidal effects, autonomic dysfunction), severe extrapyramidal symptoms even after dosage is lowered. Drug should be discontinued 48 hours before and 24 hours after myelography using metrizamide because of risk of seizures. When feasible, drug should be withdrawn slowly and gradually; many drug effects persist after withdrawal.

Overdose and treatment

CNS depression is characterized by deep, unarousable sleep and possible coma, hypotension or hypertension, extrapyramidal symptoms, dystonia, abnormal involuntary muscle movements, agitation, seizures, arrhythmias, ECG changes, hypothermia or hyperthermia, and autonomic nervous system dysfunction.

Treatment is symptomatic and supportive and includes maintaining vital signs, airway, stable body temperature, and fluid and electrolyte balance.

Do not induce vomiting: drug inhibits cough reflex and aspiration may occur. Use gastric lavage and then activated charcoal and saline cathartics; dialysis is usually ineffective. Regulate body temperature as needed. Treat hypotension with I.V. fluids; *do not give epinephrine.* Treat seizures with parenteral diazepam or barbiturates; arrhythmias with parenteral phenytoin (1 mg/kg with rate titrated to blood pressure); extrapyramidal reactions with barbiturates, benztropine, or parenteral diphenhydramine 2 mg/kg/minute.

▶ Special considerations

Besides those relevant to all *phenothiazines,* consider the following recommendations.

● When drug is given for anxiety, do not exceed 6 mg daily for longer than 12 weeks. However, some clinicians recommend against use of this drug for anything but psychosis.

● Administer I.M. injection deep in the upper outer quadrant of the buttock. Massaging the area after administration may prevent formation of abscesses. I.M. injection may cause skin necrosis; do not extravasate.

● Solution for injection may be slightly discolored. Do not use if excessively discolored or a precipitate is evident. Contact pharmacist.

● Monitor blood pressure before and after parenteral administration.

● Shake concentrate before administration.

● Worsening anginal pain has been reported in patients receiving trifluoperazine; however, ECG reactions are less frequent with this drug than with other phenothiazines.

● Liquid and injectable formulations may cause a rash after contact with skin.

● Drug may cause pink to brown discoloration of urine.

● Trifluoperazine is associated with a high incidence of extrapyramidal symptoms and photosensitivity reactions. Patient should avoid exposure to sunlight or heat lamps.

● Monitor regularly for abnormal movements (at least once every 6 months).

● Oral formulations may cause stomach upset. Administer with food or fluid.

● Concentrate must be diluted in 2 to 4 oz of liquid, preferably water, carbonated drinks, fruit juice, tomato juice, milk, or pudding.

● Protect the liquid formulation from light.

● A 5-mg dose is the therapeutic equivalent of 100 mg chlorpromazine.

Information for the patient

● Explain the risks of dystonic reactions, akathisia, and tardive dyskinesia and tell patient to report abnormal body movements.

● Explain that many drug interactions are possible. Patient should seek medical approval before taking *any* self-prescribed medication.

● Tell patient that any adverse reactions may be alleviated by a dosage reduction. Patient should report difficulty urinating, sore throat, dizziness, or fainting.

● Warn patient against hazardous activities that require alertness until the effect of the drug is established. Reassure patient that sedative effects usually subside in several weeks.

● Tell patient to avoid sun exposure and to use a sunscreen when going outdoors, to prevent photosensitivity reactions. (Explain that heat lamps and tanning beds also may cause burning of the skin or skin discoloration.)

● Warn patient to avoid extremely hot or cold baths and exposure to temperature extremes, sunlamps, and tanning beds; drug may cause thermoregulatory changes.

● Tell patient to take drug exactly as prescribed and not to double dose for missed doses, stop taking the drug abruptly, or share drug with others.

• Advise patient to store medication in a safe place, away from children.
• Tell patient to avoid alcohol and other medications that may cause excessive sedation.
• Suggest sugarless candy or chewing gum, or ice chips to relieve dry mouth.

Geriatric use
Elderly patients tend to require lower doses, titrated to effects. Such patients also are more likely to develop adverse effects, especially tardive dyskinesia and other extrapyramidal effects and hypotension.

Pediatric use
Drug is not recommended for children under age 6.

Breast-feeding
Trifluoperazine may enter breast milk. Potential benefits to the mother should outweigh the potential harm to the infant.

Anxiolytics

alprazolam
buspirone hydrochloride
chlordiazepoxide
chlordiazepoxide hydrochloride
diazepam
doxepin (See *ANTIDEPRESSANTS*.)
halazepam
hydroxyzine hydrochoride
hydroxyzine pamoate
lorazepam
meprobamate
oxazepam
prazepam
propranolol hydrochloride

Anxiolytics – used to manage anxiety states – are the most widely prescribed of all the drugs in the United States. Anxiety is a universal and human emotion often serving adaptive purposes. It is rarely a disease in itself and the specific drug chosen to treat it seems to make little difference. Nevertheless, anxiolytics enjoy clinical popularity apparently as the result of a combination of their pharmacologic effects, relative safety, and demand by doctors and patients. A wide range of these agents are available and all produce mild sedation. Certain antihistamines and an entirely new drug class, the azaspirodecanediones, are also effective. Other classes of centrally active drugs that are now virtually obsolete for treating anxiety include the propanediol carbamates, barbiturates, and pharmacologically similar nonbarbiturates.

Pharmacologic effects
● The *propanediol carbamates* (meprobamate) produce nonselective CNS depression similar to that produced by barbiturates.
● *Benzodiazepines* (alprazolam, chlordiazepoxide, clorazepate, diazepam, halazepam, lorazepam, oxazepam, prazepam) are useful as anxiolytics and sedative-hypnotics through selective depressant effects on the CNS.
● The *antihistamine* (hydroxyzine) produces sedation and reduces anxiety through supression of subcortical activity.
● The *azaspirodecanedione* (buspirone) sup-

presses conflict and aggressive behavior and inhibits conditioned avoidance responses.
● *Miscellaneous agents* (doxepin, propranolol) also exert anxiolytic effects and have adjunctive use in treatment of anxiety.

Mechanism of action
These agents' exact mechanism of anxiolytic action is unknown.
● Meprobamate and the benzodiazepines have selective depressant effects at multiple central sites including the thalamus, hypothalamus, and limbic systems. The anxiolytic effects of the benzodiazepines are mediated through the inhibitory transmitter gamma-aminobutyric acid (GABA) and, according to recent evidence, at least two benzodiazepine receptors, BZ_1 and BZ_2, may also be involved.
● Buspirone has moderate affinity for dopamine receptors and does not affect GABA binding.
● Doxepin, a tricyclic antidepressant, blocks the neural uptake of many neurotransmitters, including serotonin and norepinephrine. It is not known how this contributes to its anxiolytic effect.
● Beta-adrenergic blocking agents act on peripheral beta receptors and are more effective against somatic symptoms, which are mediated by beta-adrenergic stimulation.

Pharmacokinetics
● *Absorption and distribution:*
—Meprobamate is well absorbed from the GI tract, achieving peak plasma concentrations in 1 to 3 hours with onset of action usually in less than 1 hour. This drug is about 15% to 20% protein-bound, is distributed uniformly throughout the body, crosses the placenta, and appears in breast milk.
—Benzodiazepines are also well absorbed from the GI tract but are slowly, erratically absorbed after I.M. administration. They are highly lipid soluble, widely distributed in body tissues, and highly protein-bound (70% to 99%). They also cross the placenta and are distributed in breast milk.
—Hydroxyzine is rapidly absorbed from the GI tract with onset of action within 15 to 30 minutes.

COMPARING ANXIOLYTICS

DRUG	USUAL DAILY DOSAGE (P.O.)	HALF-LIFE OF PARENT DRUG	HALF-LIFE OF ACTIVE METABOLITES
Benzodiazepines			
alprazolam	0.75 to 4 mg	12 to 15 hours	alpha-hydroxyalprazolam: 6 hours
chlordiazepoxide hydrochloride	15 to 100 mg	5 to 30 hours	desmethylchlordiazepoxide: 6 to 20 hours demoxepam: > 20 hours desmethyldiazepam: 40 to 50 hours oxazepam: 5 to 13 hours
diazepam	4 to 40 mg	20 to 80 hours	desmethyldiazepam: 40 to 50 hours 3-hydroxydiazepam: 5 to 20 hours oxazepam: 5 to 13 hours
halazepam	60 to 160 mg	14 hours	desmethyldiazepam: 40 to 50 hours oxazepam: 5 to 13 hours
lorazepam	2 to 4 mg	10 to 20 hours	No active metabolites
oxazepam	30 to 120 mg	5 to 13 hours	No active metabolites
prazepam	20 to 60 mg	30 to 100 hours	desmethyldiazepam: 40 to 50 hours oxazepam: 5 to 13 hours
Other			
buspirone	15 mg	2 to 3 hours	1, -pyrimidinyl-piperazine: 8 to 10 hours
hydroxyzine	200 to 400 mg	approx. 30 hours	cetirizine: 25 hours
meprobamate	1.2 to 1.6 g	6 to 17 hours	No active metabolites
propranolol	10 to 80 mg	4 hours	4-hydroxypropranolol < 3 hours

— Buspirone is also rapidly absorbed from the GI tract and reaches peak plasma levels in 40 to 90 minutes. It is about 95% plasma protein bound.

• *Metabolism and excretion:*

— Approximately 80% to 92% of meprobamate is rapidly metabolized by the liver; the remainder is excreted unchanged in the urine. It can stimulate microsomal enzymes but it is unknown if it can induce its own metabolism. Plasma half-life may be 24 to 48 hours with chronic administration. Excretion is mainly through the urine, with about 10% in feces.

— Benzodiazepines undergo hepatic biotransformation and plasma half-lives vary widely depending on the agent, the active metabolites, and the individual. Most are excreted almost entirely in the urine.

— Hydroxyzine is also metabolized in the liver but the exact mechanism is unknown.

— Buspirone undergoes oxidation and is excreted in urine and feces.

Adverse reactions and toxicity

Drowsiness, fatigue, and ataxia are the most common adverse reactions produced by anxiolytics. Physical and/or psychological dependence and abuse may also occur (except with buspirone and beta-adrenergic blocking agents). Paradoxical reactions, such as hyperexcitation, anxiety, hallucinations, spasticity, insomnia, rage, and sleep disturbances, may also occur.

Acute intoxication is evidenced by exaggerated adverse reactions; treatment is symptomatic and supportive. Gastric lavage may be useful.

Clinical considerations

• Advise patients to avoid ingestion of alcohol to prevent excessive CNS depression.

---

*Canada only   †Unlabeled clinical use   Italicized adverse reactions are life-threatening.

- If paradoxical reactions occur, the drug should be discontinued immediately.
- Benzodiazepines are more effective than meprobamate or barbiturates in treating anxiety states.
- Buspirone does not have anticonvulsant, muscle relaxant, or prominent sedative effects and has no established antipsychotic activity.
- Anxiolytic effects of doxepin precede its antidepressant effects.
- Alprazolam is indicated for use in panic disorders.
- Because many anxious patients are sensitive to the effects of beta blockade, low doses of beta blocking agents are often effective in alleviating symptoms (propranolol 10 to 40 mg daily, for example).
- Elimination may be prolonged in geriatric patients and in those with liver disease.
- After prolonged therapy, benzodiazepines should be discontinued slowly to avoid withdrawal symptoms.
- When substituting buspirone for a benzodiazepine, discontinue the benzodiazepine gradually to avoid withdrawal symptoms.
- Buspirone does not show cross-tolerance with benzodiazepines.

---

alprazolam
Xanax

- Pharmacologic classification: benzodiazepine
- Therapeutic classification: anxiolytic
- Controlled substance schedule IV
- Pregnancy risk category D

How supplied
Available by prescription only
Tablets: 0.25 mg, 0.5 mg, 1 mg, 2 mg

Indications, route, and dosage
Anxiety and tension
Adults: Usual starting dose is 0.25 to 0.5 mg t.i.d. Maximum total daily dosage is 4 mg in divided doses. In elderly or debilitated patients, usual starting dose is 0.25 mg b.i.d. or t.i.d.
Panic disorder
Adults: Initially, 0.5 mg P.O. t.i.d. Increase dosage based on response at intervals of 3 to 4 days and in increments of no greater than 1 mg/day. Dosage greater than 4 mg/day may be required; some clinicians have used 6 mg/day. In controlled studies, dosage ranged from 1 to 10 mg/day.

†*Depression*
Adults: 0. 25 mg P.O. t.i.d.

Pharmacodynamics
Anxiolytic action: Alprazolam depresses the CNS at the limbic and subcortical levels of the brain. It produces an anxiolytic effect by enhancing the effect of the neurotransmitter gamma-aminobutyric acid (GABA) on its receptor in the ascending reticular activating system, which increases inhibition and blocks both cortical and limbic arousal.

Pharmacokinetics
- *Absorption:* When administered orally, alprazolam is well absorbed. Onset of action occurs within 15 to 30 minutes, with peak action in 1 to 2 hours.
- Distribution: Alprazolam is distributed widely throughout the body. Approximately 80% to 90% of an administered dose is bound to plasma protein.
- *Metabolism:* Alprazolam is metabolized in the liver equally to alpha-hydroxyalprazolam and inactive metabolites.
- *Excretion:* Alpha-hydroxyalprazolam and other metabolites are excreted in urine. Alprazolam's half-life is 12 to 15 hours.

Contraindications and precautions
Alprazolam is contraindicated in patients with known hypersensitivity to the drug; in patients with acute narrow-angle glaucoma or untreated open-angle glaucoma because of its possible anticholinergic effect; in patients in coma; and in patients with acute alcohol intoxication who have depressed vital signs because the drug will worsen CNS depression.

Use alprazolam cautiously in patients with psychoses because the drug is rarely beneficial in such patients and may induce paradoxical reactions; in patients with myasthenia gravis or Parkinson's disease because it may exacerbate the disorder; in patients with impaired renal or hepatic function, which prolongs elimination of the drug; and in elderly or debilitated patients, who are usually more sensitive to the drug's CNS effects. Abrupt withdrawal may precipitate seizures in some patients. Alprazolam may produce additive CNS depression in patients with acute alcohol intoxication.

Use cautiously in individuals prone to addiction or drug abuse.

Interactions
Alprazolam potentiates the CNS depressant effects of phenothiazines, narcotics, barbiturates,

---

alcohol, general anesthetics, antihistamines, MAO inhibitors, and antidepressants.

Concomitant use with cimetidine and possibly disulfiram diminishes hepatic metabolism of alprazolam, increasing its plasma concentration.

Heavy smoking accelerates alprazolam metabolism, thus lowering clinical effectiveness.

Benzodiazepines may decrease serum levels of haloperidol.

Effects on diagnostic tests

Alprazolam therapy may elevate liver function test results. Minor changes in EEG patterns, usually low-voltage and fast activity, may occur during and after alprazolam therapy.

Adverse reactions

● CNS: confusion, depression, drowsiness, lethargy, light-headedness, headache, confusion, hostility, hangover effect, ataxia, dizziness, syncope, nightmares, fatigue, slurred speech, tremor, vertigo.
● CV: hypotension, bradycardia, palpitations, shortness of breath.
● DERM: rash, urticaria, jaundice, flushing.
● EENT: diplopia, blurred vision, photosensitivity, nystagmus.
● GI: constipation, dry mouth, metallic taste, hiccups, nausea, vomiting, abdominal discomfort.
● GU: urinary incontinence, urine retention.
● Other: *respiratory depression,* dysarthria, hepatic dysfunction, changes in libido.

Note: Drug should be discontinued if hypersensitivity or the following paradoxical reactions occur: acute hyperexcited state, anxiety, hallucinations, increased muscle spasticity, insomnia, or rage.

Overdose and treatment

Clinical manifestations of overdose include somnolence, confusion, coma, hypoactive reflexes, dyspnea, labored breathing, hypotension, bradycardia, slurred speech, unsteady gait, and impaired coordination.

Support blood pressure and respiration until drug effects subside; monitor vital signs. Mechanical ventilatory assistance via endotracheal tube may be required to maintain a patent airway and support adequate oxygenation. As needed, I.V. fluids and vasopressors such as dopamine and phenylephrine to treat hypotension. If the patient is conscious, induce emesis. Use gastric lavage if ingestion was recent, but only if an endotracheal tube is in place to prevent aspiration. After emesis or lavage,
administer activated charcoal with a cathartic as a single dose. Dialysis is of limited value. Do not use barbiturates if excitation occurs because of possible exacerbation of excitation or CNS depression.

▶ Special considerations

Besides those relevant to all *benzodiazepines,* consider the following recommendations.
● Lower doses are effective in elderly patients and patients with renal or hepatic dysfunction.
● Anxiety associated with depression is also responsive to alprazolam.
● Store in a cool, dry place away from direct light.
● Consider the potential for abuse before prescribing alprazolam for anyone with a tendency to substance abuse.

Information for the patient

● Be sure patient understands that the potential exists for physical and psychological dependence with chronic use of alprazolam.
● Instruct patient not to alter drug regimen in any way or to discontinue the drug suddenly.
● Warn patient that sudden changes in position can cause dizziness. Advise patient to dangle legs for a few minutes before getting out of bed to prevent falls and injury.

Geriatric use

● Lower doses are usually effective in elderly patients because of decreased elimination.
● During initiation of therapy or after an increase in dose, elderly patients who receive this drug require supervision with ambulation and activities of daily living.

Pediatric use

● Closely observe a neonate for withdrawal symptoms if mother took alprazolam during pregnancy. Use of alprazolam during labor may cause neonatal flaccidity.
● Safety has not been established in children under age 18.

Breast-feeding

The breast-fed infant of a woman who uses alprazolam may become sedated, have feeding difficulties, or lose weight. Avoid use in breast-feeding women.

buspirone hydrochloride
BuSpar

- Pharmacologic classification: azaspirodecane-dione derivative
- Therapeutic classification: anxiolytic
- Pregnancy risk category B

How supplied
Available by prescription only
Tablets: 5 mg, 10 mg

Indications, route, and dosage
Management of anxiety disorders; short-term relief of anxiety
Adults: Initially, 5 mg P.O. t.i.d. Dosage may be increased at 3-day intervals. Usual maintenance dosage is 20 to 30 mg daily in divided doses.

Pharmacodynamics
Anxiolytic action: Buspirone is an azaspirode-canedione derivative with anxiolytic activity. It suppresses conflict and aggressive behavior and inhibits conditioned avoidance responses. Its precise mechanism of action has not been determined, but it appears to depend on simultaneous effects on several neurotransmitters and receptor sites: decreased serotonin neuronal activity, increased norepinephrine metabolism, and partial action as a presynaptic dopamine antagonist. Studies suggest an indirect effect on benzodiazepine gamma-aminobutyric acid (GABA)-chloride receptor complex or GABA receptors or on other neurotransmitter systems.

Buspirone is not pharmacologically related to benzodiazepines, barbiturates, or other sedatives and anxiolytics. It exhibits both a nontraditional clinical profile and is uniquely anxiolytic. It has no anticonvulsant or muscle relaxant activity and does not appear to cause physical dependence or significant sedation.

Pharmacokinetics
- *Absorption:* Buspirone is absorbed rapidly and completely after oral administration, but extensive first-pass metabolism limits absolute bioavailability to 1% to 13% of the oral dose. Food slows absorption but increases the amount of unchanged drug in systemic circulation.
- *Distribution:* The drug is 95% protein-bound; it does not displace other highly protein-bound medications such as warfarin. Onset of therapeutic effect may require 1 to 2 weeks.
- *Metabolism:* The drug is metabolized in the liver by hydroxylation and oxidation, resulting in at least one pharmacologically active metabolite – 1,-pyrimidinyl piperazine.
- *Excretion:* 29% to 63% is excreted in urine in 24 hours, primarily as metabolites; 18% to 38% is excreted in feces.

Contraindications and precautions
Buspirone is contraindicated in patients with known hypersensitivity to the drug.

The drug should be used cautiously in patients with a history of drug abuse or dependence (because of potential misuse or abuse) and in patients with impaired hepatic or renal function because impaired metabolism or excretion may result.

Interactions
When used concomitantly with MAO inhibitors, buspirone may elevate blood pressure; avoid this combination.

Buspirone may displace digoxin from serum-binding sites when the drugs are used concomitantly.

Use cautiously with alcohol or other CNS depressants because sedation may result, especially with doses greater than 30 mg per day. Buspirone does not increase alcohol-induced impairment of mental and motor performance; however, CNS effects in individuals are not predictable.

Effects on diagnostic tests
None reported.

Adverse reactions
- CNS: dizziness, drowsiness, nervousness, headache, fatigue, weakness, insomnia, lightheadedness, excitement, confusion, depression, decreased concentration, chewing movements, lip-smacking or puckering, puffing of checks or rapid, wormlike movements of tongue; tardive dyskinesia (with long-term use).
- CV: tachycardia, palpitations, nonspecific chest pain.
- EENT: blurred vision, tinnitus, sore throat, nasal congestion.
- GI: nausea, dry mouth, abdominal pain, gastric distress, diarrhea, constipation, vomiting.
- Other: hyperventilation, shortness of breath.

Overdose and treatment
Signs of overdose include severe dizziness, drowsiness, unusual constriction of pupils, and stomach upset, including nausea and vomiting.

Treatment of overdose is symptomatic and

supportive; empty stomach with immediate gastric lavage. Monitor respiration, pulse, and blood pressure. No specific antidote is known. Effect of dialysis is unknown.

▶ **Special considerations**
● Although buspirone does not appear to cause tolerance or physical or psychological dependence, the possibility exists that patients prone to drug abuse may experience these effects.
● Buspirone will not block withdrawal syndrome associated with benzodiazepines or other common sedative and hypnotic agents; therefore, these agents should be withdrawn gradually before replacement with buspirone therapy.
● Some clinicians find buspirone less effective in patients who have previously received benzodiazepines for the treatment of anxiety.
● Useful for anxiety disorder of at least 1 month's duration with three of the four diagnostic criteria for anxiety disorders (autonomic hyperactivity, apprehensive expectations, vigilance, scanning).
● Be aware that this may be the drug of choice for patients with a history of physical dependence or drug seeking behavior. No direct evidence exists that this drug causes such behavior.
● Monitor hepatic and renal function; hepatic and renal impairment will impede metabolism and excretion of the drug and may lead to toxic accumulation; dosage reduction may be necessary.

Information for the patient
● Advise patient to take drug exactly as prescribed; explain that therapeutic effect may not occur for 2 weeks or more. Warn patient not to double the dose if one is missed, but to take a missed dose as soon as possible, unless it is almost time for next dose.
● Caution patient to avoid hazardous tasks requiring alertness until effect of medication is known. The effects of alcohol and other CNS depressants (such as antihistamines, sedatives, tranquilizers, sleeping aids, prescription pain medication, barbiturates, seizure medicine, muscle relaxants, anesthetics, and medicines for colds, coughs, hay fever, or allergies) may be enhanced by additive sedation and drowsiness caused by buspirone.
● Tell patient to store drug away from heat and light and out of children's reach.
● Explain importance of regular follow-up visits to check progress. Urge patient to report adverse reactions immediately.

Breast-feeding
Reports of animal studies show that buspirone and its metabolites are excreted in the breast milk of rats; however, the extent of excretion in human milk is unknown. Buspirone should be avoided in breast-feeding women.

---

chlordiazepoxide
Libritabs

chlordiazepoxide hydrochloride
Apo-Chlordiazepoxide∗, Librium, Lipoxide, Medilium∗, Murcil, Novopoxide∗, Reposans-10, Sereen, SK-Lygen, Solium∗

● Pharmacologic classification: benzodiazepine
● Therapeutic classification: anxiolytic; anticonvulsant, sedative-hypnotic
● Controlled substance schedule IV
● Pregnancy risk category D

How supplied
Available by prescription only
Tablets: 5 mg, 10 mg, 25 mg
Capsules: 5 mg, 10 mg, 25 mg
Powder for injection: 100 mg/ampule

Indications, route, and dosage
Mild to moderate anxiety and tension
Adults: 5 to 10 mg t.i.d. or q.i.d.
Children over age 6: 5 mg P.O. b.i.d. to q.i.d. Maximum dosage is 10 mg P.O. b.i.d. to t.i.d.
Severe anxiety and tension
Adults: 20 to 25 mg t.i.d. or q.i.d.
Severe alcohol withdrawal syndrome (hypertension, tachycardia, tremor)
Adults: 50 to 100 mg P.O., I.M., or I.V. Maximum dosage is 300 mg/day.
Preoperative apprehension and anxiety
Adults: 5 to 10 mg P.O. t.i.d. or q.i.d. on day before surgery; or 50 to 100 mg I.M. 1 hour before surgery.
Note: Parenteral form is not recommended in children under age 12.

Pharmacodynamics
● *Anxiolytic action:* Chlordiazepoxide depresses the CNS at the limbic and subcortical levels of the brain. It produces an anxiolytic effect by influencing the effect of the neurotransmitter gamma-aminobutyric acid (GABA) on its receptor in the ascending reticular activating system, which increases inhibition and

blocks both cortical and limbic arousal after stimulation of the reticular formation.

• *Anticonvulsant action:* Chlordiazepoxide suppresses the spread of seizure activity produced by the epileptogenic foci in the cortex, thalamus, and limbic structures by enhancing presynaptic inhibition.

Pharmacokinetics

• *Absorption:* When given orally, chlordiazepoxide is absorbed well through the GI tract. Action begins in 30 to 45 minutes, with peak action in 1 to 3 hours. I.M. administration results in erratic absorption of the drug; onset of action usually occurs in 15 to 30 minutes. After I.V. administration, rapid onset of action occurs in 1 to 5 minutes after injection.

• *Distribution:* Chlordiazepoxide is distributed widely throughout the body. Drug is 80% to 90% protein-bound.

• *Metabolism:* Chlordiazepoxide is metabolized in the liver to several active metabolites.

• *Excretion:* Most metabolites of chlordiazepoxide are excreted in urine as glucuronide conjugates. The half-life of chlordiazepoxide is 5 to 30 hours.

Contraindications and precautions

Chlordiazepoxide is contraindicated in patients with known hypersensitivity to the drug; in patients with acute narrow-angle glaucoma or untreated open-angle glaucoma because of the drug's possible anticholinergic effect; in patients in shock or coma because the drug's hypnotic or hypotensive effect may be prolonged or intensified; in patients with acute alcohol intoxication who have depressed vital signs because the drug will worsen CNS depression; and in neonates because slow metabolism causes the drug to accumulate.

Chlordiazepoxide should be used cautiously in patients with psychoses because it is rarely beneficial in such patients and may induce paradoxical reactions; in patients with myasthenia gravis or Parkinson's disease because drug may exacerbate the disorder; in patients with impaired renal or hepatic function, which prolongs elimination of the drug; in elderly or debilitated patients, who are usually more sensitive to the drug's CNS effects; and in individuals prone to addiction or drug abuse.

Interactions

Chlordiazepoxide potentiates the CNS depressant effects of phenothiazines, narcotics, barbiturates, alcohol, antihistamines, MAO inhibitors, general anesthetics, and antidepressants. Concomitant use with cimetidine and possibly disulfiram diminishes hepatic metabolism of chlordiazepoxide, which increases its plasma concentration. Heavy smoking accelerates chlordiazepoxide's metabolism, thus lowering clinical effectiveness. Oral contraceptives may impair the metabolism of chlordiazepoxide. Antacids may delay the absorption of chlordiazepoxide. Concomitant use with levodopa may decrease the therapeutic effects of levodopa. Benzodiazepines may decrease serum levels of haloperidol.

Effects on diagnostic tests

Chlordiazepoxide therapy may elevate results of liver function tests. Minor changes in EEG patterns, usually low-voltage and fast activity, may occur during and after chlordiazepoxide therapy. Chlordiazepoxide may cause a false-positive pregnancy test, depending on method used. It may also alter urinary 17-ketosteroids (Zimmerman reaction), urine alkaloid determination (Frings thin-layer chromatography method), and urinary glucose determinations (with Clinistix and Diastix, but not Tes-Tape).

Adverse reactions

• CNS: confusion, depression, drowsiness, lethargy, hangover effect, ataxia, dizziness, syncope, nightmares, fatigue, slurred speech, tremor, vertigo, paradoxical reactions (such as hyperaggressiveness, rage).

• CV: *CV collapse,* transient hypotension, palpitations, bradycardia.

• DERM: rash, urticaria, hair loss.

• EENT: diplopia, blurred vision, nystagmus.

• GI: constipation, dry mouth, nausea, vomiting, difficulty swallowing, anorexia, abdominal discomfort.

• GU: urinary incontinence, urine retention.

• Local: pain, phlebitis, and desquamation at injection site.

• Other: *respiratory depression,* dysarthria, headache, hepatic dysfunction, changes in libido, active intermittent porphyria.

Note: Drug should be discontinued if hypersensitivity or the following paradoxical reactions occur: acute hyperexcited state, anxiety, hallucinations, increased muscle spasticity, insomnia, or rage.

Overdose and treatment

Clinical manifestations of overdose include somnolence, confusion, coma, hypoactive reflexes, dyspnea, labored breathing, hypotension, bradycardia, slurred speech, and unsteady gait or impaired coordination.

Support blood pressure and respiration until drug effects subside; monitor vital signs. Mechanical ventilatory assistance via endotracheal tube may be required to maintain a patent airway and support adequate oxygenation. Use I.V. fluids and vasopressors like dopamine and phenylephrine to treat hypotension as needed. Use gastric lavage if ingestion was recent, but only if an endotracheal tube is in place to prevent aspiration. Induce emesis if the patient is conscious. After emesis or lavage, administer activated charcoal with a cathartic as a single dose. Do not administer barbiturates if excitation occurs. Dialysis is of limited value.

▶ **Special considerations**
Besides those relevant to all *benzodiazepines*, consider the following recommendations.
● Use cautiously in patients with a potential for substance abuse.
● I.M. administration is not recommended because of erratic and slow absorption. However, if I.M. route is used, reconstitute with special diluent only. Do not use diluent if hazy. Discard unused portion. Inject I.M. deep into large muscle mass.
● For I.V. administration, drug should be reconstituted with sterile water or normal saline solution and infused slowly, directly into a large vein, at a rate not exceeding 50 mg/minute for adults. Do not infuse chlordiazepoxide into small veins. Avoid extravasation into S.C. tissue. Observe the infusion site for phlebitis. Keep resuscitation equipment nearby in case of an emergency.
● Prepare solutions for I.V. or I.M. use immediately before administration. Discard any unused portions.
● Patients should remain in bed under observation for at least 3 hours after parenteral administration of chlordiazepoxide.
● Lower doses are effective in patients with renal or hepatic dysfunction. Closely monitor renal and hepatic studies for signs of dysfunction. After long-term therapy, do not discontinue the drug abruptly because this may precipitate withdrawal syndrome.

Information for the patient
Warn patient that sudden changes in position may cause dizziness. Advise patient to dangle legs a few minutes before getting out of bed to prevent falls and injury.

Geriatric use
● Elderly patients demonstrate a greater sensitivity to the CNS depressant effects of chlor-

diazepoxide. Some may require supervision with ambulation and activities of daily living during initiation of therapy or after an increase in dose.
● Lower doses are usually effective in elderly patients because of decreased elimination.
● Parenteral administration of this drug is more likely to cause apnea, hypotension, and bradycardia in elderly patients.

Pediatric use
Safety of oral use has not been established in children under age 6; safety of parenteral use, in children under age 12.

Breast-feeding
The breast-fed infant of a woman who uses chlordiazepoxide may become sedated, have feeding difficulties, or lose weight. Do not administer drug to breast-feeding women.

---

diazepam
Apo-Diazepam∗, E-Pam∗, Meval∗, Novodipam∗, Valium, Valrelease, Vivol∗

● Pharmacologic classification: benzodiazepine
● Therapeutic classification: anxiolytic, anticonvulsant, sedative-hypnotic
● Controlled substance schedule IV
● Pregnancy risk category D

How supplied
Available by prescription only
Tablets: 2 mg, 5 mg, 10 mg
Capsules (extended-release): 15 mg
Oral solution: 5 mg/ml; 5 mg/5 ml
Oral suspension: 5 mg/5 ml
Injection: 5 mg/ml in 2-ml ampules or 10-ml vials
Disposable syringe: 2-ml Tel-E-Ject

Indications, route, and dosage
Anxiety and tension
Adults: 2 to 10 mg P.O. b.i.d. to q.i.d.; or 2 to 5 mg I.M. or I.V., repeated in 3 to 4 hours as needed.
Acute alcohol withdrawal
Adults: 10 mg P.O. t.i.d. or q.i.d. for the first 24 hours; reduce to 5 mg t.i.d. or q.i.d., if needed; or 10 mg I.M. or I.V. initially, followed by 5 to 10 mg in 3 to 4 hours, if needed.
Adjunct to seizure disorders
Adults: 2 to 10 mg b.i.d. to q.i.d.
Children over age 6 months: 1 to 2.5 mg P.O. t.i.d. or q.i.d.

Status epilepticus

Adults: 5 to 10 mg I.V., repeated at 10- to 15-minute intervals to a maximum dose of 30 mg. Repeat q 3 to 4 hours, if needed.

Infants age 1 month to children age 5: 0.2 to 0.5 mg/kg I.V. q 2 to 5 minutes to a maximum dose of 5 mg.

Children age 5 and over: 1 mg I.V. q 2 to 5 minutes to a maximum of 10 mg; repeat in 2 to 4 hours, as needed.

Note: One extended-release capsule can be substituted for oral diazepam; 5 mg t.i.d. of oral solution may be substituted for oral tablets.

Pharmacodynamics

• *Anxiolytic and sedative-hypnotic actions:* Diazepam depresses the CNS at the limbic and subcortical levels of the brain. It produces an anxiolytic effect by influencing the effect of the neurotransmitter gamma-aminobutyric acid on its receptor in the ascending reticular activating system, which increases inhibition and blocks cortical and limbic arousal.

• *Anticonvulsant action:* Diazepam suppresses the spread of seizure activity produced by epileptogenic foci in the cortex, thalamus, and limbic structures by enhancing presynaptic inhibition.

Pharmacokinetics

• *Absorption:* When administered orally, diazepam is absorbed through the GI tract. Onset of action occurs within 30 to 60 minutes, with peak action in 1 to 2 hours. I.M. administration results in erratic absorption of the drug; onset of action usually occurs in 15 to 30 minutes. After I.V. administration, rapid onset of action occurs 1 to 5 minutes after injection.

• *Distribution:* Diazepam is distributed widely throughout the body. Approximately 85% to 95% of an administered dose is bound to plasma protein.

• *Metabolism:* Diazepam is metabolized in the liver to the active metabolite desmethyldiazepam.

• *Excretion:* Most metabolites of diazepam are excreted in urine, with only small amounts excreted in feces. Duration of effect is 3 hours; this may be prolonged up to 90 hours in elderly patients and in patients with hepatic or renal dysfunction.

Contraindications and precautions

Diazepam is contraindicated in patients with known hypersensitivity to the drug; in patients with acute narrow-angle glaucoma or untreated open-angle glaucoma because of the drug's pos-sible anticholinergic effect; in patients in shock or coma because the drug's hypnotic or hypotensive effect may be prolonged or intensified; in patients with acute alcohol intoxication who have depressed vital signs because the drug will worsen CNS depression; and in neonates because slow metabolism of the drug causes it to accumulate.

Diazepam should be used cautiously in patients with psychoses because the drug is rarely beneficial in such patients and may induce paradoxical reactions; in patients with myasthenia gravis or Parkinson's disease because it may exacerbate the disorder; in patients with impaired renal or hepatic function, which prolongs elimination of the drug; in elderly or debilitated patients, who are usually more sensitive to the drug's CNS effects; and in individuals prone to addiction or drug abuse. Abrupt withdrawal of diazepam may precipitate seizures in patients with seizure disorders. Use of I.V. diazepam in patients with Lennox-Gastaut syndrome may precipitate status epilepticus.

Interactions

Diazepam potentiates the CNS depressant effects of phenothiazines, narcotics, barbiturates, alcohol, antihistamines, MAO inhibitors, general anesthetics, and antidepressants. Concomitant use with cimetidine and possibly disulfiram causes diminished hepatic metabolism of diazepam, which increases its plasma concentration.

Antacids may decrease the rate of absorption of diazepam.

Haloperidol may change the seizure patterns of patients treated with diazepam; benzodiazepines also may reduce the serum levels of haloperidol.

Diazepam reportedly can decrease digoxin clearance; monitor patients for digoxin toxicity.

Patients receiving diazepam and nondepolarizing neuromuscular blocking agents such as pancuronium and succinylcholine have intensified and prolonged respiratory depression.

Heavy smoking accelerates diazepam's metabolism, thus lowering clinical effectiveness.

Oral contraceptives may impair the metabolism of diazepam.

Diazepam may inhibit the therapeutic effect of levodopa.

Effects on diagnostic tests

Diazepam therapy may elevate liver function test results. Minor changes in EEG patterns, usually low-voltage and fast activity, may occur during and after diazepam therapy.

Adverse reactions

• CNS: confusion, depression, drowsiness, lethargy, hangover effect, ataxia, dizziness, syncope, nightmares, fatigue, slurred speech, tremor, vertigo, headache, muscle cramps, paresthesia, nervousness, euphoria.
• CV: *CV collapse,* transient hypotension, bradycardia, arrhythmias (with I.V.).
• DERM: rash, urticaria.
• EENT: diplopia, blurred vision, photosensitivity, nystagmus.
• GI: constipation, salivation changes, anorexia, metallic taste, depressed gag reflex (with I.V.), nausea, vomiting, abdominal discomfort.
• GU: urinary incontinence, urine retention.
• Local: pain, phlebitis at the injection site, desquamation of the skin at the I.V. site.
• Other: blood dyscrasias, *respiratory depression,* dysarthria, hepatic dysfunction, changes in libido, tissue necrosis (with intra-arterial administration), lactic acidosis (high-dose I.V. use).

Note: Drug should be discontinued if hypersensitivity and the following paradoxical reactions occur: acute hyperexcited state, anxiety, hallucinations, increased muscle spasticity, insomnia, or rage.

Overdose and treatment

Clinical manifestations of overdose include somnolence, confusion, coma, hypoactive reflexes, dyspnea, labored breathing, hypotension, bradycardia, slurred speech, and unsteady gait or impaired coordination.

Support blood pressure and respiration until drug effects subside; monitor vital signs. Mechanical ventilatory assistance via endotracheal tube may be required to maintain a patent airway and support adequate oxygenation. Use I.V. fluids and vasopressors such as dopamine and phenylephrine to treat hypotension as needed. If the patient is conscious, induce emesis; use gastric lavage if ingestion was recent but only if an endotracheal tube is present to prevent aspiration. After emesis or lavage, administer activated charcoal with a cathartic as a single dose. Dialysis is of limited value.

▶ Special considerations

Besides those relevant to all *benzodiazepines,* consider the following recommendations.
• To enhance taste, oral solution can be mixed with liquids or semisolid foods, such as applesauce or puddings, immediately before administration.
• Patient should not crush or chew extended-release capsule but should swallow the capsule whole.

• Shake oral suspension well before administering.
• When prescribing with opiates for endoscopic procedures, reduce opiate dose by at least one third.
• Assess gag reflex postendoscopy and before resuming oral intake to prevent aspiration.
• Parenteral forms of diazepam may be diluted in normal saline solution; a slight precipitate may form although the solution can still be used.
• Diazepam interacts with plastic. Do not store diazepam in plastic syringes or administer it in plastic administration sets, which will decrease availability of the infused drug.
• I.V. route is preferred because of rapid and more uniform absorption.
• For I.V. administration, drug should be infused slowly, directly into a large vein, at a rate not exceeding 5 mg/minute for adults or 0.25 mg/kg of body weight over 3 minutes for children. Do not inject diazepam into small veins to avoid extravasation into S.C. tissue. Observe the infusion site for phlebitis. If direct I.V. administration is not possible, inject diazepam directly into I.V. tubing at point closest to vein insertion site to prevent extravasation.
• Administration by continuous I.V. infusion is not recommended.
• Inject I.M. dose deep into deltoid muscle. Aspirate for backflow to prevent inadvertent intra-arterial administration. Use I.M. route only if I.V. or oral routes are unavailable.
• Patients should remain in bed under observation for at least 3 hours after parenteral administration of diazepam to prevent potential hazards; keep resuscitation equipment nearby.
• During prolonged therapy, periodically monitor blood counts and liver function studies. Withdraw drug gradually to avoid withdrawal reactions. Signs of withdrawal include anorexia, anxiety, irritability, or hallucinations.
• Lower doses are effective in patients with renal or hepatic dysfunction.
• Anticipate possible transient increase in frequency or severity of seizures when diazepam is used as adjunctive treatment of seizure disorders. Impose seizure precautions.
• Do not mix diazepam with any other drug in a syringe or infusion container.

Information for the patient

• Advise patient of the potential for physical and psychological dependence with chronic use.
• Warn patient that sudden changes of position can cause dizziness. Advise patient to dangle legs for a few minutes before getting out of bed to prevent falls and injury.

• Encourage patient to avoid or limit smoking to prevent increased diazepam metabolism.
• Warn female patient to notify physician immediately if she becomes pregnant.
• Warn patient to avoid alcohol while taking diazepam.

Geriatric use
• Elderly patients are more sensitive to the CNS depressant effects of diazepam. Use with caution.
• Lower doses are usually effective in elderly patients because of decreased elimination.
• Elderly patients who receive this drug require assistance with walking and activities of daily living during initiation of therapy or after an increase in dose.
• Parenteral administration of this drug is more likely to cause apnea, hypotension, and bradycardia in elderly patients.

Pediatric use
• Safe use of oral diazepam in infants less than age 6 months has not been established. Safe use of parenteral diazepam in neonates has not been established.
• Closely observe neonates of mothers who took diazepam for a prolonged period during pregnancy; the neonates may show withdrawal symptoms. Use of diazepam during labor may cause neonatal flaccidity.

Breast-feeding
Diazepam is distributed into breast milk. The breast-fed infant of a woman who uses diazepam may become sedated, have feeding difficulties, or lose weight. Avoid use in breast-feeding women.

---

halazepam
Paxipam

• Pharmacologic classification: benzodiazepine
• Therapeutic classification: anxiolytic
• Controlled substance schedule IV
• Pregnancy risk category D

How supplied
Available by prescription only
Tablets: 20 mg, 40 mg

Indications, route, and dosage
Relief of anxiety and tension
Adults: Usually, 20 to 40 mg P.O. t.i.d. or q.i.d.; optimal daily dosage is 80 to 160 mg. Daily doses up to 600 mg have been given. In elderly or debilitated patients, initial dosage is 20 mg once daily or b.i.d.

Pharmacodynamics
Anxiolytic action: Halazepam depresses the CNS at the limbic and subcortical levels of the brain. It produces an anxiolytic effect by enhancing the effect of the neurotransmitter gamma-aminobutyric acid on its receptor in the ascending reticular activating system, which increases inhibition and blocks both cortical and limbic arousal.

Pharmacokinetics
• *Absorption:* When administered orally, halazepam is absorbed through the GI tract. Peak levels occur in 1 to 3 hours.
• *Distribution:* Halazepam is distributed widely throughout the body. Drug is approximately 85% to 95% protein-bound.
• *Metabolism:* Halazepam is metabolized in the liver to the active metabolite desmethyldiazepam.
• *Excretion:* The metabolites of halazepam are excreted in urine as glucuronide conjugates. Although the half-life of halazepam is about 14 hours, the half-life of its metabolite, desmethyldiazepam, ranges from 30 to 200 hours.

Contraindications and precautions
Halazepam is contraindicated in patients with known hypersensitivity to the drug; in patients with acute narrow-angle glaucoma or untreated open-angle glaucoma because of the drug's possible anticholinergic effect; in patients in shock or coma because the drug's hypnotic or hypotensive effect may be prolonged or intensified; and in patients with acute alcohol intoxication who have depressed vital signs because the drug will worsen CNS depression.

Halazepam should be used cautiously in patients with psychoses because the drug is rarely beneficial in such patients and may induce paradoxical reactions; in patients with myasthenia gravis or Parkinson's disease because it may exacerbate the disorder; in patients with impaired renal or hepatic function, which prolongs elimination of the drug; in elderly or debilitated patients, who are usually more sensitive to the drug's CNS effects; and in individuals prone to addiction or drug abuse.

Interactions

Halazepam potentiates the CNS depressant effects of phenothiazines, narcotics, barbiturates, alcohol, antihistamines, MAO inhibitors, general anesthetics, and antidepressants.

Concomitant use with cimetidine and possibly disulfiram causes diminished hepatic metabolism of halazepam, which increases its plasma concentration.

Heavy smoking accelerates halazepam's metabolism, thus lowering clinical effectiveness.

Effects on diagnostic tests

Halazepam therapy may elevate liver function test results. Minor changes in EEG patterns, usually low-voltage and fast activity, may occur during and after halazepam therapy.

Adverse reactions

● CNS: confusion, depression, drowsiness, lethargy, hangover effect, ataxia, dizziness, syncope, nightmares, fatigue, slurred speech, tremor, vertigo, headache, euphoria, irritability.
● CV: bradycardia, *CV collapse,* transient hypotension.
● DERM: rash, urticaria.
● EENT: diplopia, blurred vision, nystagmus.
● GI: constipation, dry mouth, anorexia, nausea, vomiting, abdominal discomfort.
● GU: urinary incontinence, urine retention.
● Other: *respiratory depression,* dysarthria, hepatic dysfunction, changes in libido.

Note: Drug should be discontinued if hypersensitivity or the following paradoxical reactions occur: acute hyperexcited state, anxiety, hallucinations, increased muscle spasticity, insomnia, or rage.

Overdose and treatment

Clinical manifestations of overdose include somnolence, confusion, coma, hypoactive reflexes, dyspnea, labored breathing, hypotension, bradycardia, slurred speech, and unsteady gait or impaired coordination.

Support blood pressure and respiration until drug effects subside; monitor vital signs. Mechanical ventilatory assistance via endotracheal tube may be required to maintain a patent airway and support adequate oxygenation. Use I.V. fluids and vasopressors such as dopamine and phenylephrine to treat hypotension as needed. If patient is conscious, induce emesis with ipecac syrup. Use gastric lavage if ingestion was recent, but only if an endotracheal tube is present to prevent aspiration. After emesis or lavage, administer activated charcoal with a cathartic as a single dose. Dialysis is of limited value.

▶ Special considerations

Besides those relevant to all *benzodiazepines,* consider the following recommendations.
● Assess hepatic function periodically to ensure adequate drug metabolism.
● Lower doses are effective in patients with renal or hepatic dysfunction.
● Store in a cool, dry place away from light.
● Withdrawal symptoms may occur if drug is used for an extended period and is abruptly discontinued.
● Prescribe only a limited quantity of this drug for patient who is depressed or potentially suicidal.

Information for the patient

● Warn patient that sudden changes of position can cause dizziness. Advise patient to dangle legs for a few minutes before getting out of bed to prevent falls and injury.
● Advise patient of potential for physical and psychological dependence with chronic use.
● Advise patient to call before taking any OTC medications or making any changes in drug regimen.
● Warn patient to notify physician immediately if she becomes pregnant.

Geriatric use

● Elderly patients are more sensitive to the CNS depressant effects of halazepam. Use with caution.
● Lower doses are usually effective in elderly patients because of decreased elimination.
● Elderly patients who receive this drug require supervision with ambulation and activities of daily living during initiation of therapy or after an increase in dose.

Pediatric use

Safe use has not been established in children under age 18.

Breast-feeding

Because a breast-fed infant may become sedated, have feeding difficulties, or lose weight, avoid use in breast-feeding women.

---

hydroxyzine hydrochloride
Anxanil, Atarax, Atozine, E-Vista, Hydroxacen,
Hyzine-50, Multipax*, Quiess, Vistacon,
Vistaject-25, Vistaject-50, Vistaquel, Vistazine 50

hydroxyzine pamoate
Vamate, Vistaril

- Pharmacologic classification: antihistamine (piperazine derivative)
- Therapeutic classification: anxiolytic, sedative
- Pregnancy risk category C

How supplied
Available by prescription only
hydroxyzine hydrochloride
Capsules: 10 mg, 25 mg, 50 mg
Syrup: 10 mg/5 ml
Tablets: 10 mg, 25 mg, 50 mg, 100 mg
Injection: 25 mg/ml, 50 mg/ml
hydroxyzine pamoate
Capsules: 25 mg, 50 mg, 100 mg
Oral suspension: 25 mg/5 ml

Indications, route, and dosage
Anxiety and tension
Adults: 25 to 100 mg P.O. t.i.d. or q.i.d.
Anxiety, tension, hyperkinesia
Children over age 6: 50 to 100 mg P.O. daily in divided doses.
Children under age 6: 50 mg P.O. daily in divided doses.

Pharmacodynamics
- *Anxiolytic and sedative actions:* Hydroxyzine produces its sedative and anxiolytic effects through suppression of activity at subcortical levels; analgesia occurs at high doses.

Pharmacokinetics
- *Absorption:* Hydroxyzine is absorbed rapidly and completely after oral administration. Peak serum levels occur within 2 to 4 hours. Sedation and other clinical effects are usually noticed in 15 to 30 minutes.
- *Distribution:* The distribution of hydroxyzine in humans is not well understood.
- *Metabolism:* Hydroxyzine is metabolized almost completely in the liver.
- *Excretion:* Metabolites of hydroxyzine are excreted primarily in urine; small amounts of drug and metabolites are found in feces. Half-life of the drug is 3 hours. Sedative effects can last for

4 to 6 hours and antihistaminic effects can persist for up to 4 days.

Contraindications and precautions
Hydroxyzine is contraindicated in patients with known hypersensitivity to the drug. Hyroxyzine should be used cautiously in patients with open-angle glaucoma, urine retention, or any other condition where anticholinergic effects would be detrimental.

Interactions
Hydroxyzine may add to or potentiate the effects of opioids, barbiturates, alcohol, tranquilizers, and other CNS depressants; the dose of CNS depressants should be reduced by 50%.

Concomitant use with other anticholinergic drugs causes additive anticholinergic effects.

Hydroxyzine may block the vasopressor action of epinephrine. If a vasoconstrictor is needed, use norepinephrine or phenylephrine.

Effects on diagnostic tests
Hydroxyzine therapy causes falsely elevated urinary 17-hydroxycorticosteroid levels. It also may cause false-negative skin allergen tests by attenuating or inhibiting the cutaneous response to histamine.

Adverse reactions
- CNS: sedation, dizziness, drowsiness, ataxia, weakness, slurred speech, headache, anxiety, tremor, and *seizures* at high doses (rare).
- DERM: rash, urticaria.
- EENT: dry mouth, blurred vision, dental problems (with prolonged use).
- GI: constipation, nausea, bitter taste.
- GU: urine retention.
- Local: marked irritation, sterile abscess, and tissue induration (after S.C. administration).
- Other: hypersensitivity (tightness of chest, wheezing).
Note: Drug should be discontinued if hypersensitivity with tightness of chest, wheezing, tremor, or seizures occurs.

Overdose and treatment
Clinical manifestations of overdose include excessive sedation and hypotension; seizures may occur.

Treatment is supportive only. For recent oral ingestion, empty gastric contents through emesis or lavage. Correct hypotension with fluids and vasopressors (phenylephrine or metaraminol). Do not give epinephrine, because hydroxyzine may counteract its effect.

▶ **Special considerations**
● Observe patients for excessive sedation, especially those receiving other CNS depressants.
● Inject deep I.M. only; not for I.V., intra-arterial, or S.C. use. Aspirate injection carefully to prevent inadvertent intravascular administration.

Information for the patient
● Tell patient to avoid tasks that require mental alertness or physical coordination until the CNS effects of the drug are known; advise against use of other CNS depressants with hydroxyzine unless prescribed. Patient should avoid alcohol ingestion.
● Instruct patient to seek medical approval before taking any OTC cold or allergy preparations that contain antihistamines, which may potentiate the effects of hydroxyzine.
● Recommend use of sugarless gum or candy to help relieve dry mouth; advise drinking plenty of water to help with dry mouth or constipation.

Geriatric use
Elderly patients may experience greater CNS depression and anticholinergic effects. Lower doses are indicated.

Breast-feeding
It is unknown whether hydroxyzine passes into breast milk. Safe use has not been established in breast-feeding women.

---

lorazepam
Alzapam, Apo-Lorazepam∗, Ativan, Loraz, Novolorazem∗

● Pharmacologic classification: benzodiazepine
● Therapeutic classification: anxiolytic, sedative-hypnotic
● Controlled substance schedule IV
● Pregnancy risk category D

How supplied
Available by prescription only
Tablets: 0.5 mg, 1 mg, 2 mg
Sublingual tablets∗: 1 mg, 2 mg
Injection: 2 mg/ml, 4 mg/ml

Indications, route, and dosage
Anxiety, tension, agitation, irritability
Adults: 2 to 6 mg P.O. daily in divided doses. Maximum dosage is 10 mg/day.
Insomnia
Adults: 2 to 4 mg P.O. h.s.

Pharmacodynamics
Anxiolytic and sedative actions: Lorazepam depresses the CNS at the limbic and subcortical levels of the brain. It produces an anxiolytic effect by influencing the effect of the neurotransmitter gamma-aminobutyric acid on its receptor in the ascending reticular activating system, which increases inhibition and blocks both cortical and limbic arousal after stimulation of the reticular formation.

Pharmacokinetics
● *Absorption:* When administered orally, lorazepam is well absorbed through the GI tract. Peak levels occur in 2 hours.
● *Distribution:* Lorazepam is distributed widely throughout the body. Drug is about 85% protein-bound.
● *Metabolism:* Lorazepam has no active metabolites; glucuronide conjugation occurs in the liver.
● *Excretion:* The metabolites of lorazepam are excreted in urine as glucuronide conjugates.

Contraindications and precautions
Lorazepam is contraindicated in patients with known hypersensitivity to the drug or any ingredients in its formulation; in patients with acute narrow-angle glaucoma or untreated open-angle glaucoma because of the drug's possible anticholinergic effect; in patients in coma because the drug's hypnotic or hypotensive effect may be prolonged or intensified; and in patients with acute alcohol intoxication who have depressed vital signs because the drug will worsen CNS depression.

Lorazepam should be used cautiously in patients with psychoses because the drug is rarely beneficial in such patients and may induce paradoxical reactions; in patients with myasthenia gravis or Parkinson's disease because it may exacerbate the disorder; in patients with impaired hepatic function, which prolongs elimination of the drug; in elderly or debilitated patients, who are usually more sensitive to the drug's CNS effects; in individuals prone to addiction or drug abuse; and in patients with impaired respiratory function, such as chronic obstructive pulmonary disease.

Interactions
Lorazepam potentiates the CNS depressant effects of phenothiazines, narcotics, barbiturates, alcohol, antihistamines, MAO inhibitors, general anesthetics, and antidepressants.

Concomitant use with cimetidine and possibly disulfiram causes diminished hepatic me-

---

tabolism of lorazepam, which increases its plasma concentration.

Heavy smoking accelerates lorazepam's metabolism, thus lowering clinical effectiveness.

Combined use of parenteral lorazepam and scopolamine may be associated with an increased incidence of hallucinations, irrational behavior, and increased sedation.

Effects on diagnostic tests
None reported.

Adverse reactions
● CNS: confusion, depression, drowsiness, lethargy, hangover effect, ataxia, dizziness, syncope, nightmares, fatigue, slurred speech, tremor, vertigo, behavior problems, paradoxical excitement, weakness, headache.
● CV: bradycardia, *circulatory collapse,* transient hypotension.
● DERM: rash, urticaria.
● EENT: diplopia, blurred vision, nystagmus.
● GI: constipation, dry mouth, anorexia, difficulty swallowing, nausea, vomiting, abdominal discomfort.
● GU: urinary incontinence, urine retention.
● Other: *respiratory depression,* dysarthria, hepatic dysfunction, changes in libido.
   Note: Drug should be discontinued if hypersensitivity or the following paradoxical reactions occur: acute hyperexcited state, anxiety, hallucinations, increased muscle spasticity, insomnia, or rage.

Overdose and treatment
Clinical manifestations of overdose include somnolence, confusion, coma, hypoactive reflexes, dyspnea, labored breathing, hypotension, bradycardia, slurred speech, and unsteady gait or impaired coordination.

Treatment requires support of blood pressure and respiration until drug effects subside; monitor vital signs. Mechanical ventilatory assistance via endotracheal tube may be required to maintain a patent airway and support adequate oxygenation. Use I.V. fluids and vasopressors such as dopamine and phenylephrine to treat hypotension, if necessary. If patient is conscious, induce emesis with ipecac syrup. Use gastric lavage if ingestion was recent, but only if an endotracheal tube is present to prevent aspiration. After emesis or lavage, administer activated charcoal with a cathartic as a single dose. Dialysis is of limited value.

▶ Special considerations
Besides those relevant to all *benzodiazepines,* consider the following recommendations.
● Lorazepam is one of the preferred benzodiazepines for patients with hepatic disease. It is also useful in patients requiring parenteral therapy.
● Use lowest possible effective dose to avoid oversedation.
● After prolonged therapy, discontinue drug gradually to prevent withdrawal symptoms.
● Parenteral lorazepam appears to possess potent amnesic effects.
● Administer oral lorazepam in divided doses, with the largest dose given before bedtime.
● Arteriospasm may result from intra-arterial injection of lorazepam. Do not administer by this route.
● For I.V. administration, dilute lorazepam with an equal volume of a compatible diluent, such as dextrose 5% in water, sterile water for injection, or normal saline solution.
● Lorazepam may be injected directly into a vein or into the tubing of a compatible I.V. infusion, such as 0.9% saline solution or 5% dextrose solution. The rate of lorazepam I.V. injection should not exceed 2 mg/minute. Emergency resuscitative equipment should be available when administering I.V.
● Administer diluted lorazepam solutions immediately.
● Do not use lorazepam solutions if they are discolored or contain a precipitate.
● Administer I.M. dose of lorazepam undiluted, deep into a large muscle mass.

Information for the patient
● Caution patient not to make any changes in medication regimen without specific instructions.
● As appropriate, teach safety measures to protect from injury, such as gradual position changes and supervised walking.
● Advise patient of possible retrograde amnesia after I.V. or I.M. use.
● Advise patient to avoid large amounts of caffeine-containing products, which may interfere with lorazepam's effectiveness.
● Advise patient of potential for physical and psychological dependence with chronic use.

Geriatric use
● Elderly patients are more sensitive to lorazepam's CNS depressant effects. They may require supervision with ambulation and activities of daily living during initiation of therapy or after an increase in dose.

• Lower doses usually are effective in elderly patients because of decreased elimination.
• Parenteral administration of lorazepam is more likely to cause apnea, hypotension, bradycardia, and cardiac arrest in elderly patients.

Pediatric use
• Safe use of oral lorazepam in children under age 12 has not been established.
• Safe use of sublingual or parenteral lorazepam in children under age 18 has not been established.
• Closely observe neonate for withdrawal symptoms if the mother took lorazepam for a prolonged period during pregnancy.

Breast-feeding
Lorazepam may be excreted in breast milk. Do not administer to breast-feeding women.

---

meprobamate
Apo-Meprobamate∗, Equanil, Meditran∗, Meprospan, Miltown, Neuramate, Novomepro∗, Sedabamate, SK-Bamate, Tranmep

• Pharmacologic classification: propanediol carbamate
• Therapeutic classification: anxiolytic
• Controlled substance schedule IV
• Pregnancy risk category D

How supplied
Available by prescription only
Tablets: 200 mg, 400 mg, 600 mg
Capsules: 200 mg, 400 mg
Capsules (sustained-release): 200 mg, 400 mg

Indications, route, and dosage
Anxiety and tension
Adults: 1.2 to 1.6 g P.O. in three or four equally divided doses. Maximum dosage is 2.4 g daily.
Children ages 6 to 12: 100 to 200 mg P.O. b.i.d. or t.i.d. Not recommended for children under age 6.

Pharmacodynamics
Anxiolytic action: Although the cellular mechanism of meprobamate is unknown, the drug causes nonselective CNS depression similar to that seen with use of barbiturates. Meprobamate acts at multiple sites in the CNS, including the thalamus, hypothalamus, limbic system, and spinal cord but not the medulla or reticular activating system.

Pharmacokinetics
• *Absorption:* After oral administration, meprobamate is well absorbed; peak serum levels occur in 1 to 3 hours. Sedation usually occurs within 1 hour.
• *Distribution:* Meprobamate is distributed throughout the body; 20% is protein-bound. The drug occurs in breast milk at two to four times the serum concentration; meprobamate crosses the placenta.
• *Metabolism:* Meprobamate is metabolized rapidly in the liver to inactive glucuronide conjugates.
• *Excretion:* The metabolites of meprobamate and 10% to 20% of a single dose as unchanged drug are excreted in urine.

Contraindications and precautions
Meprobamate is contraindicated in patients with known hypersensitivity to the drug or other carbamates and in patients with intermittent porphyria. Some formulations contain tartrazine, which is contraindicated in patients allergic to aspirin (because significant cross-reactivity has been demonstrated).

Meprobamate should be used cautiously in patients with impaired renal or hepatic function and in patients with depression, suicidal tendencies, or a history of drug abuse or addiction.

Meprobamate is not useful as an anticonvulsant and may precipitate seizures or lower seizure threshold. Use cautiously, if at all, in patients with a history of seizures or an active seizure disorder.

Interactions
Meprobamate may add to or potentiate the effects of alcohol, barbiturates, antihistamines, tranquilizers, narcotics, or other CNS depressants.

Effects on diagnostic tests
Meprobamate therapy may falsely elevate urinary 17-ketosteroids (as determined by the Zimmerman reaction), and 17-hydroxycorticosteroid levels (as determined by the Glenn-Nelson technique).

Adverse reactions
• CNS: dizziness, drowsiness, ataxia, slurred speech, headache, vertigo, weakness, euphoria, paradoxical excitation.
• CV: palpitations, arrhythmias, syncope, hypotension, tachycardia.
• DERM: pruritus, urticaria, dermatitis, erythematous maculopapular rash, *exfoliative dermatitis, erythema multiforme.*

- EENT: blurred vision.
- GI: anorexia, nausea, vomiting, diarrhea, stomatitis.
- HEMA: *agranulocytosis,* thrombocytopenic purpura, *aplastic anemia,* pancytopenia (rare).
- Other: hypersensitivity (eosinophilia, hyperpyrexia, chills, *bronchospasm,* angioedema, *Stevens-Johnson syndrome, anaphylaxis).*

Note: Drug should be discontinued if hypersensitivity, paradoxical excitation with EEG changes, severe prolonged hypotension, skin rash, sore throat, or unusual bleeding or bruising occurs.

Overdose and treatment
Clinical manifestations of overdose are similar to those seen after barbiturate overdose and include drowsiness, lethargy, ataxia, coma, hypotension, shock, and respiratory depression.

Treatment of overdose is supportive and symptomatic including maintaining adequate ventilation and a patent airway, with mechanical ventilation if needed.

Treat hypotension with fluids and vasopressors as needed. Empty gastric contents by emesis or lavage if ingestion was recent, followed by activated charcoal and a cathartic. Treat seizures with parenteral diazepam. Peritoneal and hemodialysis may effectively remove the drug. Serum levels greater than 100 mcg/ml may be fatal.

▶ Special considerations
- Many clinicians consider meprobamate no longer useful because it has been replaced by other safer, more effective drugs, such as benzodiazepines.
- Assess level of consciousness and vital signs frequently.
- Impose safety precautions, such as raised bed rails, especially for elderly patients, when initiating treatment or increasing the dose. Patient may need assistance when walking.
- Periodic evaluation of complete blood count is recommended during long-term therapy.
- The possibility of abuse and addiction exists.
- Discontinue drug gradually; otherwise, withdrawal symptoms may occur if patient has been taking the drug for a long time. Observe patient closely for 48 hours after discontinuation.

Information for the patient
- Tell patient to avoid other CNS depressants, such as antihistamines, narcotics, and tranquilizers, while taking this drug, unless prescribed. Tell patient to avoid alcoholic beverages while on drug.
- Advise patient not to increase the dose or frequency and not to abruptly discontinue or decrease the dose unless prescribed.
- Tell patient to avoid tasks that require mental alertness or physical coordination until the drug's CNS effects are known.
- Advise patient that sugarless candy or gum or ice chips can help relieve dry mouth.
- Advise patient to report any sore throat, fever, or unusual bleeding or bruising.
- Advise patient of the potential for physical or psychological dependence with chronic use.

Geriatric use
Elderly patients may have more pronounced CNS effects. Use lowest dose possible.

Pediatric use
Safety has not been established in children under age 6.

Breast-feeding
The drug is found in breast milk at two to four times the serum concentration. Do not use in breast-feeding women.

---

oxazepam
Apo-Oxazepam∗, Novoxapam∗, Ox-Pam∗, Serax, Zapex∗

- Pharmacologic classification: benzodiazepine
- Therapeutic classification: anxiolytic, sedative-hypnotic
- Controlled substance schedule IV
- Pregnancy risk category D

How supplied
Available by prescription only
Tablets: 15 mg
Capsules: 10 mg, 15 mg, 30 mg

Indications, route, and dosage
Alcohol withdrawal
Adults: 15 to 30 mg P.O. t.i.d. or q.i.d.
Severe anxiety; anxiety associated with depression
Adults: 10 to 30 mg P.O. t.i.d. or q.i.d.
Tension, mild to moderate anxiety
Adults: 10 to 15 mg P.O. t.i.d. or q.i.d.

Pharmacodynamics
Anxiolytic and sedative-hypnotic action: Oxazepam depresses the CNS at the limbic and subcortical levels of the brain. It produces an anx-

iolytic effect by enhancing the effect of the neurotransmitter gamma-aminobutyric acid on its receptor in the ascending reticular activating system, which increases inhibition and blocks both cortical and limbic arousal.

Pharmacokinetics
● *Absorption:* When administered orally, oxazepam is well absorbed through the GI tract. Peak levels occur in 1 to 4 hours. Onset of action occurs at 60 to 120 minutes.
● *Distribution:* Oxazepam is distributed widely throughout the body. Drug is 85% to 95% protein-bound.
● *Metabolism:* Oxazepam has no active metabolites; glucuronide conjugation occurs in the liver.
● *Excretion:* The metabolites of oxazepam are excreted in urine as glucuronide conjugates. The half-life of oxazepam ranges from 5 to 13 hours.

Contraindications and precautions
Oxazepam is contraindicated in patients with known hypersensitivity to the drug; in patients with acute narrow-angle glaucoma or untreated open-angle glaucoma because of the drug's possible anticholinergic effects; in patients in coma because the drug's hypnotic effect may be prolonged or intensified; and in patients with acute alcohol intoxication who have depressed vital signs because the drug will worsen CNS depression. Oxazepam tablets contain tartrazine, which may induce allergic reaction in hypersensitive individuals. Patients allergic to aspirin exhibit a high incidence of cross-sensitivity.

Oxazepam should be used cautiously in patients with psychoses because the drug is rarely beneficial in such patients and may induce paradoxical reactions; in patients with myasthenia gravis or Parkinson's disease because it may exacerbate the disorder; in patients with impaired renal or hepatic function, which prolongs elimination of the drug; in elderly or debilitated patients, who are usually more sensitive to the drug's CNS effects; and in individuals prone to addiction or drug abuse.

Interactions
Oxazepam potentiates the CNS depressant effects of phenothiazines, narcotics, antihistamines, MAO inhibitors, barbiturates, alcohol, general anesthetics, and antidepressants.

Concomitant use with cimetidine and possibly disulfiram causes diminished hepatic metabolism of oxazepam, which increases its plasma concentration.

Heavy smoking accelerates oxazepam metabolism, thus lowering clinical effectiveness.

Antacids may decrease the rate of oxazepam absorption.

Oxazepam may inhibit the therapeutic effects of levodopa.

Effects on diagnostic tests
Oxazepam therapy may increase liver function test results. Changes in EEG patterns, usually low-voltage and fast activity, may occur during and after oxazepam therapy.

Adverse reactions
● CNS: confusion, depression, drowsiness, lethargy, hangover effect, ataxia, dizziness, syncope, nightmares, fatigue, slurred speech, tremor, vertigo, headache, behavior problems.
● CV: bradycardia, *circulatory collapse,* transient hypotension.
● DERM: rash, urticaria.
● EENT: diplopia, blurred vision, nystagmus.
● GI: constipation, dry mouth, anorexia, nausea, vomiting, abdominal discomfort.
● GU: urinary incontinence, urine retention.
● Other: *respiratory depression,* dysarthria, hepatic dysfunction, changes in libido.
Note: Drug should be discontinued if the following paradoxical reactions occur: acute hyperexcited state, anxiety, hallucinations, increased muscle spasticity, insomnia, or rage.

Overdose and treatment
Clinical manifestations of overdose include somnolence, confusion, coma, hypoactive reflexes, dyspnea, labored breathing, hypotension, bradycardia, slurred speech, and unsteady gait or impaired coordination.

Support blood pressure and respiration until the drug effects have subsided; monitor vital signs. Mechanical ventilatory assistance via endotracheal tube may be required to maintain a patent airway and support adequate oxygenation. As needed, use I.V. fluids and vasopressors such as dopamine and phenylephrine to treat hypotension. If the patient is conscious, induce emesis. Use gastric lavage if ingestion was recent, but only if an endotracheal tube is present to prevent aspiration. After emesis or lavage, administer activated charcoal with a cathartic as a single dose. Dialysis is of limited value.

▶ **Special considerations**
Besides those relevant to all *benzodiazepines,* consider the following recommendations.
● Monitor hepatic and renal function studies to ensure normal function.

- Oxazepam tablets contain tartrazine dye; check patient's history for allergy to this substance.
- Store in a cool, dry place away from light.

Information for the patient
- Advise patient not to change any part of medication regimen without medical approval.
- Instruct patient in safety measures, such as gradual position changes and supervised ambulation, to prevent injury.
- Sleepiness may not occur for up to 2 hours after taking oxazepam; tell patient to wait before taking an additional dose.
- Advise patient of potential for physical and psychological dependence with chronic use of oxazepam.

Geriatric use
- Elderly patients are more susceptible to the CNS depressant effects of oxazepam. Some may require supervision with ambulation and activities of daily living during initiation of therapy or after an increase in dose.
- Lower doses are usually effective in elderly patients because of decreased elimination.

Pediatric use
Safe use in children under age 12 has not been established. Closely observe neonate for withdrawal symptoms if mother took oxazepam for a prolonged period during pregnancy.

Breast-feeding
The breast-fed infant of a woman who uses oxazepam may become sedated, have feeding difficulties, or lose weight; avoid use in breast-feeding women.

---

prazepam
Centrax

- Pharmacologic classification: benzodiazepine
- Therapeutic classification: anxiolytic
- Controlled substance schedule IV
- Pregnancy risk category D

How supplied
Available by prescription only
Tablets: 10 mg
Capsules: 5 mg, 10 mg, 20 mg

Indications, route, and dosage
Anxiety
Adults: 30 mg P.O. daily in divided doses. Dosage range is 20 to 60 mg/day. May be administered as single daily dose h.s. with an initial dose of 20 mg.

Pharmacodynamics
Anxiolytic action: Prazepam depresses the CNS at the limbic and subcortical levels of the brain. It produces an anxiolytic effect by enhancing the effect of the neurotransmitter gamma-aminobutyric acid on its receptor in the ascending reticular activating system, which increases inhibition and blocks both cortical and limbic arousal.

Pharmacokinetics
- *Absorption:* When administered orally, prazepam is well absorbed through the GI tract. Peak levels occur in 2½ to 6 hours. Prazepam undergoes nearly complete first-pass metabolism to desmethyldiazepam after absorption.
- *Distribution:* Prazepam is distributed widely throughout the body. Drug is 85% to 95% protein-bound.
- *Metabolism:* Prazepam is metabolized in the liver to desmethyldiazepam and oxazepam.
- *Excretion:* The metabolites of prazepam are excreted in urine as glucuronide conjugates. The half-life of desmethyldiazepam ranges from 30 to 200 hours; oxazepam, from 5 to 15 hours.

Contraindications and precautions
Prazepam is contraindicated in patients with known hypersensitivity to the drug; in those with acute narrow-angle glaucoma or untreated open-angle glaucoma because of the drug's possible anticholinergic effect; in patients in coma because the drug's hypnotic or hypotensive effect may be prolonged or intensified; and in patients with acute alcohol intoxication who have depressed vital signs because the drug will worsen CNS depression.

Prazepam should be used cautiously in patients with psychoses because the drug is rarely beneficial in such patients and may induce paradoxical reactions; in patients with myasthenia gravis or Parkinson's disease because it may exacerbate the disorder; in patients with impaired renal or hepatic function, which prolongs elimination of the drug; in elderly or debilitated patients, who are usually more sensitive to the drug's CNS effects; and in individuals prone to addiction or drug abuse.

Interactions

Prazepam potentiates the CNS depressant effects of phenothiazines, narcotics, antihistamines, MAO inhibitors, barbiturates, alcohol, general anesthetics, and antidepressants.

Concomitant use with cimetidine and possibly disulfiram causes diminished hepatic metabolism of prazepam, which increases its plasma concentration.

Heavy smoking accelerates prazepam's metabolism, thus lowering clinical effectiveness.

Antacids may delay the absorption of prazepam. Prazepam may antagonize levodopa's therapeutic effects.

Effects on diagnostic tests

Prazepam therapy may elevate liver function test results. Minor changes in EEG patterns, usually low-voltage and fast activity, may occur during and after prazepam therapy.

Adverse reactions

● CNS: confusion, depression, drowsiness, lethargy, hangover effect, ataxia, dizziness, syncope, nightmares, fatigue, slurred speech, tremor, vertigo, behavior problems, headache.
● CV: bradycardia, *circulatory collapse,* transient hypotension.
● DERM: rash, urticaria.
● EENT: diplopia, blurred vision, nystagmus.
● GI: constipation, dry mouth, anorexia, nausea, vomiting, abdominal discomfort.
● GU: urinary incontinence, urine retention.
● Other: *respiratory depression,* dysarthria, hepatic dysfunction, changes in libido.

Note: Drug should be discontinued if hypersensitivity or the following paradoxical reactions occur: acute hyperexcited state, anxiety, hallucinations, increased muscle spasticity, insomnia, or rage.

Overdose and treatment

Clinical manifestations of overdose include somnolence, confusion, coma, hypoactive reflexes, dyspnea, labored breathing, hypotension, bradycardia, slurred speech, and unsteady gait or impaired coordination.

Support blood pressure and respiration until drug effects subside; monitor vital signs. Mechanical ventilatory assistance via endotracheal tube may be required to maintain a patent airway and support adequate oxygenation. Use I.V. fluids and vasopressors such as dopamine and phenylephrine to treat hypotension, as needed. If patient is conscious, induce emesis with ipecac syrup. Use gastric lavage if ingestion was recent but only if an endotracheal tube is present to prevent aspiration. After emesis or lavage, administer activated charcoal with a cathartic as a single dose. Dialysis is of limited value.

▶ Special considerations

Besides those relevant to all *benzodiazepines,* consider the following recommendations.
● Use lowest possible effective dose. Gradually increase dose as necessary to avoid adverse reactions.
● Lower doses are effective in patients with renal or hepatic dysfunction.
● Monitor hepatic function studies periodically to prevent toxicity.
● Do not discontinue drug suddenly if patient is on long-term therapy.

Information for the patient

● As necessary, teach patient safety measures to prevent injury, such as gradual position changes and supervised ambulation.
● Caution patient to seek medical approval before making any changes in drug regimen.
● Advise patient of the potential for physical and psychological dependence with chronic use.
● Do not discontinue drug suddenly if patient has received long-term therapy.

Geriatric use

● Lower doses usually are effective in elderly patients because of decreased elimination.
● Elderly patients are more susceptible to the CNS depressant effects of prazepam. Use with caution.
● Elderly patients who receive this drug require supervision with ambulation and activities of daily living during initiation of therapy or after an increase in dose.

Pediatric use

● Safe use in patients under age 18 has not been established.
● Closely observe a neonate for withdrawal symptoms if mother took prazepam during pregnancy. Use of prazepam during labor may cause neonatal flaccidity.

Breast-feeding

Prazepam is excreted in breast milk. A breast-fed infant may become sedated, have feeding difficulties, or lose weight. Avoid use in breast-feeding women.

---

propranolol hydrochloride
Inderal, Inderal LA

- Pharmacologic classification: beta-adrenergic blocker
- Therapeutic classification: antihypertensive, antianginal, antiarrhythmic, anxiolytic
- Pregnancy risk category C

How supplied
Available by prescription only
Tablets: 10 mg, 20 mg, 40 mg, 60 mg, 80 mg, 90 mg
Capsules (extended-release): 80 mg, 120 mg, 160 mg
Injection: 1 mg/ml

Indications, route, and dosage
Prevention of frequent, severe, uncontrollable, or disabling migraine or vascular headache
Adults: Initially, 80 mg daily in divided doses or one sustained-release capsule once daily. Usual maintenance dosage is 160 to 240 mg daily, divided t.i.d. or q.i.d.
†*Adjunctive treatment of anxiety*
Adults: 10 to 80 mg P.O. 1 hour before anxiety-provoking activity.
†*Treatment of essential, familial, or senile movement tremor*
Adults: 40 mg P.O. t.i.d. or q.i.d. as tolerated and needed.
†*Intermittent explosive disorder;* †*symptoms of acute panic;* †*uncontrolled aggression as a sequela to traumatic brain injury*
Adults: Initially, 40 mg P.O. q.i.d. Titrate dosage as needed to a maximum of 360 mg/day.
†*Tardive dyskinesia*
Adults: 30 to 80 mg P.O. daily in divided doses.

Pharmacodynamics
- *Anxiolytic action:* The mechanism by which propranolol decreases anxiety is unknown. As a beta-adrenergic blocker, it decreases cardiac output and may reduce sympathetic outflow from the CNS. It acts peripherally to reduce skeletal muscle tremor. The drug lowers blood pressure and heart rate and may inhibit some of the physical symptoms of anxiety. Some clinicians believe that if the physical symptoms of anxiety are not perceived, anxiety is not reinforced.

Pharmacokinetics
- *Absorption:* Propranolol is absorbed almost completely from the GI tract. Absorption is enhanced when given with food. Peak plasma concentrations occur 60 to 90 minutes after administration of regular-release tablets. After I.V. administration, peak concentrations occur in about 1 minute, with virtually immediate onset of action.
- *Distribution:* Propranolol is distributed widely throughout the body; drug is more than 90% protein-bound.
- *Metabolism:* Hepatic metabolism is almost total; oral dosage form undergoes extensive first-pass metabolism.
- *Excretion:* Approximately 96% to 99% of a given dose of propranolol is excreted in urine as metabolites; remainder is excreted in feces as unchanged drug and metabolites. Biological half-life is about 4 hours.

Contraindications and precautions
Propranolol is contraindicated in patients with known hypersensitivity to the drug; in patients with overt cardiac failure, sinus bradycardia, second- or third-degree AV block, bronchial asthma, cardiogenic shock, and Raynaud's syndrome, because drug may worsen these conditions.

Propranolol should be used cautiously in patients with coronary insufficiency because beta-adrenergic blockade may precipitate CHF; in patients with pulmonary disease; in patients with diabetes mellitus, hypoglycemia, or hyperthyroidism because propranolol may mask tachycardia (it does not mask dizziness and sweating caused by hypoglycemia); and in patients with impaired hepatic function. Propranolol may also mask common signs of shock.

Interactions
Concomitant use with cardiac glycosides potentiates bradycardia and myocardial depressant effects of propranolol; cimetidine may decrease clearance of propranolol via inhibition of hepatic metabolism and thus also enhance its beta blocking effects.

Propranolol may potentiate antihypertensive effects of other antihypertensive agents, especially catecholamine-depleting agents such as reserpine.

Propranolol may antagonize beta-adrenergic stimulating effects of sympathomimetic agents such as isoproterenol and of MAO inhibitors; use with epinephrine causes severe vasoconstriction.

Atropine, tricyclic antidepressants, and other

---

drugs with anticholinergic effects may antagonize propranolol-induced bradycardia; nonsteroidal anti-inflammatory drugs may antagonize its hypotensive effects.

High doses of propranolol may potentiate neuromuscular blocking effect of tubocurarine and related compounds.

Concomitant use with insulin or hypoglycemic agents can alter dosage requirements in previously stable diabetic patients.

Effects on diagnostic tests
Propranolol may elevate serum transaminase, alkaline phosphatase, and lactate dehydrogenase levels and may elevate BUN levels in patients with severe heart disease.

Adverse reactions
- CNS: fatigue, lethargy, vivid dreams, hallucinations.
- CV: bradycardia, hypotension, *CHF,* peripheral vascular disease.
- DERM: rash.
- GI: nausea, vomiting, diarrhea.
- GU: impotence.
- Metabolic: hypoglycemia without tachycardia.
- Other: *bronchospasm,* fever, arthralgia.
  Note: Drug should be discontinued if signs of heart failure or bronchospasm develop.

Overdose and treatment
Clinical signs of overdose include severe hypotension, bradycardia, heart failure, and bronchospasm.

After acute ingestion, induce emesis or empty stomach by gastric lavage; follow with activated charcoal to reduce absorption, and administer symptomatic and supportive care. Treat bradycardia with atropine (0.25 to 1 mg); if no response, administer isoproterenol cautiously. Treat cardiac failure with digitalis and diuretics and hypotension with vasopressors: epinephrine is preferred. Treat bronchospasm with isoproterenol and aminophylline.

▶ **Special considerations**
Propranolol also has been used to treat aggression and rage, stage fright, recurrent GI bleeding in cirrhotic patients, and menopausal symptoms.

Information for the patient
Advise patient to take drug with meals because food increases absorption.

Geriatric use
Elderly patients may require lower maintenance doses of propranolol because of increased bioavailability or delayed metabolism; they also may experience enhanced adverse reactions.

Pediatric use
The safety of propranolol as an anxiolytic in children has not been established.

Breast-feeding
Propranolol is distributed into breast milk; an alternate feeding method is recommended during therapy.

CNS stimulants

amphetamine sulfate
benzphetamine hydrochloride
dextroamphetamine sulfate
diethylproprion hydrochloride
fenfluramine
mazindol
methamphetamine hydrochloride
methylphenidate hydrochloride
pemoline
phendinmetrazine tartrate
phenmetrazine hydrochloride
phentermine hydrochloride

CNS stimulants increase the activity of portions of the brain or spinal cord and are among the most commonly prescribed for hyperactivity, minimal brain dysfunction, and attention deficit disorders in children. They are divided into two groups: analeptics and anorexiants.

CNS stimulants have sometimes dramatic pharmacologic effects but are less important therapeutically than the CNS depressants. The effectiveness of stimulants is related to their ability to enhance excitation of the CNS, which increases motor activity, enhances mental alertness, brightens mood, and combats mental fatigue. They were once used to treat drug-induced central depression, postanesthesia respiratory depression or apnea, and acute chronic obstructive pulmonary disease associated with hypercapnea; however, in most cases, mechanical ventilator support is more effective.

Pharmacologic effects
● *Analeptics* (amphetamine, dextroamphetamine, methamphetamine, methylphenidate, pemolin) are useful in treating hyperactive behavior in children or narcolepsy in adults.
● *Anorexiants* (benzphetamine, diethylpropion, fenfluramine, mazindol, phendimetrazine, phenmetrazine, phentermine) are used as short-term adjuncts in weight reduction.

Mechanism of action
The analeptics have sympathomimetic activity, but their exact mechanism of action in producing CNS stimulation has not been determined. Anorexiants are indirect-acting sympathomimetic amines with an unknown mechanism of action. It is thought, however, that their effect on appetite may result from direct stimulation of the satiety centers in the hypothalamus and limbic areas.

Pharmacokinetics
● *Absorption and distribution:* All CNS stimulants are well absorbed. They achieve peak levels as follows: psychostimulants, within 3 hours after oral dosage, and anorexiants, 4 to 6 hours after oral dosage (except mazindol, 8 to 15 hours). All are widely distributed and most cross the blood-brain barrier and the placenta.
● *Metabolism and excretion:* All CNS stimulants are metabolized in the liver and excreted in urine as unchanged drug and/or metabolites. Urinary acidification results in more rapid excretion.

Adverse reactions and toxicity
Adverse reactions result from CNS stimulation and most commonly include insomnia, restlessness, muscular tremor, headaches, light-headedness, palpitations, diuresis, and overstimulation. After prolonged use, withdrawal symptoms may occur if the drug is stopped abruptly; the severity and duration of withdrawal symptoms vary depending on the drug.

Treatment of overdose is symptomatic and supportive and may include gastric lavage.

Clinical considerations
● Patients should be advised to take CNS stimulants early in the day to avoid nighttime insomnia and warned not to take more frequently than prescribed.
● For weight reduction, clinicians recommend a 3- to 6-week treatment followed by a discontinuation for half the original treatment period.

---

*Canada only   †Unlabeled clinical use   Italicized adverse reactions are life-threatening.

COMPARING CNS STIMULANTS

DRUG	USUAL ADULT DOSAGE	HALF-LIFE	COMMENTS
amphetamine	5 mg t.i.d.	5 to 21 hours	Very high abuse potential; Drug Enforcement Agency (DEA) schedule II
			Excretion is pH dependent. When urine pH is < 5.6, half-life is 7 to 8 hours when urine pH is raised to > 7, half-life increases to 18 to 30 hours.
benzphetamine	25 to 50 mg daily	4 hours	High abuse potential; DEA schedule III
dextroamphetamine	5 mg t.i.d.	5 to 21 hours	Very high abuse potential; DEA schedule II
			Excretion is pH dependent. When urine pH is < 5.6, half-life is 7 to 8 hours; when urine pH is raised to > 7, half-life increases to 18 to 30 hours.
diethylproprion	25 mg t.i.d.	Data unavailable	DEA schedule IV
fenfluramine	20 mg t.i.d.	18 hours	DEA schedule IV
			Excretion is pH dependent; when urine pH is < 6, half-life is reduced to 11 hours.
mazindol	1 mg t.i.d.	36 hours	DEA schedule IV
methamphetamine	5 mg daily	12 to 20 hours	Very high abuse potential; DEA schedule II
			Excretion is pH dependent; decreasing urine pH to < 6 greatly reduces half-life
methylphenidate	20 to 30 mg daily	1 to 3 hours	Very high abuse potential; DEA schedule II
pemoline	56.25 to 75 mg daily	12 hours	DEA schedule IV
			Children may exhibit shorter plasma half-life (8 hours)
phendimetrazine	35 mg b.i.d.	2 to 10 hours	High abuse potential; DEA schedule III
phenmetrazine	75 mg daily	Data unavailable	Very high abuse potential; DEA schedule II
phentermine	8 mg t.i.d.	Data unavailable	DEA schedule IV

■■■■■■■■■■

amphetamine sulfate

- Pharmacologic classification: amphetamine
- Therapeutic classification: CNS stimulant, short-term adjunctive anorexigenic agent, sympathomimetic amine
- Controlled substance schedule II
- Pregnancy risk category D

How supplied
Available by prescription only
Tablets: 5 mg, 10 mg
Capsules: 5 mg, 10 mg

Indications, route, and dosage
Attention deficit disorder with hyperactivity

Children ages 6 and older: 5 mg P.O. daily. Increase at 5-mg increments weekly until desired response. Dosage rarely exceeds 40 mg/day.
Children ages 3 to 5: 2.5 mg P.O. daily. Increase at 2.5-mg increments weekly until desired response.
Narcolepsy
Adults: 5 to 60 mg P.O. daily in divided doses.
Children over age 12: 10 mg P.O. daily. Increase at 10-mg increments weekly p.r.n.

Children ages 6 to 12: 5 mg P.O. daily. Increase at 5-mg increments weekly p.r.n.

Children under age 6: Dosage seldom exceeds 40 mg daily.

Short-term adjunct in exogenous obesity

Adults: 5 to 30 mg P.O. daily in divided doses 30 to 60 minutes before meals. Not recommended for children under age 12.

†**Short-term treatment of depression in patients intolerant of tricyclic antidepressants**

Adults: 5 to 10 mg P.O. b.i.d. 30 minutes before meals.

Pharmacodynamics

● *CNS stimulant action:* Amphetamines are sympathomimetic amines with CNS stimulant activity; in hyperactive children, they have a paradoxical calming effect. Amphetamines are used to treat narcolepsy and as adjuncts to psychosocial measures in attention deficit disorder in children. The cerebral cortex and reticular activating system appear to be their primary sites of activity; amphetamines release nerve terminal stores of norepinephrine, promoting nerve impulse transmission. At high dosages, effects are mediated by dopamine.

Pharmacokinetics

● *Absorption:* Amphetamine sulfate is absorbed completely within 3 hours after oral administration; therapeutic effects persist for 4 to 24 hours.

● *Distribution:* Amphetamine sulfate is distributed widely throughout the body, with high concentrations in the brain. Therapeutic plasma levels are 5 to 10 mcg/dl.

● *Metabolism:* Amphetamine sulfate is metabolized by hydroxylation and deamination in the liver.

● *Excretion:* Amphetamine sulfate is excreted in urine.

Contraindications and precautions

Amphetamines are contraindicated in patients with hypersensitivity or idiosyncratic reaction to sympathomimetic amines; in those with symptomatic CV disease, hyperthyroidism, nephritis, angina pectoris, hypertension, glaucoma, advanced arteriosclerosis, or agitated states; and in patients with a history of drug or alcohol abuse. They also are contraindicated for concomitant use with or within 14 days of discontinuing MAO inhibitors.

Amphetamines should be used with caution in patients with diabetes mellitus; in elderly, debilitated, or hyperexcitable patients; and in children with Gilles de la Tourette's syndrome. Avoid long-term therapy, when possible, because of the risk of physical or psychological dependence.

Interactions

Concomitant use with MAO inhibitors (or drugs with MAO-inhibiting effects, such as furazolidone) or within 14 days of such therapy may cause hypertensive crisis; concomitant use with antihypertensives may antagonize their hypertensive effects.

Concomitant use with antacids, sodium bicarbonate, or acetazolamide may enhance reabsorption of amphetamines and prolong their duration of action, whereas concomitant use with ammonium chloride or ascorbic acid enhances amphetamine excretion or shortens duration of action. Use with phenothiazines or haloperidol decreases amphetamine effects; barbiturates counteract amphetamines by CNS depression, whereas caffeine or other CNS stimulants produce additive effects.

Amphetamines may alter insulin requirements.

Effects on diagnostic tests

Amphetamines may elevate plasma corticosteroid levels and also may interfere with urinary steroid determinations.

Adverse reactions

● CNS: restlessness, tremor, hyperactivity, talkativeness, insomnia, irritability, dizziness, headache, chills, overstimulation, dysphoria, psychosis, paranoid ideation.

● CV: tachycardia, palpitations, hypertension, hypotension.

● GI: nausea, vomiting, cramps, dry mouth, diarrhea, constipation, metallic taste, anorexia, weight loss.

● GU: changes in libido, impotence.

● Other: urticaria, tolerance, physical and psychological dependence.

Note: Drug should be discontinued if signs of hypersensitivity or idiosyncrasy occur.

Overdose and treatment

Symptoms of acute overdose include increasing restlessness, irritability, insomnia, tremor, hyperreflexia, diaphoresis, mydriasis, flushing, confusion, hypertension, tachypnea, fever, delirium, self-injury, arrhythmias, seizures, coma, circulatory collapse, and death.

Treat overdose symptomatically and supportively: if ingestion is recent (within 4 hours) use gastric lavage or emesis with ipecac syrup;

---

activated charcoal, saline catharsis, and urinary acidification may enhance excretion. Forced fluid diuresis may help. In massive ingestion, hemodialysis or peritoneal dialysis may be needed. Keep patient in a cool room, monitor his temperature, and minimize external stimulation. Haloperidol may be used for psychotic symptoms; diazepam, for hyperactivity.

▶ Special considerations
Recommendations for administration of amphetamine sulfate, for care and teaching of the patient during therapy, and for use in elderly or breast-feeding patients are the same as those for all *amphetamines.*
● Avoid administration late in the day (after 4 p.m.) to prevent insomnia.
● The first dose is usually given upon awakening, additional doses at 4- to 6-hour intervals.
● Amphetamines are not recommended for the treatment of obesity because their effectiveness in appetite suppression is transient.

Pediatric use
Amphetamines are not recommended for weight reduction in children under age 12; use of amphetamines for hyperactivity is contraindicated in children under age 3. Temporary suppression of normal growth has followed long-term use of amphetamines; such use must be monitored carefully.

---

benzphetamine hydrochloride
Didrex

● Pharmacologic classification: amphetamine
● Therapeutic classification: short-term adjunctive anorexigenic agent for refractory exogenous obesity, sympathomimetic amine
● Controlled substance schedule III
● Pregnancy risk category X

How supplied
Available by prescription only
Tablets: 25 mg, 50 mg

Indications, route, and dosage
Short-term adjunct in exogenous obesity
Adults: 25 to 50 mg P.O. daily b.i.d. or t.i.d., preferably b.i.d., given midmorning and midafternoon.

Pharmacodynamics
Anorexigenic action: The precise mechanism of action for appetite control is unknown; anorexigenic effects are thought to occur in the hypothalamus, where decreased smell and taste acuity decreases appetite. The cerebral cortex and reticular activating system appear to be the primary sites of activity; amphetamines release nerve terminal stores of norepinephrine, promoting nerve impulse transmission. At high doses, effects are mediated by dopamine.

Benzphetamine is used as an adjunct in the short-term control of refractory obesity, with caloric restriction and behavior modification.

Pharmacokinetics
● *Absorption:* Benzphetamine is readily absorbed from the GI tract; effects persist for about 4 hours after oral administration.
● *Distribution:* Widely distributed throughout the body.
● *Metabolism:* Metabolized by the liver.
● *Excretion:* Excreted in urine.

Contraindications and precautions
Benzphetamine is contraindicated in patients with hypersensitivity or idiosyncratic reaction to sympathomimetic amines; in those with hyperthyroidism, nephritis, glaucoma, any degree of hypertension, angina pectoris, other symptomatic CV disease, arteriosclerosis-induced parkinsonism, advanced arteriosclerosis, or agitated states; and in patients with a history of substance abuse. It also is contraindicated for concomitant use with or within 14 days of discontinuing MAO inhibitors.

The 25-mg tablet contains tartrazine and is contraindicated in patients with asthma or aspirin allergy. Benzphetamine should be used with caution in patients with diabetes mellitus and in elderly, debilitated, or hyperexcitable patients.

Interactions
Concomitant use of benzphetamine with MAO inhibitors (or drugs with MAO-inhibiting activity, such as furazolidone) or within 14 days of such therapy may cause hypertensive crisis; use with antihypertensives may antagonize the antihypertensive effects.

Concomitant use with antacids, sodium bicarbonate, or acetazolamide enhances renal reabsorption of benzphetamine and prolongs its duration of action. Use with phenothiazines or haloperidol may decrease benzphetamine effects. Concomitant use with barbiturates antagonize benzphetamine, resulting in CNS de-

---

pression; use with caffeine or other CNS stimulants produces additive effects.

Amphetamines may alter insulin requirements.

Effects on diagnostic tests
Benzphetamine may elevate plasma corticosteroid levels and may interfere with urinary steroid determinations.

Adverse reactions
• CNS: restlessness, tremor, hyperactivity, talkativeness, insomnia, irritability, dizziness, headache, chills, overstimulation, dysphoria, paranoid ideation.
• CV: tachycardia, palpitations, hypertension, hypotension.
• DERM: urticaria.
• GI: nausea, vomiting, cramps, dry mouth, diarrhea, constipation, metallic taste, anorexia, weight loss.
• GU: changes in libido, impotence.
• Other: tolerance, physical and psychological dependence.
Note: Drug should be discontinued if signs of hypersensitivity or idiosyncrasy occur.

Overdose and treatment
Clinical manifestations of overdose include flushing, pallor, palpitations, changing pulse rate and blood pressure levels, heart block, chest pain, hyperpyrexia, confusion, delirium, psychoses, and hallucinations.

Treat overdose symptomatically and supportively: if ingestion is recent (within 4 hours), use gastric lavage or emesis with ipecac syrup and sedate with barbiturate; monitor vital signs and fluid and electrolyte balance. Urinary acidification may enhance excretion. Specific treatment to lower body temperature or intracranial pressure may be necessary.

▶ Special considerations
Recommendations for administration of benzphetamine, for care and teaching of patient during therapy, and for use in elderly or breastfeeding patients are the same as those for all amphetamines.
• The use of benzamphetamine for weight control is highly controversial because the drug's appetite suppression effects are transient.
• In managing benzphetamine withdrawal, place patient in a quiet room with low stimulation and allow him to sleep. Monitor vital signs; institute suicide precautions.

Pediatric use
Benzphetamine is not recommended for weight reduction in children.

---

dextroamphetamine sulfate
Dexedrine, Oxydess II, Spancap No. 1

• Pharmacologic classification: amphetamine
• Therapeutic classification: CNS stimulant, sympathomimetic amine
• Controlled substance schedule II
• Pregnancy risk category C

How supplied
Available by prescription only
Tablets: 5 mg, 10 mg
Capsules (sustained-release): 5 mg, 10 mg, 15 mg
Elixir: 5 mg/5 ml

Indications, route, and dosage
Narcolepsy
Adults: 5 to 30 mg P.O. daily in divided doses. Long-acting dosage forms allow once-daily dosing.
Children over age 12: 10 mg P.O. daily. Increase at 10-mg increments weekly p.r.n.
Children ages 6 to 12: 5 mg P.O. daily. Increase at 5-mg increments weekly p.r.n.
Attention deficit disorder with hyperactivity
Children age 6 and older: 5 mg once daily or b.i.d. Increase at 5-mg increments weekly p.r.n.
Children ages 3 to 5: 2.5 mg P.O. daily. Increase at 2.5-mg increments weekly p.r.n.; not recommended for children under age 3.

Pharmacodynamics
• *CNS stimulant action:* Amphetamines are sympathomimetic amines with CNS stimulant activity; in hyperactive children, they have a paradoxical calming effect. Amphetamines are used to treat narcolepsy and as adjuncts to psychosocial measures in attention deficit disorder in children.

The cerebral cortex and reticular activating system appear to be the primary sites of activity; amphetamines release nerve terminal stores of norepinephrine, promoting nerve impulse transmission. At high dosages, effects are mediated by dopamine.

Pharmacokinetics
- *Absorption:* Dextroamphetamine is rapidly absorbed from the GI tract; peak serum concentrations occur 2 to 4 hours after oral administration; long-acting capsules are absorbed more slowly and have a longer duration of action.
- *Distribution:* Dextroamphetamine is distributed widely throughout the body. It crosses the placenta.
- *Metabolism:* Hepatic.
- *Excretion:* Excreted in urine.

Contraindications and precautions
Dextroamphetamine is contraindicated in patients with hypersensitivity or idiosyncratic reaction to amphetamines; in patients with hyperthyroidism, angina pectoris, glaucoma, any degree of hypertension, or other severe CV disease; and in patients with a history of substance abuse. It also is contraindicated for concomitant use with or within 14 days of discontinuing MAO inhibitors.

It should be used with caution in patients with diabetes mellitus; in elderly, debilitated, or hyperexcitable patients; and in children with Gilles de la Tourette's syndrome. Amphetamine-induced CNS stimulation superimposed on CNS depression can cause seizures. Some formulations (Dexedrine) contain tartrazine, which may induce allergic reactions in hypersensitive individuals.

Interactions
Concomitant use with MAO inhibitors (or drugs with MAO-inhibiting activity, such as furazolidone) or within 14 days of such therapy may cause hypertensive crisis; use with antihypertensives may antagonize antihypertensive effects.

Concomitant use with antacids, sodium bicarbonate, or acetazolamide enhances reabsorption of dextroamphetamine and prolongs duration of action; use with ascorbic acid enhances dextroamphetamine excretion and shortens duration of action.

Concomitant use with phenothiazines or haloperidol decreases dextroamphetamine effects; barbiturates antagonize dextroamphetamine by CNS depression; use with theophylline, caffeine, or other CNS stimulants produces additive effects.

Dextroamphetamine may alter insulin requirements.

Effects on diagnostic tests
Dextroamphetamine may elevate plasma corticosteroid levels and may interefere with urinary steroid determinations.

Adverse reactions
- CNS: euphoria, restlessness, tremor, hyperactivity, talkativeness, insomnia, irritability, dizziness, headache, chills, overstimulation, dysphoria, psychosis.
- CV: tachycardia, palpitations, hypertension, hypotension.
- DERM: urticaria.
- GI: nausea, vomiting, cramps, dry mouth, diarrhea, constipation, metallic taste, anorexia, weight loss.
- GU: impotence, changes in libido.
- Other: tolerance, physical and psychological dependence.

Note: Drug should be discontinued if signs of hypersensitivity or idiosyncrasy occur.

Overdose and treatment
Individual responses to overdose vary widely. Toxic symptoms may occur at 15 mg and 30 mg and can cause severe reactions; however, doses of 400 mg or more have not always proved fatal.

Symptoms of overdose include restlessness, compulsive stereotyped behavior, tremor, hyperreflexia, tachypnea, confusion, aggressiveness, hallucinations, panic, and psychosis; fatigue and depression usually follow excitement stage. Other symptoms may include arrhythmias, shock, alterations in blood pressure, nausea, vomiting, diarrhea, and abdominal cramps; death is usually preceded by seizures and coma.

Treat overdose symptomatically and supportively: if ingestion is recent (within 4 hours), use gastric lavage or emesis with ipecac syrup and sedate with a barbiturate; monitor vital signs and fluid and electrolyte balance. Protect the airway; oxygen and artificial ventilation may be necessary. Urinary acidification may enhance excretion. Saline catharsis (magnesium citrate) may hasten GI evacuation of unabsorbed sustained-release drug. In severe overdose, hemodialysis or peritoneal dialysis may be useful.

▶ Special considerations
Besides those relevant to all *amphetamines,* consider the following recommendations.
- Amphetamines are not recommended for the treatment of obesity because their effectiveness on appetite suppression is transient.
- To minimize insomnia, avoid giving within 6 hours of bedtime.

● Check vital signs regularly. Observe patient for signs of excessive stimulation.
● Monitor blood and urine glucose levels. Drug may alter daily insulin requirement in patients with diabetes.
● For narcolepsy, patient should take first dose on awakening.
● Discontinuing amphetamines after prolonged use can produce hypersomnolence, increased appetite, and depression.
● Observe patient frequently for signs of aggressive behavior. Frequently assess anxiety level to prevent onset of physical aggression as anxiety increases.

Information for the patient
● Tell patient to avoid drinks containing caffeine, which increases stimulant effects of the drug.
● Warn patient to avoid hazardous activities that require alertness until CNS response to drug is determined.
● Patient should take drug early in the day to minimize insomnia.
● Sustained-release capsules should be swallowed whole, not opened or mixed with food.
● Diabetic patients should monitor blood sugar as ordered. Changes in food intake, body weight, or level of activity may necessitate changes in hypoglycemic drug regimen.
● Patients should be aware of the risks of physical or psychological dependence before beginning therapy.

Geriatric use
Lower doses are recommended for use in elderly patients.

Breast-feeding
Safety has not been established. Alternate feeding method is recommended during therapy with dextroamphetamine.

diethylpropion hydrochloride
Nobesine-75, Nu-Dispoz, Regibon, Ro-Diet, Tenuate, Tepanil

● Pharmacologic classification: amphetamine
● Therapeutic classification: short-term adjunctive anorexigenic agent, sympathomimetic amine
● Controlled substance schedule IV
● Pregnancy risk category C

How supplied
Available by prescription only
Tablets: 25 mg
Tablets (controlled-release): 75 mg

Indications, route, and dosage
Short-term adjunct in exogenous obesity
Adults: 25 mg P.O. t.i.d. before meals or 75 mg controlled-release tablet P.O. at midmorning. An additional 25-mg dose may be added in the evening to control night hunger.

Pharmacodynamics
Anorexigenic action: The precise mechanism of action for appetite control is unknown; anorexigenic effects are thought to occur in the hypothalamus, where decreased smell and taste acuity decreases appetite. The cerebral cortex and reticular activating system appear to be the primary sites of activity; amphetamines release nerve terminal stores of norepinephrine, promoting nerve impulse transmission.

Diethylpropion is used adjunctively with caloric restriction and behavior modification to control appetite in exogenous obesity. Diethylpropion is a sympathomimetic amine and is considered the safest of its class for potential use in patients with mild to moderate hypertension.

Pharmacokinetics
● *Absorption:* Diethylpropion is readily absorbed after oral administration; therapeutic effects persist for 4 hours with regular tablets, longer with controlled-release preparation.
● *Distribution:* Widely distributed throughout the body. Crosses the placenta and enters breast milk.
● *Metabolism:* Metabolized in the liver.
● *Excretion:* Excreted in urine.

Contraindications and precautions

Diethylpropion is contraindicated in patients with hypersensitivity or idiosyncratic reaction to sympathomimetic amines; in patients with severe CV disease, hyperthyroidism, moderate to severe hypertension, or advanced arteriosclerosis; and in patients with a history of substance abuse.

Diethylpropion also is contraindicated for use with MAO inhibitors or within 14 days of such use. It should be used with caution in patients with seizure disorders because it may increase seizures and in patients with diabetes mellitus or hyperexcitability states. Habituation or psychic dependence may occur.

Interactions

Concomitant use with MAO inhibitors (or drugs with MAO-inhibiting effects, such as furazolidone), or within 14 days of such therapy may cause hypertensive crisis.

Diethylpropion may decrease antihypertensive effects of guanethidine; it may also decrease insulin requirements in diabetic patients as a result of weight loss. Diethylpropion may increase the effects of antidepressants; excessive concomitant use of caffeine produces additive CNS stimulation. Barbiturates antagonize diethylpropion by CNS depression and may decrease its effects.

Effects on diagnostic tests

None reported.

Adverse reactions

● CNS: headache, nervousness, dizziness, restlessness, overstimulation.
● CV: tachycardia, palpitations, rise in blood pressure.
● DERM: urticaria.
● EENT: blurred vision.
● GI: nausea, abdominal cramps, dry mouth, diarrhea, constipation.
● GU: impotence, changes in libido, menstrual upset.
● Other: physical or psychological dependence.
Note: Drug should be discontinued if signs of hypersensitivity or idiosyncrasy occur.

Overdose and treatment

Symptoms of acute overdose include restlessness, tremor, hyperreflexia, tachypnea, confusion, aggressive behavior, hallucinations, blood pressure changes, arrhythmias, nausea, vomiting, diarrhea, and cramps. Fatigue and depression usually follow initial stimulation; seizures and coma may follow.

Treat overdose symptomatically and supportively: if ingestion is recent (within 4 hours), use gastric lavage or emesis with ipecac syrup. Treatment may require administration of a sedative and, if acute hypertension develops, I.V. phentolamine. Monitor vital signs and fluid and electrolyte balance.

▶ Special considerations

Besides those relevant to all *amphetamines*, consider the following recommendations.
● Diethylpropion can be used to stop nighttime overeating. Drug rarely causes insomnia.
● Do not crush controlled-release tablets.

Information for the patient

● Tell patient to avoid drinks containing caffeine to prevent overstimulation.
● Tell patient to swallow controlled-release tablet whole and not to chew or crush it.
● Warn patient against exceeding prescribed dosage.
● Tell patient drug may color urine pink to brown. This is not harmful.
● Warn patient not to stop taking the drug abruptly to avoid withdrawal reactions.

Geriatric use

In elderly patients, lower dosages may be effective because of diminished renal function.

Pediatric use

Diethylpropion is not recommended for weight reduction in children under age 12.

Breast-feeding

Diethylpropion is excreted in breast milk; alternate feeding method is recommended during therapy with this drug.

---

fenfluramine hydrochloride
Pondimin

● Pharmacologic classification: amphetamine congener
● Therapeutic classification: short-term adjunctive anorexigenic agent, indirect-acting sympathomimetic amine
● Controlled substance schedule IV
● Pregnancy risk category C

How supplied

Available by prescription only
Tablets: 20 mg

Indications, route, and dosage
Short-term adjunct in exogenous obesity
Adults: Initially, 20 mg P.O. t.i.d. before meals; maximum of 40 mg t.i.d. Adjust dosage according to patient's response.
†*Autism*
Children: Dosage varies with treatment protocol. Some studies have employed doses of 1.5 mg/kg P.O. daily in a single dose or divided doses, not to exceed the usual adult dose.

Pharmacodynamics
Anorexigenic action: The mechanism of fenfluramine's anorexigenic effects is incompletely understood; it appears to involve stimulation of the hypothalamus and may be related to brain serotonin levels or to increased glucose use.

Fenfluramine differs from other sympathomimetics in that it usually depresses the CNS. As an anorexigenic, it is considered a second-line drug. However, because of its depressant effects, it may be especially useful for tense, nervous patients and others who should avoid CNS stimulation; it can also be used to help prevent nighttime snacking if taken before the evening meal.

Fenfluramine may *improve* glucose tolerance and is considered the anorexigenic agent of choice in patients with type II (non-insulin-dependent) diabetes; it also has a slightly hypotensive effect.

Fenfluramine is used adjunctively with caloric restriction and behavior modification to control appetite in patients with exogenous obesity.
Autism treatment adjunct action: The mechanism of action whereby fenfluramine decreases stereotypical behavior and increases attention span in children with autism is unknown. The drug lowers plasma serotonin levels, but this does not appear to be a quantitative or reliable predictor of response.

Fenfluramine is being investigated as a means to improve intellectual functioning in patients with autism. It reduces excessive serotonergic activity in these patients, but has variable effects on social behavior and attention span.

Pharmacokinetics
• *Absorption:* Fenfluramine is well absorbed after oral administration; maximal anorexia occurs at 2 to 4 hours.
• *Distribution:* Fenfluramine is distributed widely throughout the body, including the CNS.
• *Metabolism:* Fenfluramine is metabolized in the liver.
• *Excretion:* Most drug and metabolites are excreted in urine; rate of elimination is pH-dependent.

Contraindications and precautions
Fenfluramine is contraindicated in patients with hypersensitivity or idiosyncratic reaction to sympathomimetic amines; in depressed or alcoholic patients; in patients with symptomatic CV disease; and in patients with a history of substance abuse. Fenfluramine also is contraindicated for use with MAO inhibitors or within 14 days of such use.

Fenfluramine should be used with caution in patients with hypertension, diabetes mellitus, or a history of depressive disorder. Habituation or psychological dependence may occur with prolonged use.

Fenfluramine should be used with caution in patients undergoing general anesthesia; fatal cardiac arrest has been reported. Therefore, when possible, fenfluramine should be discontinued for 1 week before surgery; if surgery cannot be postponed, full cardiac monitoring and resuscitative equipment must be available.

Fenfluramine is not recommended for intermittent courses of therapy in weight control.

Drug interactions
Concomitant use with MAO inhibitors (or drugs with MAO-inhibiting effects, such as furazolidone) and use within 14 days of such therapy may cause hypertensive crisis. Fenfluramine may increase hypotensive effects of other drugs, especially guanethidine, methyldopa, and reserpine; concomitant use with other CNS depressants will produce additive effects.

Effects on diagnostic tests
None reported.

Adverse reactions
• CNS: drowsiness, dizziness, incoordination, headache, euphoria or depression, anxiety, insomnia, weakness or fatigue, agitation, hallucinations.
• CV: palpitations, hypotension, hypertension, chest pain.
• DERM: rashes, urticaria, burning sensation.
• EENT: eye irritation, blurred vision.
• GI: diarrhea, dry mouth, nausea, vomiting, abdominal pain, constipation.
• GU: changes in libido, dysuria, increased urinary frequency, impotence.
• Other: sweating, chills, fever.
Note: Drug should be discontinued if signs of hypersensitivity or idiosyncrasy occur or if pulmonary hypertension develops.

Overdose and treatment
Symptoms of acute overdose include nystagmus, jaw tremor, confusion, sweating, abdominal pain, hyperventilation, and dilated, nonreactive pupils. Higher doses may cause seizures, coma, and arrhythmias leading to cardiac arrest.

Treat overdose symptomatically and supportively. If ingestion is recent (within 4 hours), use gastric lavage or emesis; avoid drug-induced emesis, as subsequent development of coma may cause aspiration. Treatment may include use of I.V. beta blockers for tachycardia and other arrhythmias, and diazepam or phenobarbital for seizures. Monitor vital signs and fluid and electrolyte balance.

▶ Special considerations
Besides those relevant to all *amphetamines,* consider the following recommendations.
• Because of possible hypoglycemia, patients with diabetes may have altered insulin or sulfonylurea requirements. Monitor glucose levels.
• Fenfluramine should not be discontinued abruptly; severe mental depression may result.
• After discontinuation of fenfluramine in autistic children, rebound increases in plasma serotonin levels have been reported.

Information for the patient
• Tell patient to avoid use of alcohol, caffeine, or other stimulants.
• Warn patient not to discontinue drug abruptly.
• Encourage patient to report palpitations, nervousness, or dizziness.

Geriatric use
Lower doses are recommended for elderly patients.

Pediatric use
Fenfluramine is not recommended for weight reduction in children under age 12.

mazindol
Mazanor, Sanorex

• Pharmacologic classification: imidazoisoindol
• Therapeutic classification: anorexigenic agent
• Controlled substance schedule IV
• Pregnancy risk category C

How supplied
Available by prescription only
Tablets: 1 mg, 2 mg

Indications, route, and dosage
Short-term adjunct in exogenous obesity
Adults: 1 mg P.O. t.i.d. 1 hour before meals or 2 mg daily 1 hour before lunch. Use lowest effective dosage.
†*Treatment adjunct in cocaine abusers*
Adults: 1 to 3 mg P.O. daily.
†*Narcolepsy*
Adults: 0.5 to 4 mg P.O. daily.

Pharmacodynamics
Stimulant action: Mazindol's chemical structure is different from that of amphetamines or other anorexigenics; it appears to act in the limbic system, inhibiting norepinephrine and dopamine uptake. Mazindol does not appear to produce euphoria and, therefore, has a low potential for abuse. Its appetite suppressant activity is comparable to that of amphetamines and diethylpropion.

Pharmacokinetics
• *Absorption:* Mazindol is absorbed readily after oral administration; onset of action is 30 to 60 minutes. Duration of action is 8 to 15 hours, permitting once-daily dosing.
• *Distribution:* Mazindol enters the CNS.
• *Metabolism:* Unknown.
• *Excretion:* Mazindol is excreted unchanged in urine.

Contraindications and precautions
Mazindol is contraindicated in patients with known hypersensitivity to the drug; in patients with glaucoma because it can exacerbate the disease; in patients with a history of substance abuse; in agitated states; and for use with MAO inhibitors or within 14 days of such use.

Mazindol should be used with caution in patients with hypertension, severe CV disease, or diabetes mellitus and in hyperexcitability states.

Habituation or psychic dependence may follow prolonged use.

Interactions
Concomitant use with MAO inhibitors or within 14 days of such therapy may cause hypertensive crisis. Mazindol may decrease hypotensive effects of guanethidine and other antihypertensive agents; it also may alter insulin requirements in diabetic patients.

Concomitant use with pressor amines (norepinephrine or isoproterenol) during treatment for shock may cause hypertension; initiate therapy with lower doses, titrate slowly, and monitor blood pressure frequently.

Mazindol reportedly (one case) has increased lithium toxicity.

Concomitant use of mazindol and fenfluramine may increase risk of cardiac toxicity. Avoid concomitant use. Concomitant use with caffeine or caffeinated beverages may enhance adverse CNS effects. Avoid concomitant use.

Effects on diagnostic tests
None reported.

Adverse reactions
- CNS: nervousness, restlessness, dizziness, insomnia, dysphoria, headache, depression, drowsiness, weakness, tremor.
- CV: palpitations, tachycardia.
- DERM: rash, clamminess, pallor.
- GI: dry mouth, nausea, constipation, diarrhea, unpleasant taste.
- GU: difficulty initiating micturition, impotence.
- Other: shivering, excessive sweating, tolerance, physical and psychological dependence.

Note: Drug should be discontinued if signs of hypersensitivity occur.

Overdose and treatment
No data exist on acute overdose with mazindol in humans. However, anticipated symptoms include restlessness, tremor, hyperreflexia, fever, tachypnea, dizziness, nausea, vomiting, diarrhea, cramps, hypertension, tachycardia, and circulatory collapse.

Treat overdose supportively: monitor vital signs and fluid and electrolyte balance. Acidifying the urine may enhance mazindol excretion.

▶ Special considerations
- Administer mazindol with meals instead of 1 hour before meals if GI irritation occurs.

- Drug may alter insulin requirements. Monitor blood glucose levels.
- Tolerance or dependence may develop, but abuse potential is lower than that of other CNS stimulants.
- Concomitant use of mazindol and fenfluramine may increase risk of cardiac toxicity and should be avoided.
- Concomitant use with caffeine or caffeinated beverages may enhance CNS effects and should be avoided.

Information for the patient
- Instruct patient to take last daily dose at least 6 hours before bedtime to avoid insomnia.
- Tell patient to take drug with meals to prevent GI distress.

Geriatric use
Use with caution in elderly patients.

Pediatric use
Mazindol is not recommended for children under age 12.

Breast-feeding
Safety in breast-feeding has not been established. Alternate feeding method is recommended during therapy.

---

methamphetamine hydrochloride
Desoxyn, Desoxyn Gradumets

- Pharmacologic classification: amphetamine
- Therapeutic classification: CNS stimulant, short-term adjunctive anorexigenic agent, sympathomimetic amine
- Controlled substance schedule II
- Pregnancy risk category C

How supplied
Available by prescription only
Tablets: 5 mg, 10 mg
Tablets (long-acting): 5 mg, 10 mg, 15 mg

Indications, route, and dosage
Attention deficit disorder with hyperactivity
Children age 6 and older: 2.5 to 5 mg P.O. once daily or b.i.d. Increase at 5-mg increments weekly p.r.n. Usual effective dosage is 20 to 25 mg daily.

Short-term adjunct in exogenous obesity
Adults: 2.5 to 5 mg P.O. once daily to t.i.d. 30 minutes before meals; or one long-acting 5- to 15-mg tablet daily before breakfast.

Pharmacodynamics

● *CNS stimulant action:* Amphetamines are sympathomimetic amines with CNS stimulant activity; in hyperactive children, they have a paradoxical calming effect.

● *Anorexigenic action:* Anorexigenic effects are thought to occur in the hypothalamus, where decreased smell and taste acuity decreases appetite; they may involve other systemic and metabolic effects. They may be tried for short-term control of refractory obesity, with caloric restriction and behavior modification.

The cerebral cortex and reticular activating system appear to be the primary sites of activity; amphetamines release nerve terminal stores of norepinephrine, promoting nerve impulse transmission. At high dosages, effects are mediated by dopamine.

Amphetamines are used to treat narcolepsy and as adjuncts to psychosocial measures in attention deficit disorder in children. The precise mechanisms of action in these conditions are unknown.

Pharmacokinetics

● *Absorption:* Methamphetamine is rapidly absorbed from the GI tract after oral administration; effects last 6 to 12 hours.

● *Distribution:* Widely distributed throughout the body. Crosses the placenta and enters breast milk.

● *Metabolism:* Metabolized in the liver to at least seven metabolites.

● *Excretion:* Excreted in urine.

Contraindications and precautions

Methamphetamine is contraindicated in patients with hypersensitivity or idiosyncratic reaction to sympathomimetic amines; in patients with hyperthyroidism, glaucoma, angina pectoris, or any degree of hypertension or other severe CV disease because it may cause hazardous arrhythmias and changes in blood pressure; and in patients with a history of substance abuse. They also are contraindicated for concomitant use with MAO inhibitors or within 14 days of discontinuing such therapy.

Methamphetamine should be used with caution in patients with diabetes mellitus; in patients who are elderly, debilitated, asthenic, or psychopathic; in patients who have a history of suicidal or homicidal tendencies, and in children

with Gilles de la Tourette's syndrome. Amphetamine-induced CNS stimulation superimposed on CNS depression can cause seizures. Some formulations (Desoxyn Gradumets, 15 mg) may contain tartrazine, which may precipitate an allergic reaction in sensitive individuals.

Interactions

Concomitant use with MAO inhibitors (or drugs with MAO-inhibiting effects, such as furazolidone), or within 14 days of such therapy may cause hypertensive crisis; use with antihypertensives may antagonize their effects.

Concomitant use with antacids, sodium bicarbonate, or acetazolamide enhances reabsorption of methamphetamine and prolongs duration of action, whereas use with ascorbic acid enhances methamphetamine excretion and shortens duration of action. Use with phenothiazines or haloperidol decreases methamphetamine effects; barbiturates antagonize methamphetamine by CNS depression, whereas caffeine or other CNS stimulants produce additive effects.

Patients using methamphetamine have an increased risk of arrhythmias during general anesthesia.

Methamphetamine may alter insulin requirements.

Effects on diagnostic tests

Methamphetamine may elevate plasma corticosteroid levels and may interfere with urinary steroid determinations.

Adverse reactions

● CNS: nervousness, insomnia (common), irritability, talkativeness, dizziness, headache, hyperexcitability, tremor, *psychosis.*
● CV: *hypertension* or hypotension, *tachycardia,* palpitations, *arrhythmias.*
● DERM: urticaria.
● EENT: blurred vision, mydriasis.
● GI: nausea, vomiting, abdominal cramps, diarrhea or constipation, dry mouth, anorexia, metallic aftertaste.
● GU: impotence, changes in libido.
● Other: exacerbation of tics, tolerance, physical and psychological dependence.

Note: Drug should be discontinued if signs of hypersensitivity or idiosyncrasy occur.

Overdose and treatment

Symptoms of overdose include increasing restlessness, tremor, hyperreflexia, tachypnea, confusion, aggressiveness, hallucinations, and panic; fatigue and depression usually follow the excitement stage. Other symptoms may include arrhythmias, shock, alterations in blood pressure, nausea, vomiting, diarrhea, and abdominal cramps; death is usually preceded by seizures and coma.

Treat overdose symptomatically and supportively: if ingestion is recent (within 4 hours), use gastric lavage or emesis and sedate with barbiturate; monitor vital signs and fluid and electrolyte balance. Urinary acidification may enhance excretion. Saline catharsis (magnesium citrate) may hasten GI evacuation of unabsorbed long-acting forms. Hemodiaylsis or peritoneal dialysis may be effective in severe cases.

▶ **Special considerations**
Besides those relevant to all *amphetamines*, consider the following recommendations.
● Methamphetamine is not recommended for first-line treatment of obesity because its effectiveness on appetite suppression is usually transient.
● Do not crush long-acting dosage forms.
● When treating behavioral disorders in children, consider a periodic discontinuation of the drug to evaluate effectiveness and the need for continued therapy.
● Rapid withdrawal after prolonged use may lead to depression, somnolence, and increased appetite.

Information for the patient
● Warn patient that potential for abuse is high. Discourage use to combat fatigue.
● Advise patient to avoid caffeine-containing drinks and alcohol, to take drug 1 hour before next meal, and to take last daily dose at least 6 hours before bedtime to prevent insomnia.
● Warn patient not to increase dosage unless prescribed.

Geriatric use
Elderly or debilitated patients may be especially sensitive to methamphetamine's effects. Drug should be used with caution.

Pediatric use
Methamphetamine is not recommended for weight reduction in children under age 12.

---

methylphenidate hydrochloride
Ritalin, Ritalin-SR

● Pharmacologic classification: piperidine derivative
● Therapeutic classification: CNS stimulant
● Controlled substance schedule II
● Pregnancy risk category C

How supplied
Available by prescription only
Tablets: 5 mg, 10 mg, 20 mg
Tablets (sustained-release): 20 mg

Indications, route, and dosage
Attention deficit disorder with hyperactivity
Children age 6 and older: Initially, 5 to 10 mg P.O. daily before breakfast and lunch. Increase at 5- to 10-mg increments weekly p.r.n. until an optimum daily dosage of 2 mg/kg is reached, not to exceed 60 mg/day. The usual effective dosage is 10 to 20 mg/day.
Narcolepsy
Adults: 10 mg P.O. b.i.d. or t.i.d. ½ hour before meals. Dosage varies with patient needs; average dose is 20 to 30 mg/day (range 5 to 60 mg/day).

Pharmacodynamics
Analeptic action: The cerebral cortex and reticular activating system appear to be the primary sites of activity; methylphenidate releases nerve terminal stores of norepinephrine, promoting nerve impulse transmission. At high doses, effects are mediated by dopamine.

Methylphenidate is used to treat narcolepsy and as an adjunctive to psychosocial measures in attention deficit disorder in children. Like amphetamines, it has a paradoxical calming effect in hyperactive children.

Pharmacokinetics
● *Absorption:* Methylphenidate is absorbed rapidly and completely after oral administration; peak plasma concentrations occur at 1 to 2 hours. Duration of action is usually 4 to 6 hours (with considerable individual variation); sustained-release tablets may act for up to 8 hours.
● *Distribution:* Unknown.
● *Metabolism:* Methylphenidate is metabolized by the liver.
● *Excretion:* Methylphenidate is excreted in urine.

Contraindications and precautions

Methylphenidate is contraindicated in patients with known hypersensitivity to sympathomimetic amines; in patients with symptomatic CV disease, hyperthyroidism, angina pectoris, moderate to severe hypertension, or advanced arteriosclerosis because it may cause dangerous arrhythmias and blood pressure changes; in patients with severe exogenous or endogenous depression, glaucoma, parkinsonism, or agitated states; in patients with a history of marked anxiety, tension, or agitation because it can exacerbate such conditions; or in patients with a history of substance abuse.

Methylphenidate should be used with caution in patients with a history of diabetes mellitus, CV disease, motor tics, seizures, or Gilles de la Tourette's syndrome (drug may precipitate disorder); and in elderly, debilitated, or hyperexcitable patients.

Interactions

Concomitant use with caffeine may decrease efficacy of methylphenidate in attention deficit disorder; use with MAO inhibitors (or drugs with MAO-inhibiting effects, such as furazolidone) or within 14 days of such therapy may cause severe hypertension.

Methylphenidate may inhibit metabolism and increase the serum levels of anticonvulsants (phenytoin, phenobarbital, primidone), coumarin anticoagulants, phenylbutazone, and tricyclic antidepressants; it also may decrease the hypotensive effects of guanethidine and bretylium.

Caffeine may enhance the CNS stimulant effects of methylphenidate. Avoid concomitant use.

Effects on diagnostic tests

None reported.

Adverse reactions

● CNS: nervousness, insomnia, dizziness, headache, akathisia, dyskinesia, Gilles de la Tourette's syndrome.
● CV: palpitations, angina, tachycardia, changes in blood pressure and pulse rate, arrhythmias.
● DERM: rash, urticaria, *exfoliative dermatitis,* erythema multiforme.
● EENT: difficulty with accommodation, blurred vision.
● GI: nausea, dry throat, abdominal pain, anorexia, weight loss.
● Other: growth suppression, tolerance, physical and psychological dependence.
Note: Drug should be discontinued if signs of hypersensitivity or seizures occur or if no improvement is noticed within 1 month at maintenance dosage level.

Overdose and treatment

Symptoms of overdose may include euphoria, confusion, delirium, coma, toxic psychosis, agitation, headache, vomiting, dry mouth, mydriasis, self-injury, fever, diaphoresis, tremor, hyperreflexia, muscle twitching, seizures, flushing, hypertension, tachycardia, palpitations, and arrhythmias.

Treat overdose symptomatically and supportively: use gastric lavage or induce emesis with ipecac syrup in patients with intact gag reflex. Maintain airway and circulation. Closely monitor vital signs and fluid and electrolyte balance. Maintain patient in cool room, monitor temperature, minimize external stimulation, and protect him against self-injury. External cooling blankets may be needed.

▶ Special considerations

● Methylphenidate is the drug of choice for attention deficit disorder. Therapy is usually discontinued after puberty.
● Monitor initiation of therapy closely; drug may precipitate Gilles de la Tourette's syndrome.
● Check vital signs regularly for increased blood pressure or other signs of excessive stimulation; avoid late-day or evening dosing, especially of long-acting dosage forms, to minimize insomnia.
● Monitor blood and urine glucose levels in diabetic patients; drug may alter insulin requirements.
● Drug may decrease seizure threshold in seizure disorders.
● Monitor complete blood count, differential, and platelet counts when patient is taking drug long-term.
● Intermittent drug-free periods when stress is least evident (weekends, school holidays) may help prevent development of tolerance and permit decreased dosage when drug is resumed. Sustained-release form allows convenience of single, at-home dosing for school children.
● Drug has abuse potential; discourage use to combat fatigue. Some abusers dissolve tablets and inject drug.
● After high-dose and long-term use, abrupt withdrawal may unmask severe depression. Lower dosage gradually to prevent acute rebound depression.
● Methylphenidate impairs ability to perform tasks requiring mental alertness.
● Be sure patient obtains adequate rest; fatigue may result as drug wears off.

● Monitor height and weight; drug has been associated with growth suppression.

● Discourage methylphenidate use for analeptic effect; CNS stimulation superimposed on CNS depression may cause neuronal instability and seizures.

Information for the patient

● Explain rationale for therapy and the risks and benefits that may be anticipated.

● Tell patient to avoid drinks containing caffeine to prevent added CNS stimulation and not to alter dosage unless prescribed.

● Advise narcoleptic patient to take first dose on awakening; advise patient with attention deficit disorder to take last dose several hours before bedtime to avoid insomnia.

● Tell patient not to chew or crush sustained-release dosage forms.

● Warn patient not to use drug to mask fatigue, to be sure to obtain adequate rest, and to call if excessive CNS stimulation occurs.

● Advise diabetic patients to monitor blood glucose levels, as drug may alter insulin needs.

● Advise patient to avoid hazardous activities that require mental alertness until degree of sedative effect is determined.

Pediatric use

Methylphenidate is not recommended for attention deficit disorder in children under age 6. Drug has been associated with growth suppression; all patients should be monitored.

---

pemoline
Cylert

● Pharmacologic classification: oxazolidinedione derivative, CNS stimulant
● Therapeutic classification: analeptic
● Controlled substance schedule IV
● Pregnancy risk category B

How supplied
Available by prescription only
Tablets: 18.75 mg, 37.5 mg, 75 mg
Tablets (chewable and containing povidine): 37.5 mg

Indications, route, and dosage
Attention deficit disorder
Children age 6 and older: Initially, 37.5 mg P.O. given in the morning. Daily dosage can be raised by 18.75 mg weekly. Effective dosage range is

56.25 to 75 mg daily; maximum is 112.5 mg daily.
Narcolepsy
Adults: 50 to 200 mg daily divided b.i.d. after breakfast and lunch.
†*Mild stimulant in elderly patients*
Adults: 40 to 50 mg P.O. daily b.i.d. in divided doses after breakfast and lunch.

Pharmacodynamics
Analeptic action: Pemoline differs structurally from methylphenidate and amphetamines; however, like those drugs, pemoline has a paradoxical calming effect in children with attention deficit disorder.

Pemoline's mechanism of action is unknown; it may be mediated by enhanced cerebral neurotransmission.

Pemoline is used primarily to treat attention deficit disorder in children over age 6; investigationally, its CNS stimulant effect has been studied in narcolepsy in adults, in fatigue, in depressed and schizophrenic states, and in elderly patients.

Pharmacokinetics
● *Absorption:* Pemoline is well absorbed after oral administration. Peak therapeutic effects occur at 4 hours and persist about 8 hours.
● *Distribution:* Distribution is unknown. Drug is 50% protein-bound.
● *Metabolism:* Metabolized by the liver to active and inactive metabolites.
● *Excretion:* Pemoline and its metabolites are excreted in urine; 75% of an oral dose is excreted within 24 hours.

Contraindications and precautions
Pemoline is contraindicated in patients with hypersensitivity to pemoline; in those with impaired hepatic function because it may have an adverse effect on liver function; and in children under age 6. It should be used with caution in patients with decreased renal function and in patients with a history of Gilles de la Tourette's syndrome because it may precipitate this disorder.

Interactions
Concomitant use with caffeine may decrease efficacy of pemoline in attention deficit disorder; concomitant use with anticonvulsants may decrease the seizure threshold.

Effects on diagnostic tests
Pemoline may cause abnormalities in liver function test results.

Adverse reactions

● CNS: insomnia, malaise, irritability, fatigue, mild depression, dizziness, headache, drowsiness, hallucinations, nervousness (large doses), *seizures*, nystagmus, oculogyric crisis, unusual facial movement, Gilles de la Tourette's syndrome, psychosis.
● CV: tachycardia (with large doses).
● DERM: rash.
● GI: anorexia, abdominal pain, nausea, diarrhea.
● GU: prostatic hyperplasia.
● Hepatic: liver enzyme elevations, jaundice.
● Other: weight loss on initial therapy; weight gain after 3 to 6 months, tolerance, physical and psychological dependence.

Note: Drug should be discontinued if signs of hypersensitivity occur or if markedly elevated liver function test results and jaundice occur concurrently.

Overdose and treatment

Symptoms of overdose may include irregular respiration, hyperreflexia, restlessness, tachycardia, hallucinations, excitement, and agitation.

Treat overdose symptomatically and supportively: use gastric lavage if symptoms are not severe (hyperexcitability or coma). Monitor vital signs and fluid and electrolyte balance. Maintain patient in a cool room, monitor temperature, and minimize external stimulation; protect patient from self-injury. Chlorpromazine or haloperidol usually can reverse CNS stimulation. Hemodialysis may help.

▶ Special considerations

● Monitor initiation of therapy closely; drug may precipitate Gilles de la Tourette's syndrome.
● Check vital signs regularly for increased blood pressure or other signs of excessive stimulation.
● Give drug in a single morning dose for maximum daytime benefit and to minimize insomnia.
● Monitor blood and urine glucose levels in diabetic patients; drug may alter insulin requirement.
● Monitor complete blood counts, differential, and platelet counts while patient is on long-term therapy.
● Explain that therapeutic effects may not appear for 3 to 4 weeks and that intermittent drug-free periods when stress is least evident (weekends, school holidays) may help prevent development of tolerance and permit decreased dosage when drug is resumed.

● Monitor height and weight; drug has been associated with growth suppression.
● Abrupt withdrawal after high-dose and long-term use may unmask severe depression. Lower dosage gradually to prevent acute rebound depression.
● Pemoline impairs ability to perform tasks requiring mental alertness.
● Be sure patient obtains adequate rest; fatigue may result as drug wears off.
● Discourage pemoline use for analeptic effect, as drug has abuse potential; CNS stimulation superimposed on CNS depression may cause neuronal instability and seizures.
● Carefully follow manufacturer's directions for reconstitution, storage, and administration of all preparations. Pemoline has been used to treat narcolepsy (50 to 200 mg divided b.i.d.), depression, and schizophrenia in adults, but these uses are controversial.

Information for the patient

● Explain rationale for therapy and the anticipated risks and benefits; teach signs and symptoms of adverse reactions and need to report these.
● Tell patient to avoid drinks containing caffeine, to prevent added CNS stimulation, and not to alter dosage without medical approval.
● Warn patient not to use drug to mask fatigue, to be sure to obtain adequate rest, and to report excessive CNS stimulation.
● Advise diabetic patients to monitor blood glucose levels, as drug may alter insulin needs.
● Advise patient to avoid tasks that require mental alertness until degree of sedative effect is determined.

Pediatric use

Pemoline is not recommended for attention deficit disorder in children under age 6.

phendimetrazine tartrate
Adipost, Anorex, Bacarate, Bontril PDM, Obalan, Obezine, Phenzine, Prelu-2, Sprx-1, Sprx-2, Sprx-3, Statobex, Trimtabs, Wehless-105 Timecelles

- Pharmacologic classification: amphetamine congener
- Therapeutic classification: short-term anorexigenic agent for exogenous obesity, indirect-acting sympathomimetic amine
- Controlled substance schedule III
- Pregnancy risk category C

How supplied
Available by prescription only
Tablets: 35 mg
Capsules: 35 mg
Capsules (sustained-release): 105 mg

Indications, route, and dosage
Short-term adjunct in exogenous obesity
Adults: 35 mg P.O. b.i.d. or t.i.d. 1 hour before meals. Maximum dosage is 70 mg t.i.d. Use lowest effective dosage adjusted to individual response. Dosage for sustained-release capsule is 105 mg once daily in the morning 1 hour before breakfast.

Pharmacodynamics
Anorexigenic action: Phendimetrazine is an indirect-acting sympathomimetic amine; it is considered a second-line drug for weight control because it causes euphoria, has a high abuse potential, and often causes unacceptable CNS stimulation. Anorexigenic effects are thought to follow direct stimulation of the hypothalamus and may involve other CNS and metabolic effects.

Pharmacokinetics
- *Absorption:* Phendimetrazine is absorbed readily after oral administration; therapeutic effects persist for 4 hours with regular tablets, longer with the sustained-release preparation.
- *Distribution:* Phendimetrazine is distributed widely throughout the body.
- *Metabolism:* Phendimetrazine is metabolized by the liver.
- *Excretion:* Phendimetrazine is excreted in urine. Half-life ranges from 2 hours for the regular dosage forms to 10 hours for the sustained-release capsules.

Contraindications and precautions
Phendimetrazine is contraindicated in patients with known hypersensitivity to phendimetrazine; in patients with hyperthyroidism, all degrees of hypertension, angina pectoris or other severe CV disease, glaucoma, and advanced arteriosclerosis; in agitated or highly nervous patients; and in patients with a history of drug abuse.

Phendimetrazine also is contraindicated for use with MAO inhibitors or within 14 days of such use because this combination may cause hypertensive crisis; or with other CNS stimulants. Some phendimetrazine formulations may contain tartrazine and are contraindicated in patients with asthma or aspirin allergy.

It should be used with caution in patients with known hypersensitivity to sympathomimetic amines and in hyperexcitability states. Habituation or psychological dependence may occur with prolonged use.

Interactions
Concomitant use with MAO inhibitors (or drugs with MAO-inhibiting effects, such as furazolidone) or within 14 days of such therapy may cause hypertensive crisis.

Phendimetrazine may decrease hypotensive effects of guanethidine and other antihypertensive agents; it also may alter insulin requirements in diabetic patients. Concomitant use with excessive caffeine may cause additive CNS stimulation; use with general anesthetics may result in arrhythmias.

Use with antacids, sodium bicarbonate, or acetazolamide increases renal reabsorption of phendimetrazine and prolongs its duration of action; use with phenothiazines or haloperidol decreases effects of phendimetrazine.

Effects on diagnostic tests
None reported.

Adverse reactions
- CNS: nervousness, dizziness, insomnia, tremor, headache, euphoria, overstimulation.
- CV: tachycardia, palpitations, *arrhythmias, hypertension.*
- EENT: blurred vision.
- GI: dry mouth, nausea, abdominal cramps, diarrhea or constipation, glossitis, stomatitis.
- GU: dysuria, changes in libido.
- Other: tolerance, physical and psychological dependence.

Note: Drug should be discontinued if signs of hypersensitivity occur.

Overdose and treatment

Symptoms of acute overdose include restlessness, tremor, hyperreflexia, fever, tachypnea, dizziness, confusion, aggressive behavior, hallucinations, panic, blood pressure changes, arrhythmias, nausea, vomiting, diarrhea, and cramps. Fatigue and depression usually follow CNS stimulation; seizures, coma, and death may follow.

Treat overdose symptomatically and supportively: treatment may include sedation with barbiturates. Acidification of urine may hasten excretion. Monitor vital signs and fluid and electrolyte balance.

▶ Special considerations

Besides those relevant to all *amphetamines,* consider the following recommendations.
● Give morning dose 2 hours after breakfast.
● Give last daily dose at least 6 hours before bedtime to prevent insomnia.
● Abrupt discontinuation may lead to extreme fatigue and depression.

Information for the patient

● Tell patient to avoid caffeine-containing drinks, not to take drug more frequently than prescribed, and to take last dose at least 6 hours before bedtime to prevent insomnia.
● Advise patient to call if palpitations occur.

Geriatric use

Lower dosages may be indicated for elderly patients.

Pediatric use

Phendimetrazine is not recommended for children under age 12.

---

phenmetrazine hydrochloride

Preludin Endurets

● Pharmacologic classification: amphetamine congener
● Therapeutic classification: short-term anorexigenic agent, indirect-acting sympathomimetic amine
● Controlled substance schedule II
● Pregnancy risk category C

How supplied

Available by prescription only
Tablets: (sustained-release): 75 mg

Indications, route, and dosage
Short-term adjunct in exogenous obesity

Adults: 75-mg sustained-release tablet daily at midmorning.

Pharmacodynamics

Anorexigenic action: Phenmetrazine is an indirect-acting sympathomimetic amine; it is considered a second-line drug for weight control. Its precise mechanism of action for appetite control has not been established; anorexigenic effects are thought to follow direct stimulation of the hypothalamus. Other CNS and metabolic effects may be involved.

Phenmetrazine is equally effective for continuous or intermittent use.

Pharmacokinetics

● *Absorption:* Phenmetrazine is absorbed readily after oral administration; therapeutic effects persist for 4 to 6 hours or longer.
● *Distribution:* Phenmetrazine is distributed widely throughout the body.
● *Metabolism:* Unknown.
● *Excretion:* Phenmetrazine is excreted in urine.

Contraindications and precautions

Phenmetrazine is contraindicated in patients with known hypersensitivity to phenmetrazine; in patients with hyperthyroidism, all degrees of hypertension, angina pectoris or other severe CV disease, glaucoma, or advanced arteriosclerosis; in agitated states; and in patients with a history of drug addiction. Phenmetrazine also is contraindicated for use with MAO inhibitors or within 14 days of such therapy; and with other CNS stimulants. Some phenmetrazine formulations (Preludin Endurets) contain tartrazine and may induce allergic responses in patients with asthma or aspirin allergy.

Phenmetrazine should be used with caution in patients with known hypersensitivity to sympathomimetic amines; in hyperexcitability states; in patients with diabetes; and in those with a history of substance abuse. Habituation or psychological dependence may occur with prolonged use.

Interactions

Concomitant use with MAO inhibitors (or drugs with MAO-inhibiting effects, such as furazolidone) or within 14 days of such therapy may cause hypertensive crisis. Phenmetrazine may decrease hypotensive effects of guanethidine and other antihypertensive agents; it also may alter insulin requirements in diabetic patients. Concomitant use with excessive caffeine may

---

cause additive CNS stimulation; use with general anesthetics may result in cardiac arrhythmias.

Antacids, sodium bicarbonate, and acetazolamide increase renal reabsorption of phenmetrazine and prolong its duration of action; phenothiazines and haloperidol decrease phenmetrazine effects.

Effects on diagnostic tests
None reported.

Adverse reactions
● CNS: nervousness, dizziness, insomnia, headache, fainting, euphoria.
● CV: tachycardia, palpitations, increased blood pressure, arrhythmias.
● DERM: urticaria, rash, hair loss, burning sensation.
● EENT: blurred vision.
● GI: dry mouth, nausea, abdominal cramps, constipation.
● GU: changes in libido, impotence, dysuria, menstrual changes.
● HEMA: bone marrow depression.
● Other: dyspnea, gynecomastia, sweating, chills, fever, physical and psychological dependence, tolerance.
   Note: Drug should be discontinued if signs of hypersensitivity occur.

Overdose and treatment
Symptoms of acute overdose include restlessness, tremor, hyperreflexia, fever, tachypnea, dizziness, confusion, aggressive behavior, hallucinations, panic, blood pressure changes, arrhythmias, nausea, vomiting, diarrhea, and cramps. Fatigue and depression usually follow CNS stimulation; seizures, coma, and death may follow.

Treat overdose symptomatically and supportively: sedation may be necessary. Treatment with chlorpromazine may antagonize CNS stimulation. Acidification of urine may hasten excretion. Monitor vital signs and fluid and electrolyte balance.

▶ **Special considerations**
Besides those relevant to all *amphetamines,* consider the following recommendations.
● Check vital signs regularly. Observe for signs of excessive stimulation.
● Urinary acidification enhances renal excretion; urinary alkalinization enhances renal reabsorption and recycling.
● Tolerance or dependence may develop; drug

has a high abuse potential. Not advised for prolonged use.
● Be sure patient also is following a weight-reduction program.
● Fatigue may result as drug effects wear off. Patient will need more rest.
● Intermittent courses of therapy (6 weeks on, 4 weeks off) are equally effective as continuous use.
● Greatest weight loss occurs in first few weeks of therapy, decreasing in succeeding weeks. When tolerance develops, it is best to discontinue the drug rather than increase the dosage.
● Do not crush sustained-release tablets.
● Give morning dose 2 hours after breakfast.

Information for the patient
● Tell patient to avoid drinks containing caffeine, which increases the effects of amphetamines and related amines.
● Advise patient to take last dose at least 6 hours before bedtime to avoid insomnia.
● Warn patient that drug may produce dizziness and fatigue and to use caution while driving or performing other hazardous tasks.
● Tell patient not to take drug more frequently than prescribed, not to crush or chew sustained-release tablets, and to avoid concurrent caffeine use.
● Advise patient to call if palpitations occur.

Geriatric use
Lower dosages may be effective because of decreased renal function.

Pediatric use
Phenmetrazine is not recommended for children under age 12.

---

phentermine hydrochloride
Adipex-P, Anoxine-AM, Dapex-37.5, Fastin,
Ionamin, Obe-Nix, Obephen, Obermine,
Parmine, Phentrol 2, Phentrol 4, Phentrol 5,
Wilpowr

- Pharmacologic classification: amphetamine
  congener
- Therapeutic classification: short-term adjunctive anorexigenic agent, indirect-acting sympathomimetic amine
- Controlled substance schedule IV
- Pregnancy risk category C

How supplied
Available by prescription only
Capsules and tablets: 8 mg, 15 mg, 18.75 mg,
30 mg, 37.5 mg
Capsules (resin complex, sustained-release): 15
mg, 30 mg

Indications, route, and dosage
*Short-term adjunct adjunct in exogenous
obesity*
Adults: 8 mg. P.O. t.i.d. ½ hour before meals;
or 15 to 37.5 mg daily before breakfast (sustained-release).

Pharmacodynamics
Anorexigenic action: Phentermine is an indirect-
acting sympathomimetic amine; it causes fewer
and less severe adverse reactions from CNS
stimulation than do amphetamines, and its potential for addiction is lower.
  Anorexigenic effects are thought to follow direct stimulation of the hypothalamus; they may
involve other CNS and metabolic effects.

Pharmacokinetics
- *Absorption:* Phentermine is absorbed readily
  after oral administration; therapeutic effects
  persist for 4 to 6 hours.
- *Distribution:* Phentermine is distributed
  widely throughout the body.
- *Metabolism:* Unknown.
- *Excretion:* Phentermine is excreted in urine.

Contraindications and precautions
Phentermine is contraindicated in patients with
known hypersensitivity to phentermine, and in
patients with hyperthyroidism, all degrees of
hypertension, angina pectoris or other severe
CV disease, glaucoma, or advanced arteriosclerosis. Phentermine also is contraindicated for

use with MAO inhibitors or within 14 days of
such use.
  It should be used with caution in patients with
known hypersensitivity to sympathomimetic
amines; in hyperexcitability and agitated states;
and in patients with a history of substance
abuse. Habituation or psychological dependence may follow prolonged use.

Interactions
Concomitant use with MAO inhibitors (or drugs
with MAO-inhibiting effects, such as furazoli-
dine) or within 14 days of such therapy may
cause hypertensive crisis. Phentermine may decrease hypotensive effects of guanethidine and
other antihypertensive agents; it also may alter
insulin requirements in diabetic patients. Concomitant use with excessive amounts of caffeine
may cause additive CNS stimulation.
  Concomitant use with general anesthetics may
result in cardiac arrhythmias. Antacids, sodium
bicarbonate, and acetazolamide increase renal
reabsorption of phentermine and prolong its duration of action. Phenothiazines and haloperidol
decrease phentermine effects.

Effects on diagnostic tests
None reported.

Adverse reactions
- CNS: nervousness, dizziness, insomnia, fainting, euphoria, depression.
- CV: palpitations, tachycardia, increased blood
  pressure, arrhythmias.
- DERM: urticaria, rash, burning sensation, hair
  loss.
- GI: dry mouth, unpleasant taste, nausea, constipation, diarrhea.
- GU: changes in libido, impotence, polyuria,
  menstrual changes.
- HEMA: bone marrow depression.
- Other: dyspnea, blurred vision, gynecomastia,
  sweating, chills, physical and psychological dependence.
  Note: Drug should be discontinued if signs
of hypersensitivity occur.

Overdose and treatment
Symptoms of acute overdose include restlessness, tremor, hyperreflexia, fever, tachypnea,
dizziness, confusion, aggressive behavior, hallucinations, blood pressure changes, arrhythmias, nausea, vomiting, diarrhea, and cramps.
Fatigue and depression usually follow CNS stimulation; seizures, coma, and death may follow.
  Treat overdose symptomatically and supportively; monitor cardiac function. Sedation

---

may be necessary. Chlorpromazine may antagonize CNS stimulation. Acidification of urine may hasten excretion. Monitor vital signs and fluid and electrolyte balance.

▶ **Special considerations**
Besides those relevant to all *amphetamines*, consider the following recommendations.
• Intermittent courses of treatment (6 weeks on, followed by 4 weeks off) are equally effective as continuous use.
• Greatest weight loss occurs in the first weeks of therapy and diminishes in succeeding weeks. When such tolerance to drug effect develops, drug should be discontinued instead of increasing the dosage.
• Do not crush sustained-release dosage forms.
• Give morning dose 2 hours after breakfast.

Information for the patient
• Advise patient to take morning dose 2 hours after breakfast, not to crush or chew sustained-release products, and to avoid caffeine-containing drinks.
• Tell patient to take last daily dosage at least 6 hours before bedtime to prevent insomnia.
• Warn patient not to take drug more frequently than prescribed.
• Tell patient to call if palpitations occur.
• Tell diabetic patients to closely monitor blood glucose. Changes in eating habits, body weight, and activity may require adjustment of hypoglycemic drug regimen.

Pediatric use
Phentermine is not recommended for children under age 12.

Sedative-hypnotics

amobarbital
amobarbital sodium
aprobarbital
butabarbital sodium
chloral hydrate
diazepam (See *ANTICONVULSANTS.*)
estazolam
ethchlorvynol
ethinamate
flurazepam hydrochloride
glutethimide
lorazepam (See *ANXIOLYTICS.*)
methyprylon
pentobarbital sodium
phenobarbital
phenobarbital sodium
quazepam
secobarbital sodium
temazepam
triazolam

Sedative-hypnotics, which produce widespread CNS depression, are used primarily to produce drowsiness and to promote sleep. They have also been useful preoperatively to allay anxiety and facilitate induction of anesthesia.

A sedative decreases CNS activity, resulting in a quieting effect accompanied by relaxation and rest without inducing sleep. A hypnotic produces drowsiness and facilitates onset and maintenance of sleep. A single drug can have both sedative and hypnotic properties; the response is dose-related.

Pharmacologic effects
● *Barbiturates* (amobarbital, aprobarbital, butabarbital, pentobarbital, phenobarbital, secobarbital) were once the drugs of choice for the management of anxiety or insomnia. Except for phenobarbital's use as an anticonvulsant, they have been replaced by the benzodiazepines.
● *Benzodiazepines* (estazolam, flurazepam, quazepam, temazepam, triazolam) are used in the treatment of insomnia and anxiety. Some are useful anticonvulsants; others are used to provide preoperative sedation.
● *Miscellaneous sedative-hypnotics* (chloral hydrate, ethchlorvynol, ethinamate, glutethimide, methyprylon), once widely used as hypnotic agents, are rarely used today.

Mechanism of action
Barbiturates act on the CNS through an unknown mechanism. Apparently, they reversibly decrease the activity of all excitable tissues, particularly in the CNS. They induce an imbalance in central inhibitory and facilitory mechanisms of the cerebral cortex and reticular formation, but the significance of this effect on neurotransmitters is unknown. They are capable of producing all levels of CNS alteration; used in low doses, they depress the sensory cortex, decrease motor activity, alter cerebral function, and produce drowsiness, sedation, and hypnosis.

Benzodiazepines are also capable of producing all levels of CNS depression. Their exact mechanism of action is unknown but appears to be mediated through the inhibitory transmitter gamma-aminobutyric acid.

Miscellaneous sedative-hypnotics require larger dosages to effect hypnosis. They have CNS depressant effects similar to barbiturates but their mechanisms of action are unknown.

Pharmacokinetics
● *Absorption and distribution:* Barbiturates are absorbed in varying degrees but the absorption rate is increased if the drug is taken on an empty stomach. They are rapidly distributed to all tissues and fluids with concentrations in brain, liver, and kidney. The benzodiazepines are well-absorbed from the GI tract and are widely distributed in the body. Glutethimide is irregularly absorbed with extensive localization in adipose tissue. Ethinamate and chloral hydrate are rapidly and almost completely absorbed but distribution in the body is unknown. Ethchlorvynol is rapidly absorbed with extensive localization in adipose tissue.

● *Metabolism and excretion:* All three groups of sedative-hypnotics are metabolized in the liver. Repeated dosage of some agents produces accumulation of the parent compound and active metabolites. They are excreted primarily in the urine as unchanged drug and/or metabolites.

COMPARING SEDATIVE-HYPNOTICS

CLASS AND DRUG	USUAL ADULT DOSAGE	HALF-LIFE	CLINICAL CONSIDERATIONS
barbiturates			
amobarbital	65 to 200 mg	20 hours	Duration of action is 6 to 8 hours
aprobarbital	40 mg	14 to 40 hours	Available only as an elixir; alcohol content is 20%.
butabarbital	15 to 30 mg	34 to 42 hours	Hypnotic dose is 50 to 100 mg
pentobarbital	100 mg	35 to 50 hours	Short duration of action (1 to 4 hours)
phenobarbital	30 to 120 mg/day	2 to 6 days	Hypnotic dose is 100 to 320 mg
secobarbital	100 mg	15 to 40 hours	Short duration of action (1 to 4 hours)
benzodiazepines			
estazolam	1 to 2 mg	10 to 24 hours	No active metabolites
flurazepam	15 to 30 mg	Short	Active metabolite desalkylflurazepam forms rapidly; half-life is 50 to 100 hours
lorazepam	2 to 4 mg	10 to 20 hours	No active metabolites
quazepam	7.5 to 15 mg	39 hours	Two active metabolites: 2-oxoquazepam (half-life is 39 hours) and N-desalkyl-2-oxo-quazepam (half-life is > 700 hours)
temazepam	15 to 30 mg	10 to 17 hours	No active metabolites
triazolam	0.125 to 0.25 mg	1.5 to 5.5 hours	No active metabolites
Other			
chloral hydrate	500 mg to 1 g	Short	Rapidly metabolized to trichloroethanol (half-life is 8 hours)
ethchlorvynol	500 mg to 1 g	10 to 20 hours	Drug accumulates in body fat
glutethimide	250 to 500 mg	10 to 12 hours	Drug accumulates in body fat
methyprylon	200 to 400 mg	3 to 6 hours	Drug accumulates in body fat

Adverse reactions and toxicity

Most common adverse reactions include drowsiness, GI irritation, nausea, vomiting, constipation, residual sedation or hangover, and skin rash. Tolerance and physical and psychological dependence may develop after prolonged use; withdrawal symptoms may follow sudden discontinuation. Treatment of overdosage is mainly supportive and symptomatic. Hemodialysis may not be useful, particularly with glutethimide overdosage.

Clinical considerations

- Use with caution in patients with liver disease.
- Avoid concurrent use with tricyclic antidepressants, MAO inhibitors, alcohol, and other CNS depressants.
- Sedative-hypnotics are frequently used preoperatively to allay anxiety and apprehension.
- The sedative agent chosen should depend on the severity of the insomnia, which may not require therapy. When treatment is appropriate, barbiturates are usually avoided in favor of safer alternatives. For example, in a

patient who needs a stronger effect than that produced by benzodiazepines, low-dose treatment with chloral hydrate could be useful.

- The risk of dependence varies among these agents and requires close medical supervision.
- Severe withdrawal symptoms may follow abrupt discontinuation if drug is stopped after prolonged use of standard dosage.
- Advise patient to avoid alcohol during treatment because the cumulative CNS effects are potentially hazardous.
- Elderly patients may react to usual dosage with disorientation, confusion, hallucinations, depression, or excitement.
- Barbiturate-induced hypothermia may occur more frequently in elderly patients.
- Many sedative-hypnotics cross the placental barrier. Chronic use in pregnancy may cause withdrawal effects in the neonate.

---

amobarbital, amobarbital sodium
Amytal

- Pharmacologic classification: barbiturate
- Therapeutic classification: sedative-hypnotic, anticonvulsant
- Controlled substance schedule II
- Pregnancy risk category D

How supplied
Available by prescription only
Tablets: 30 mg, 50 mg, 100 mg
Capsules: 65 mg, 200 mg
Powder for injection: 250 mg, 500 mg/vial
Powder (bulk): 15 g, 30 g

Indications, route, and dosage
Sedation
Adults: Usually 30 to 50 mg P.O. b.i.d. or t.i.d. but may range from 15 to 120 mg b.i.d. to q.i.d.
Children: 3 to 6 mg/kg P.O. daily divided into four equal doses.
Insomnia
Adults: 65 to 200 mg P.O. or deep I.M. h.s.; I.M. injection not to exceed 5 ml in any one site. Maximum dosage is 500 mg.
Children over age 6: 3 to 5 mg/kg deep I.M. h.s.; I.M. injection not to exceed 5 ml in any one site.
Preanesthetic sedation
Adults and children over age 6: 200 mg P.O. or I.M. 1 to 2 hours before surgery.

Adjunct in psychology – "amobarbital interview"
Adults: 50 mg/minute by slow, cautious I.V. infusion. Continue until the patient shows drowsiness or sustained rapid lateral nystagmus (commonly after 150 to 350 mg). Proceed with interview using supplemental doses of 25 to 50 mg q 5 minutes.
Seizures
Adults: 65 to 500 mg by slow I.V. injection (rate not exceeding 100 mg/minute). Maximum dose is 1 g.
Children under age 6: 3 to 5 mg/kg slowly I.V.

Pharmacodynamics
- *Anticonvulsant action:* The exact cellular site and mechanism(s) of action are unknown. Parenteral amobarbital suppresses the spread of seizure activity produced by epileptogenic foci in the cortex, thalamus, and limbic systems by enhancing the effect of gamma-aminobutyric acid (GABA). Both presynaptic and postsynaptic excitability are decreased.
- *Sedative-hypnotic action:* Amobarbital acts throughout the CNS as a nonselective depressant with an intermediate onset and duration of action. Particularly sensitive to this drug is the mesencephalic reticular activating system, which controls CNS arousal. Amobarbital decreases both presynaptic and postsynaptic membrane excitability by facilitating the action of GABA.

Pharmacokinetics
- *Absorption:* Amobarbital is absorbed well after oral administration. Absorption after I.M. administration is 100%. Onset of action is 45 to 60 minutes.
- *Distribution:* Well distributed throughout body tissues and fluids.
- *Metabolism:* Metabolized in the liver by oxidation to a tertiary alcohol.
- *Excretion:* Less than 1% of a dose is excreted unchanged in the urine. The rest is excreted as metabolites. The half-life is biphasic, with a first phase half-life of about 40 minutes and a second phase of about 20 hours. Duration of action is 6 to 8 hours.

Contraindications and precautions
Amobarbital is contraindicated in patients with known hypersensitivity to barbiturates and in patients with bronchopneumonia, status asthmaticus, or other severe respiratory distress because of the potential for respiratory depression.

Amobarbital should not be used in patients who are depressed or have suicidal ideation be-

---

cause the drug can worsen depression; in patients with uncontrolled acute or chronic pain because paradoxical excitement can occur; or in patients with porphyria because the drug can trigger symptoms of this disease.

Amobarbital should be used cautiously in patients who must perform hazardous tasks requiring mental alertness because the drug causes drowsiness. Administer parenteral amobarbital slowly and with extreme caution to patients with hypotension or severe pulmonary or cardiovascular disease because of potential adverse hemodynamic effects. Because tolerance and physical or psychological dependence may occur, prolonged use of high doses should be avoided.

Use cautiously in patients with renal or hepatic disease, as drug accumulation may occur. CNS depression may be exacerbated in patients with shock or uremia. Prenatal exposure to barbiturates is associated with an increased incidence of fetal abnormalities and possibly brain tumors. Use of barbiturates in the third trimester may be associated with physical dependence in neonates. Risk to benefit ratio must be considered.

Interactions

Amobarbital may add to or potentiate CNS and respiratory depressant effects of other sedative-hypnotics, antihistamines, narcotics, antidepressants, MAO inhibitors, tranquilizers, and alcohol.

Amobarbital enhances the enzymatic degradation of warfarin and other oral anticoagulants; patients may require increased doses of the anticoagulants. Amobarbital also enhances hepatic metabolism of digitoxin (not digoxin), corticosteroids, theophylline and other xanthines, oral contraceptives and other estrogens, and doxycycline. Amobarbital impairs the effectiveness of griseofulvin by decreasing absorption from the GI tract. Amobarbital may cause unpredictable fluctuations in serum phenytoin levels.

Valproic acid, phenytoin, MAO inhibitors, and disulfiram decrease the metabolism of amobarbital and can increase its toxicity.

Rifampin may decrease amobarbital levels by increasing metabolism.

Effects on diagnostic tests

Amobarbital may cause a false-positive phentolamine test. The physiologic effects of amobarbital may impair the absorption of cyanocobalamin ^{57}Co; it may decrease serum bilirubin concentrations in neonates, patients with

seizure disorders, and patients with congenital nonhemolytic unconjugated hyperbilirubinemia. EEG patterns are altered, with a change in low-voltage and fast activity; changes persist for a time after discontinuation of therapy.

Adverse reactions

● CNS: drowsiness, lethargy, vertigo, headache, CNS depression, mental depression, paradoxical excitement; confusion and agitation (especially in elderly patients); rebound insomnia, increased dreams or nightmares, and possibly *seizures* (after acute withdrawal or reduction in dosage).

● CV: hypotension (after rapid I.V. administration), bradycardia, syncope, *circulatory collapse.*

● DERM: urticaria, rash, *exfoliative dermatitis, Stevens-Johnson syndrome.*

● EENT: laryngospasm, *bronchospasm,* miosis, mydriasis (with severe toxicity).

● GI: nausea, vomiting, diarrhea, constipation, epigastric pain.

● Local: thrombophlebitis, pain and possible tissue damage at extravascular injection site.

● Other: *respiratory depression,* blood dyscrasias, physical and psychological dependence. Vitamin K deficiency and bleeding have occurred in neonates of mothers treated during pregnancy. Hyperalgesia occurs with low doses or in patients with chronic pain.

Note: Drug should be discontinued if hypersensitivity reaction, profound CNS or respiratory depression, or skin eruption occurs.

Overdose and treatment

Clinical manifestations of overdose include unsteady gait, slurred speech, sustained nystagmus, somnolence, confusion, respiratory depression, pulmonary edema, areflexia, and coma. Oliguria, jaundice, hypothermia, fever, and shock with tachycardia and hypotension may occur.

Maintain and support ventilation as necessary; support circulation with vasopressors and I.V. fluids as needed.

Treatment is aimed to maintain and support ventilation and pulmonary function as necessary; support cardiac function and circulation with vasopressors and I.V. fluids as needed. If patient is conscious with a functioning gag reflex and ingestion has been recent, then induce emesis by administering ipecac syrup. Gastric lavage may be performed if a cuffed endotracheal tube is in place to prevent aspiration when emesis is inappropriate. Follow with administration of activated charcoal or saline cathartic.

---

*Canada only   †Unlabeled clinical use   Italicized adverse reactions are life-threatening.

Measure fluid intake and output, vital signs, and laboratory parameters. Maintain body temperature.

Alkalinization of urine may be helpful in removing amobarbital from the body; hemodialysis may be useful in severe overdose.

▶ **Special considerations**
Besides those relevant to all *barbiturates,* consider the following recommendations.
• Not commonly used as a sedative or aid to sleeping; barbiturates have been replaced by safer alternatives (such as benzodiazepines).
• Administer oral amobarbital before meals or on an empty stomach to enhance the rate of absorption.
• Reconstitute powder for injection with sterile water for injection. Roll vial in hands; do not shake. Use 2.5 or 5 ml (for 250 or 500 mg of amobarbital) to make 10% solution. For I.M. use, prepare 20% solution by using 1.25 or 2.5 ml of sterile water for injection.
• Administer reconstituted parenteral solution within 30 minutes after opening the vial.
• Do not administer any amobarbital solution that is cloudy or forms a precipitate after 5 minutes of reconstitution.
• Administer I.V. dose at a rate no greater than 100 mg/minute in adults or 60 mg/m^2/minute in children to prevent possible hypotension and respiratory depression. Have emergency resuscitative equipment available.
• Administer I.M. dose deep into large muscle mass, giving no more than 5 ml in any one injection site. Sterile abscess or tissue damage may result from inadvertent superficial I.M. or S.C. injection.
• Administering full loading doses over short periods of time to treat status epilepticus may require ventilatory support in adults.
• Assess cardiopulmonary status frequently for possible alterations. Monitor blood counts for potential adverse reactions.
• Assess renal and hepatic laboratory studies to ensure adequate drug removal.
• Monitor prothrombin times carefully when patient on amobarbital starts or ends anticoagulant therapy. Anticoagulant dosage may need to be adjusted.

Information for the patient
Warn patient of possible physical or psychological dependence with prolonged use.

Geriatric use
Elderly patients usually require lower doses. Confusion, disorientation, and excitability may occur in elderly patients. Use with caution.

Pediatric use
Safe use in children under age 6 has not been established. Use of amobarbital may cause paradoxical excitement in some children.

Breast-feeding
Amobarbital passes into breast milk and may cause drowsiness in the infant. If so, dosage adjustment or discontinuation of drug or of breast-feeding may be necessary. Use with caution.

aprobarbital
Alurate

• Pharmacologic classification: barbiturate
• Therapeutic classification: sedative-hypnotic
• Controlled substance schedule III
• Pregnancy risk category D

How supplied
Available by prescription only
Elixir: 40 mg/5 ml

Indications, route, and dosage
Sedation
Adults: 40 mg P.O. t.i.d.
Mild insomnia
Adults: 40 to 80 mg P.O. h.s.
Severe insomnia
Adults: 80 to 160 mg P.O. h.s.

Pharmacodynamics
Sedative action: The exact cellular site and mechanism(s) of action are unknown. Aprobarbital acts throughout the CNS as a nonselective depressant with intermediate onset and duration of action. Particularly sensitive to this drug is the recticular activating system, which controls CNS arousal. Aprobarbital decreases both presynaptic and postsynaptic membrane excitability by facilitating the action of gamma-aminobutyric acid.

Pharmacokinetics
• *Absorption:* Aprobarbital is absorbed well after oral administration. Peak serum levels are reached within 3 hours, and onset of action occurs 45 to 60 minutes after dosing.

● *Distribution:* Aprobarbital is distributed widely throughout body tissues and fluids. Drug is 35% protein-bound.

● *Metabolism:* Aprobarbital is metabolized in the liver by oxidation to inactive metabolites.

● *Excretion:* Aprobarbital and metabolites are eliminated in urine; about 15% to 25% of a dose is excreted as unchanged drug. Half-life ranges from 14 to 34 hours. Its duration of action is 6 to 8 hours.

Contraindications and precautions

Aprobarbital is contraindicated in patients with known hypersensitivity to barbiturates and in patients with bronchopneumonia, status asthmaticus, or other severe respiratory distress because of the potential for respiratory depression. Aprobarbital should not be used in patients who are depressed or have suicidal ideation because the drug can worsen depression; in patients with uncontrolled acute or chronic pain because paradoxical excitement can occur; or in patients with porphyria because the drug can trigger symptoms of this disease.

Aprobarbital should be used cautiously in patients who must perform hazardous tasks requiring mental alertness because the drug causes drowsiness and in patients with impaired renal function because up to 25% of aprobarbital is excreted unchanged in urine. Prolonged use of high doses should be avoided because tolerance and physical or psychological dependence may occur.

Prenatal exposure to barbiturates is associated with an increased incidence of fetal abnormalities and, possibly, brain tumors. Use of barbiturates in the third trimester may be associated with physical dependence in neonates. Risk-benefit must be considered.

Interactions

Concomitant use with other sedative-hypnotics, antihistamines, narcotics, antidepressants, tranquilizers, and alcohol may potentiate or add to their CNS and respiratory depressant actions.

Aprobarbital enhances the enzymatic degradation of warfarin and other oral anticoagulants; patients may require increased doses of the anticoagulants. Drug also enhances hepatic metabolism of digitoxin (not digoxin), corticosteroids, theophylline and other xanthines, oral contraceptives and other estrogens, and doxycycline. Aprobarbital may inhibit absorption of griseofulvin.

Valproic acid, phenytoin, disulfiram, and MAO inhibitors decrease the metabolism of aprobarbital and can increase its toxicity; rifampin may

decrease aprobarbital levels by increasing metabolism.

Effects on diagnostic tests

Aprobarbital may cause a false-positive phentolamine test. The physiologic effects of the drug may impair the absorption of cyanocobalamin ^{57}Co; it may decrease serum bilirubin concentrations in neonates, patients with seizure disorders, and patients with congenital nonhemolytic unconjugated hyperbilirubinemia. EEG patterns are altered, with a change in low-voltage and fast activity; changes persist for a time after discontinuation of therapy.

Adverse reactions

● CNS: drowsiness, lethargy, vertigo, headache, CNS depression, mental depression, paradoxical excitement; confusion and agitation (especially in elderly patients); rebound insomnia, increased dreams or nightmares, and possibly *seizures* (after acute withdrawal or reduction in dosage).

● CV: bradycardia, hypotension, syncope.

● DERM: urticaria, rash, *exfoliative dermatitis, Stevens-Johnson syndrome.*

● EENT: laryngospasm or *bronchospasm,* miosis.

● GI: nausea, vomiting, diarrhea, constipation.

● Other: *respiratory depression,* blood dyscrasias, physical and psychological dependence. Vitamin K deficiency and bleeding have occurred in neonates of mothers treated during pregnancy. Hyperalgesia may occur with the use of low doses or in patients with chronic pain.

Note: Drug should be discontinued if hypersensitivity reaction, profound CNS or respiratory depression, or skin eruption occurs.

Overdose and treatment

Clinical manifestations of overdose include somnolence, confusion, respiratory depression, pulmonary edema, areflexia, and coma. Typical shock syndrome with tachycardia and hypotension may occur. Jaundice, oliguria and hypothermia may occur, followed by fever, unsteady gait, slurred speech, and sustained nystagmus.

Maintain and support ventilation and pulmonary function, as necessary; support cardiac function and circulation with vasopressors and I.V. fluids, as needed. If patient is conscious with a functioning gag reflex and ingestion is recent, induce emesis by administering ipecac syrup. Gastric lavage may be performed as long as a cuffed endotracheal tube is in place to prevent aspiration when emesis is inappropriate. Follow by administering activated charcoal or saline cathartic. Measure intake and output, vital signs, and laboratory parameters. Maintain body temperature. Alkalinization of urine may be helpful in removing drug from the body; hemodialysis may be useful in severe overdose.

▶ **Special considerations**
Besides those relevant to all *barbiturates,* consider the following recommendations.
● Generally, barbiturates have been replaced by benzodiazepines and other safer alternatives for the treatment of insomnia.
● Elixir contains alcohol 20%.
● Assess cardiopulmonary status frequently. Monitor vital signs and report any changes.
● Assess renal and hepatic function studies and blood counts to detect abnormalities.
● Monitor prothrombin times carefully when patient on aprobarbital starts or ends anticoagulant therapy. Anticoagulant dosage may need to be adjusted.
● Watch for signs of barbiturate toxicity (coma, pupillary constriction, cyanosis, clammy skin, hypotension). Overdose can be fatal.

Information for the patient
● Warn patient not to change dose or frequency of use or to discontinue drug abruptly without medical approval. Rebound insomnia, increased dreams or nightmares, or seizures may occur.
● Warn patient that physical and psychological dependence may follow prolonged use.
● Warn patient about the dangers of combining this drug with alcohol. An additive effect is possible even if the drug was taken the evening before drinking alcohol.

Geriatric use
● Elderly patients usually require lower doses.
● Elderly patients are more susceptible to CNS depressant effects of aprobarbital. Confusion, disorientation, and excitability may occur.

Pediatric use
Barbiturates may cause paradoxical excitement in children. Use with caution.

Breast-feeding
Aprobarbital passes into breast milk and may cause drowsiness in the infant. If so, dosage adjustment or discontinuation of the drug or of breast-feeding may be necessary. Use with caution.

butabarbital sodium
Barbased, Butalan, Butisol, Sarisol No. 2

● Pharmacologic classification: barbiturate
● Therapeutic classification: sedative-hypnotic
● Controlled substance schedule III
● Pregnancy risk category D

How supplied
Available by prescription only
Tablets: 15 mg, 30 mg, 50 mg, 100 mg
Capsules: 15 mg, 30 mg
Elixir: 30 mg/5 ml, 33.3 mg/5 ml

Indications, route, and dosage
Sedation
Adults: 15 to 30 mg P.O. t.i.d. or q.i.d.
Children: 2 mg/kg P.O. divided t.i.d. or 60 mg/m² t.i.d.
Preoperative sedation
Adults: 50 to 100 mg P.O. 60 to 90 minutes before surgery.
Children: 2 to 6 mg/kg; up to a maximum of 100 mg/dose.
Insomnia
Adults: 50 to 100 mg P.O. h.s.
Children: Dosage must be individualized.

Pharmacodynamics
Sedative action: The exact cellular site and mechanism(s) of action are unknown. Butabarbital acts throughout the CNS as a nonselective depressant with an intermediate onset and duration of action. Particularly sensitive to the drug is the reticular activating system, which controls CNS arousal. Butabarbital decreases both presynaptic and postsynaptic membrane excitability by facilitating the action of gamma-aminobutyric acid.

Pharmacokinetics
● *Absorption:* Butabarbital is absorbed well after oral administration, with peak concentrations occurring in 3 to 4 hours. Onset of action occurs in 45 to 60 minutes. Serum concentrations needed for sedation and hypnosis are 2 to 3 mcg/ml and 25 mcg/ml, respectively.
● *Distribution:* Butabarbital is distributed well throughout body tissues and fluids.
● *Metabolism:* Butabarbital is metabolized extensively in the liver by oxidation. Its duration of action is 6 to 8 hours.
● *Excretion:* Inactive metabolites of butabarbital are excreted in urine. Only 1% to 2% of

an oral dose is excreted in urine unchanged. The terminal half-life ranges from 30 to 40 hours.

Contraindications and precautions

Butabarbital is contraindicated in patients with known hypersensitivity to barbiturates and in patients with bronchopneumonia, status asthmaticus, or other severe respiratory distress because of the potential for respiratory depression. Butabarbital should not be used in patients who are depressed or have suicidal ideation because the drug can worsen depression; in patients with uncontrolled acute or chronic pain because exacerbation of pain or paradoxical excitement can occur; or in patients with porphyria because the drug can trigger symptoms of this disease. Some butabarbital preparations contain tartrazine, which may precipitate an allergic reaction. Do not administer butabarbital to patients with a tartrazine sensitivity.

Butabarbital should be used cautiously in patients who must perform hazardous tasks requiring mental alertness because the drug causes drowsiness. Prolonged use of high doses should be avoided because tolerance and physical or psychological dependence may occur.

Prenatal exposure to barbiturates is associated with an increased incidence of fetal abnormalaities, including brain tumors. Use of barbiturates in the third trimester may be associated with physical dependence in neonates. Risk-benefit must be considered.

Use cautiously in patients with renal or hepatic dysfunction because of the risk of drug accumulation.

Interactions

Butabarbital may add to or potentiate the CNS and respiratory depressant effects of other sedative-hypnotics, antihistamines, narcotics, antidepressants, tranquilizers, and alcohol. Butabarbital enhances the enzymatic degradation of warfarin and other oral anticoagulants; patients may require increased doses of the anticoagulants. Drug also enhances hepatic metabolism of some drugs, including digitoxin (not digoxin), corticosteroids, oral contraceptives and other estrogens, theophylline and other xanthines, and doxycycline. Butabarbital impairs the effectiveness of griseofulvin by decreasing absorption from the GI tract.

Valproic acid, phenytoin, disulfiram, and MAO inhibitors decrease the metabolism of butabarbital and can increase its toxicity. Rifampin may decrease butabarbital levels by increasing hepatic metabolism.

Effects on diagnostic tests

Butabarbital may cause a false-positive phentolamine test. The physiologic effects of the drug may impair the absorption of cyanocobalamin ^{57}Co; it may decrease serum bilirubin concentrations in neonates, patients with seizure disorders, and patients with congenital nonhemolytic unconjugated hyperbilirubinemia. EEG patterns are altered, with a change in low-voltage and fast activity; changes persist for a time after discontinuation of therapy. Barbiturates may increase sulfobromophthalein retention.

Adverse reactions

● CNS: drowsiness, lethargy, vertigo, headache, CNS depression, paradoxical excitement; confusion and agitation (especially in elderly patients); rebound insomnia, increased dreams and nightmares, and possibly *seizures* (after acute withdrawal or reduction in dosage).
● CV: hypotension, bradycardia, syncope, *circulatory collapse.*
● DERM: urticaria, rash, *exfoliative dermatitis, Stevens-Johnson syndrome.*
● EENT: miosis.
● GI: epigastric pain, nausea, vomiting, diarrhea, constipation.
● Other: laryngospasm, *bronchospasm,* blood dyscrasias, physical and psychological dependency. Vitamin K deficiency and bleeding have been reported in neonates of mothers treated during pregnancy. Hyperalgesia occurs with low doses or in patients with chronic pain.

Note: Drug should be discontinued if hypersensitivity reaction, profound CNS or respiratory depression, or skin eruption occurs.

Overdose and treatment

Clinical manifestations of overdose include unsteady gait, slurred speech, sustained nystagmus, somnolence, confusion, respiratory depression, pulmonary edema, areflexia, and coma. Jaundice, hypothermia followed by fever, oliguria, and typical shock syndrome with tachycardia and hypotension may occur.

To treat, maintain and support ventilation and pulmonary function, as necessary; support cardiac function and circulation with vasopressors and I.V. fluids, as needed. If patient is conscious with a functioning gag reflex and ingestion was recent, induce emesis by administering ipecac syrup. If emesis is contraindicated, perform gastric lavage while a cuffed endotracheal tube is in place, to prevent aspiration. Follow by administering activated charcoal or saline cathartic. Measure intake and output, vital signs, and laboratory parameters. Maintain body tem-

---

perature. Alkalinization of urine may be helpful in removing drug from the body; hemodialysis may be useful in severe overdose.

▶ **Special considerations**
Besides those relevant to all *barbiturates,* consider the following recommendations.
● Barbiturates have been replaced by benzodiazepines and other safer alternatives to provide sedation and treat insomnia.
● Tablet may be crushed and mixed with food or fluid if patient has difficulty swallowing. Capsule may be opened and contents mixed with food or fluids to aid in swallowing.
● Assess cardiopulmonary status frequently; monitor vital signs for significant changes.
● Monitor patients for possible allergic reaction resulting from tartrazine sensitivity.
● Periodically evaluate blood counts and renal and hepatic studies for abnormalities and adverse reactions.
● Monitor prothrombin times carefully when patient on butabarbital starts or ends anticoagulant therapy. Anticoagulant dosage may need to be adjusted.
● Watch for signs of barbiturate toxicity (coma, pupillary constriction, cyanosis, clammy skin, hypotension). Overdose can be fatal.
● Prolonged administration is not recommended; drug has not been shown to be effective after 14 days. A drug-free interval of at least 1 week is advised between dosing periods.

Information for the patient
● Tell patient to avoid driving and other hazardous activities that require alertness because the drug may cause drowsiness.
● Warn patient that prolonged use can cause physical or psychological dependence.
● Warn patient about the dangers of combining this drug with alcohol. An additive effect is possible even if the drug was taken the evening before drinking alcohol.

Geriatric use
● Elderly patients are more susceptible to the CNS depressant effects of butabarbital. Confusion, disorientation, and excitability may occur.
● Elderly patients usually require lower doses.

Pediatric use
Butabarbital may cause paradoxical excitement in children. Dosage is dependent on age and weight of child and degree of sedation required. Use with caution.

Breast-feeding
Butabarbital passes into breast milk; avoid use in breast-feeding women.

---

chloral hydrate
Aquachloral Supprettes, Noctec, Novochlorhydrate

● Pharmacologic classification: general CNS depressant
● Therapeutic classification: sedative-hypnotic
● Controlled substance schedule IV
● Pregnancy risk category C

How supplied
Available by prescription only
Capsules: 250 mg, 500 mg
Syrup: 250 mg/5 ml, 500 mg/5 ml
Suppositories: 325 mg, 500 mg, 650 mg

Indications, route, and dosage
Sedation
Adults: 250 mg P.O. or rectally t.i.d. after meals.
Children: 8 mg/kg P.O. t.i.d. Maximum dosage is 500 mg t.i.d.
Insomnia
Adults: 500 mg to 1 g P.O. or rectally 15 to 30 minutes before bedtime.
Children: 50 mg/kg single dose. Maximum dosage is 1 g.
Premedication for EEG
Children: 25 mg/kg single dose. Maximum dosage is 1 g.
Hypnosis
Children: 50 mg/kg P.O. or 1.5 g/m² as a single dose.

Pharmacodynamics
Sedative-hypnotic action: Chloral hydrate has CNS depressant activities similar to those of the barbiturates. Nonspecific CNS depression occurs at hypnotic doses; however, respiratory drive is only slightly affected. The drug's primary site of action is the reticular activating system, which controls arousal. The cellular site(s) of action are not known.

Pharmacokinetics
● *Absorption:* Chloral hydrate is absorbed well after oral and rectal administration. Sleep occurs 30 to 60 minutes after a 500-mg to 1-g dose.
● *Distribution:* Chloral hydrate and its active metabolite trichloroethanol are distributed

---

throughout the body tissue and fluids. Tri-chloroethanol is 35% to 41% protein-bound.

● *Metabolism:* Chloral hydrate is metabolized rapidly and nearly completely in the liver and erythrocytes to the active metabolite trichloroethanol. It is further metabolized in the liver and kidneys to trichloroacetic acid and other inactive metabolites.

● *Excretion:* The inactive metabolites of chloral hydrate are excreted primarily in urine. Minor amounts are excreted in bile. The half-life of trichloroethanol is 8 to 10 hours.

Contraindications and precautions

Chloral hydrate is contraindicated in patients with known hypersensitivity to chloral derivatives; in patients with severe cardiac disease; and in patients with marked renal or hepatic failure because elimination of the drug will decrease.

Chloral hydrate should be used cautiously in patients with signs and symptoms of depression, suicidal ideation, or history of drug abuse or addiction because the drug depresses CNS function and in patients who need to perform hazardous tasks requiring mental alertness or physical coordination. Do not administer oral forms of chloral hydrate to patients with esophagitis, gastritis, or gastric or duodenal ulcers because the drug is irritating to the GI tract. Rectal chloral hydrate may exacerbate proctitis or ulcerative colitis.

Interactions

Concomitant use with alcohol, sedative-hypnotics, narcotics, antihistamines, tranquilizers, tricyclic antidepressants, or other CNS depressants will add to or potentiate their effects. Concomitant use with alcohol may cause vasodilation, tachycardia, sweating, and flushing in some patients.

Administration of chloral hydrate followed by I.V. furosemide may cause a hypermetabolic state by displacing thyroid hormone from binding sites, resulting in sweating, hot flashes, tachycardia, and variable blood pressure.

Chloral hydrate may displace oral anticoagulants such as warfarin from protein-binding sites, causing increased hypoprothrombinemic effects.

Effects on diagnostic tests

Chloral hydrate therapy may produce false-positive results for urine glucose with tests using cupric sulfate, such as Benedict's reagent and possibly Clinitest. It does not interfere with Clinistix or Tes-Tape results. It will interfere with fluorometric tests for urine catecholamines; do not use drug for 48 hours before the test. Drug may also interfere with Reddy-Jenkins-Thorn test for urinary 17-hydroxycorticosteroids. It also may cause a false-positive phentolamine test.

Adverse reactions

● CNS: hangover, headache, ataxia, confusion, hallucinations, disorientation, excitement, nightmares, paranoia.
● DERM: rash, urticaria, erythema, eczematoid dermatitis, scarlatiniform exanthema.
● GI: gastric irritation, nausea, vomiting, diarrhea, flatulence, altered taste.
● GU: ketonuria.
● HEMA: leukopenia, eosinophilia.
● Other: physical or psychological dependence.
   Note: Drug should be discontinued if hypersensitivity occurs, if patient becomes incoherent or disoriented, or if patient exhibits paranoid behavior.

Overdose and treatment

Clinical manifestations of overdose include stupor, coma, respiratory depression, pinpoint pupils, hypotension, and hypothermia. Esophageal stricture may follow gastric necrosis and perforation. GI hemorrhage has also been reported. Hepatic damage and jaundice may occur.

Treatment is supportive of respiration (including mechanical ventilation if needed), blood pressure, and body temperature. If the patient is conscious, empty stomach by emesis using ipecac syrup or gastric lavage. Hemodialysis will remove chloral hydrate and its metabolite, trichloroethanol. Peritoneal dialysis is ineffective.

▶ **Special considerations**

● Not a first-line drug because of potential for adverse or toxic effects.
● Assess level of consciousness before administering drug to ensure appropriate baseline level.
● Give chloral hydrate capsules with a full glass of water to lessen GI upset; dilute syrup in a half glass of water or juice before administration to improve taste.
● Monitor vital signs frequently.
● Store in dark container away from heat and moisture to prevent breakdown of medicine. Store suppositories in refrigerator.

Information for the patient
● Advise patient to take with a full glass of water, and to dilute syrup with juice or water before taking.
● Instruct patient in proper administration of drug form prescribed.
● Warn patient not to attempt tasks that require mental alertness or physical coordination until the CNS effects of the drug are known.
● Tell patient to avoid alcohol and other CNS depressants.
● Instruct patient to call before using any OTC allergy or cold preparations.
● Warn patient not to increase the dose or stop the drug except as prescribed.

Geriatric use
Elderly patients may be more susceptible to the drug's CNS depressant effects because of decreased elimination. Lower doses are indicated.

Pediatric use
Chloral hydrate is safe and effective as a premedication for EEG and other procedures.

Breast-feeding
Small amounts pass into the breast milk and may cause drowsiness in breast-fed infants of mothers taking chloral hydrate; avoid use in breast-feeding women.

---

estazolam
ProSom

● Pharmacologic classification: benzodiazepine
● Therapeutic classification: hypnotic
● Controlled substance schedule IV
● Pregnancy risk category X

How supplied
Available by prescription only
Tablets: 1 mg, 2 mg

Indications, route, and dosage
Short-term management of insomnia characterized by difficulty in falling asleep, frequent nocturnal awakenings, and/or early morning awakenings
Adults: Initially, 1 mg P.O. h.s.; may increase to 2 mg as needed and tolerated.
Elderly patients: 1 mg P.O. h.s.
Small or debilitated older adults: Initially, 0.5 mg P.O. h.s.; may increase with care to 1 mg if needed.

Pharmacodynamics
Hypnotic action: Estazolam depresses the CNS at the limbic and subcortical levels of the brain. It produces a sedative-hypnotic effect by potentiating the effect of the neurotransmitter gamma-aminobutyric acid on its receptor in the ascending reticular activating system, which increases inhibition and blocks both cortical and limbic arousal.

Pharmacokinetics
● *Absorption:* Estazolam is rapidly and completely absorbed through the GI tract in 1 to 3 hours. Peak levels occur within 2 hours (range is 0.5 to 6 hours)
● *Distribution:* Estazolam is 93% protein-bound.
● *Metabolism:* Estazolam is extensively metabolized in the liver.
● *Excretion:* Metabolites are excreted primarily in the urine. Less than 5% is excreted in urine as unchanged drug; 4% of a 2-mg dose is excreted in feces. Elimination half-life ranges from 10 to 24 hours; clearance is accelerated in smokers.

Contraindications and precautions
Estazolam is contraindicated in patients with history of hypersensitivity to benzodiazepines and during pregnancy because of the risk of fetal damage. Use with caution in elderly, debilitated patients and in patients with hepatic impairment, compromised respiratory function, depression, impaired renal function, and sleep apnea.

Interactions
Estazolam potentiates CNS depressant effects of phenothiazines, narcotics, antihistamines, MAO inhibitors, barbiturates, alcohol, general anesthetics, and antidepressants. Concurrent use with cimetidine, disulfiram, oral contraceptives, and isoniazid may result in diminished hepatic metabolism resulting in increased plasma concentrations of estazolam and increased CNS depressant effects. Heavy smoking accelerated estazolam's metabolism, resulting in diminished clinical efficacy. As with other benzodiazepines, estazolam increases phenytoin and digoxin levels, possibly resulting in toxicity. Use with probenecid results in more rapid onset and more prolonged benzodiazepine effect. Theophyllines antagonize estazolam's pharmacologic effects. Rifampin increases clearance and decreases half-life of estazolam.

Effects on diagnostic tests
AST (SGOT) levels may be increased.

Adverse reactions
● CNS: headache, abnormal coordination, nervousness, apprehension, malaise, confusion, somnolence, irritability, drowsiness, hypokinesia, amnesia, lethargy, hangover effect, ataxia, dizziness, euphoria, talkativeness, apathy, hostility, weakness, tremor, depression, syncope, nightmares, slurred speech, daytime sedation, restlessness. Hallucinations and paradoxical reactions may occur in elderly patients.
● CV: palpitations, chest pain, hypotension (rare), tachycardia.
● GI: nausea, vomiting, diarrhea, constipation, dry mouth, taste aberrations, anorexia, abdominal discomfort, heartburn, dyspepsia, flatulence.
● DERM: rash, urticaria, sweating, flushes, acne (rare), dry skin (rare).
● EENT: abnormal vision, ear pain, eye irritation, eye pain, eye swelling, photophobia, tinnitus, diplopia (rare), decreased hearing (rare).
● GU: urinary frequency and urgency, urinary hesitancy, menstrual cramps, decreased libido, vaginal discharge and itching, penile discharge, nocturia.
● Respiratory: cold, flulike symptoms, pharyngitis, asthma, cough, dyspnea, sinusitis, epistaxis, hyperventilation.
● Other: lower extremity pain, back pain, body pain, muscle stiffness, myalgia, allergic reaction, swollen lymph nodes, edema, weight gain.

Overdose and treatment
Somnolence, confusion with reduced or absent reflexes, respiratory depression, apnea, hypotension, impaired coordination, slurred speech, seizures, or coma can occur following benzodiazepine overdose. If excitation occurs, do not use barbiturates. Remember that multiple agents may have been ingested. Gastric evacuation and lavage should be performed immediately. Monitor respiration, pulse rate, and blood pressure. Use symptomatic and supportive measures. Maintain airway and administer fluids.

▶ **Special considerations**
Besides those relevant to all *benzodiazepines,* consider the following:
● Remove all potential safety hazards, such as cigarettes, from patient's reach.
● Periodically perform blood counts, urinalysis, and blood chemistry analyses.
● Withdraw drug slowly after prolonged use.
● Encourage good sleep habits, including regular exercise, and the avoidance of caffeine or other stimulants, especially late in the day.

Information for the patient
● Avoid alcohol and other CNS depressants while taking this medication. If you take the drug in the evening, avoid alcohol the following day.
● Tell physician what medications you are taking and about usual alcohol consumption.
● May cause drowsiness. Use care while driving or operating hazardous machinery until adverse CNS effects of theh drug are known.
● Nocturnal sleep may be disturbed for 1 or 2 nights after stopping the drug.
● Inform physician if you are pregnant, plan to become pregnant, or become pregnant while taking this drug.
● Do not discontinue abruptly after taking drug daily for prolonged period.
● Do not vary dosage or increase dose unless directed by physician.
● Do not use if you are nursing; estazolam is excreted in breast milk.

Geriatric use
Elderly patients may be more susceptible to CNS depressant effects of estazolam. Use with caution. Lower dosage may be required. Supervision of the patient during ambulation and daily living activities is recommended at the start of treatment and after an increase in dosage.

Pediatric use
Safety and efficacy have not been established.

Breast-feeding
Estazolam is excreted in breast milk. Avoid use in patients who are breast-feeding.

■■■■■■■■■■■■■■■■■■■■■

ethchlorvynol
Placidyl

● Pharmacologic classification: chlorinated tertiary acetylenic carbinol
● Therapeutic classification: sedative-hypnotic
● Controlled substance schedule IV
● Pregnancy risk category C

How supplied
Available by prescription only
Capsules: 200 mg, 500 mg, 750 mg (contains tartrazine)

Indications, route, and dosage
Sedation
Adults: 100 to 200 mg P.O. b.i.d. or t.i.d.

Insomnia
Adults: 500 mg to 1 g P.O. h.s. May repeat 100 to 200 mg if awakened in early morning.

Pharmacodynamics
Sedative-hypnotic action: The activity of ethchlorvynol is similar to that of the barbiturates. It causes nonspecific depression of the CNS, particularly the reticular activating system. Low doses do not significantly depress respiration. The cellular mechanism is unknown.

Pharmacokinetics
● *Absorption:* Ethchlorvynol is absorbed completely and rapidly after oral administration. Peak serum concentrations occur within 2 hours. Action begins in 15 to 60 minutes.
● *Distribution:* Drug distributes throughout the body, including the CNS, and is extensively stored in fatty tissue.
● *Metabolism:* Ethchlorvynol is metabolized primarily in the liver; however, significant metabolism occurs in the kidney as well. In overdose, the metabolic pathways can be saturated.
● *Excretion:* Inactive metabolites of the drug are excreted in urine. Half-life is 10 to 20 hours, but the duration of sleep is about 5 hours.

Contraindications and precautions
Ethchlorvynol is contraindicated in patients with known hypersensitivity to the drug; in patients with porphyria; and in patients with persistent pain and insomnia unless the insomnia persists after the pain is controlled because the drug increases sensitivity to pain. The 750-mg dosage form is contraindicated in individuals allergic to aspirin because it contains tartrazine and because significant cross-reactivity has been demonstrated.

Because drug depresses the CNS, administer ethchlorvynol cautiously to patients who are depressed or who have suicidal tendencies and to those with a history of drug abuse or addiction.

Ethchlorvynol should be used cautiously in patients with hepatic or renal dysfunction because decreased elimination of the drug may lead to accumulation and toxicity and in patients who have shown unpredictable or paradoxical reactions to barbiturates or chloral hydrate because drug may cause a similar reaction.

Interactions
When used concomitantly, ethchlorvynol will decrease the effect of oral anticoagulants (warfarin) by increasing hepatic metabolism. Ethchlorvynol will add to or potentiate the CNS depressant effects of barbiturates, benzodiazepines, alcohol, antihistamines, narcotics, tranquilizers, and other CNS depressants. Concomitant use with MAO inhibitors may cause increased sedation.

Effects on diagnostic tests
Ethchlorvynol may cause a false-positive phentolamine test.

Adverse reactions
● CNS: hangover, dizziness, facial numbness, ataxia, fatigue, nightmares, prolonged hypnosis, excitement, hysteria.
● CV: hypotension.
● DERM: rash, urticaria.
● EENT: blurred vision.
● GI: nausea, vomiting, gastric upset, unpleasant aftertaste.
● HEMA: thrombocytopenia.
● Hepatic: cholestatic jaundice.
● Other: muscle weakness, syncope without hypotension, hypersensitivity, physical or psychological dependence.
Note: Drug should be discontinued if profound weakness, excitement, hysteria, hypotension, or hypersensitivity occurs.

Overdose and treatment
Clinical manifestations of overdose include stupor, coma, and severe respiratory depression. Hypotension, hypothermia, areflexia, and bradycardia may occur.

Treatment is supportive, with emphasis on improving respiratory function and preventing possible pulmonary edema. Empty stomach by emesis using ipecac syrup or performing gastric lavage. Hemoperfusion is the most effective means of increasing elimination; hemodialysis and peritoneal dialysis, especially with aqueous solutions, are of limited value.

▶ Special considerations
● Monitor level of consciousness and vital signs to prevent possible adverse reactions.
● Administer with food to reduce ataxia, giddiness, or stomach upset.
● Patients who are suicidal or depressed or who have a history of drug abuse should be observed to prevent hoarding or self-dosing. Overdose is difficult to treat and carries a high mortality rate.
● Discontinue drug after 1 week; drug is effective only for short-term use.
● Monitor prothrombin times of patient on an

oral anticoagulant to determine effectiveness of drug.

● Slight darkening of liquid in the capsules from exposure to air and light does not affect safety or potency. Store in tight, light-resistant container to avoid possible deterioration.

Information for the patient

● Advise patient to take the medication with food to avoid or lessen giddiness, ataxia, or GI upset.

● Warn patient not to attempt tasks that require mental alertness or physical coordination before the CNS effects of the drug are known and to avoid alcohol and the use of other CNS depressants or antidepressants unless prescribed.

● Tell patient not to change the dose or frequency or discontinue the drug without medical approval.

● Tell patient to promptly report muscle weakness, excitability, or syncope.

● Advise patient of potential for physical and psychological dependence with chronic use.

● Warn patient about the risks of combining this drug with alcohol. An additive effect is possible even if the drug was taken the evening before drinking alcohol.

Geriatric use

Elderly patients, especially those with hepatic dysfunction, will show an increased response and sensitivity. Use lowest dose possible.

Pediatric use

Not recommended for use in children; safety has not been established.

Breast-feeding

Safety of ethchlorvynol in breast-feeding women has not been established.

---

ethinamate
Valmid

● Pharmacologic classification: alicyclic alcohol derivative
● Therapeutic classification: hypnotic
● Controlled substance schedule IV
● Pregnancy risk category C

How supplied
Capsules: 500 mg

Indications, route, and dosage
Insomnia
Adults: 500 mg to 1 g P.O. 20 minutes before bedtime.

Pharmacodynamics
Hypnotic action: Mechanism is unknown. Probably acts similarly to barbiturates to produce CNS depressant effects.

Pharmacokinetics
● *Absorption:* Ethinamate is rapidly and completely absorbed from the GI tract; plasma levels for hypnotic action have not been determined.
● *Distribution:* Unknown.
● *Metabolism:* Hepatic; the primary metabolites are hydroxyethinamate and glucoronide conjugate
● *Excretion:* In the urine. About 36% excreted in 24 hours; only metabolites are found in the urine. Half-life is about 2.5 hours.

Contraindications and precautions
Contraindicated in patient's hypersensitive to the drug and in patients with uncontrolled pain. Use cautiously in patients with a history of mental depression, suicidal ideation, or drug abuse.

Interactions
Concomitant use with alcohol and other CNS depressants may cause excessive CNS depression.

Effects on diagnostic tests
May cause false elevations of urine 17-ketosteroid determinations using the modified Zimmerman reaction and 17-hydroxycorticosteroid levels using the Porter-Silber test.

Adverse reactions
● DERM: rash.
● GI: nausea, GI upset.
● Other: allergic reactions, fever, physical and psychological dependence.

Overdose and treatment
Signs and symptoms of overdose are similar to those following barbiturate overdose: CNS depression, lethargy, coma, circulatory collapse, and respiratory failure. In contrast to other CNS depressants, the CNS depression may be of short duration. Transient hepatic failure may result in jaundice.

Treatment is supportive. Maintain adequate airway and circulation; intubate if necessary. Perform gastric lavage to remove residual drug in the stomach. Hemodialysis may be useful.

▶ Special considerations

● As with many other hypnotic agents, discontinue use is associated with diminished effectiveness. Treatment for longer than 7 days is not recommended.

● After prolonged use, discontinue the drug gradually to avoid withdrawal symptoms. Hospitalize patient and decrease dose by 500 mg to 1 g every 2 to 3 days until the drug is completely withdrawn.

● Especially in elderly patients, walking during treatment should be supervised.

Information for the patient

● Warn patient that prolonged use is associated with physical and psychological dependence.

● Warn patient about the dangers of combining this drug with alcohol. An additive effect is possible even if the drug is taken the evening before drinking alcohol.

Geriatric use

Use cautiously in elderly patients. Starting dose should be 500 mg at bedtime.

Pediatric use

Not recommended for use in children under age 15 because paradoxical excitement has been reported.

Breast-feeding

It is unknown if the drug is excreted in breast milk. Use with caution in breast-feeding women.

---

flurazepam hydrochloride

Apo-Flurazepam∗, Dalmane, Durapam, Novoflupam∗, Som-Pam∗

● Pharmacologic classification: benzodiazepine
● Therapeutic classification: sedative-hypnotic
● Controlled substance schedule IV
● Pregnancy risk category D

How supplied

Available by prescription only
Capsules: 15 mg, 30 mg

Indications, route, and dosage
Insomnia

Adults: 15 to 30 mg P.O. h.s. May repeat dose once after 1 hour (but not after 2 a.m.).
Adults over age 65: 15 mg P.O. h.s.

Pharmacodynamics

Sedative action: Flurazepam depresses the CNS at the limbic and subcortical levels of the brain. It produces a sedative effect by potentiating the effect of the neurotransmitter gamma-aminobutyric acid on its receptor in the ascending reticular activating system, which increases inhibition and blocks both cortical and limbic arousal.

Pharmacokinetics

● *Absorption:* When administered orally, flurazepam is absorbed rapidly through the GI tract. Onset of action occurs within 20 minutes, with peak action in 1 to 2 hours. The duration of action is 7 to 10 hours.

● *Distribution:* Distributed widely throughout the body. Approximately 97% of an administered dose is bound to plasma protein.

● *Metabolism:* Metabolized in the liver to the active metabolite desalkylflurazepam.

● *Excretion:* Desalkylflurazepam is excreted in urine. It has a half-life of 50 to 100 hours.

Contraindications and precautions

Flurazepam is contraindicated in patients with known hypersensitivity to the drug; in patients with acute narrow-angle glaucoma or untreated open-angle glaucoma because of the drug's possible anticholinergic effect; in patients in shock or coma because the drug's hypnotic or hypotensive effect may be prolonged or intensified; and in patients with acute alcohol intoxication who have depressed vital signs because the drug will worsen CNS depression. Do not use in patients who are depressed or have suicidal tendencies.

Flurazepam should be used cautiously in patients with psychoses because the drug is rarely beneficial in such patients and may induce paradoxical reactions; in patients with myasthenia gravis or Parkinson's disease because it may exacerbate the disorder; in patients with impaired renal or hepatic function, which prolongs elimination of the drug; in elderly or debilitated patients, who are usually more sensitive to the drug's CNS effects; and in individuals prone to addiction or drug abuse.

Interactions

Flurazepam potentiates the CNS depressant effects of phenothiazines, narcotics, barbiturates, alcohol, antihistamines, MAO inhibitors, general anesthetics, and antidepressants.

Concomitant use with cimetidine and possibly disulfiram causes diminished hepatic me-

---

tabolism of flurazepam, which increases its plasma concentration.

Heavy smoking accelerates flurazepam's metabolism, thus lowering clinical effectiveness.

Benzodiazepines may decrease plasma levels of haloperidol.

Flurazepam may decrease the therapeutic effects of levodopa.

Effects on diagnostic tests

Flurazepam therapy may elevate liver function test results. Minor changes in EEG patterns, usually low-voltage and fast activity, may occur during and after flurazepam therapy.

Adverse reactions

● CNS: confusion, depression, drowsiness, lethargy, daytime sedation, disturbed coordination, hangover effect, ataxia, dizziness, syncope, nightmares, fatigue, slurred speech, tremor, vertigo, headache.
● CV: palpitations, chest pains, tachycardia, hypotension (rare).
● DERM: rash (rare), flushing, sweating, urticaria.
● EENT: diplopia, blurred vision, nystagmus.
● GI: constipation, dry mouth, taste alterations, anorexia, nausea, vomiting, abdominal discomfort.
● GU: urinary incontinence, urine retention.
● HEMA: leukopenia, granulocytopenia (rare).
● Hepatic: hepatic dysfunction.
● Other: *respiratory depression,* dysarthria, changes in libido, physical or psychological dependence.

Note: Drug should be discontinued if hypersensitivity or the following paradoxical reactions occur: acute hyperexcited state, anxiety, hallucinations, increased muscle spasticity, insomnia, or rage.

Overdose and treatment

Clinical manifestations of overdose include somnolence, confusion, hypoactive reflexes, dyspnea, labored breathing, hypotension, bradycardia, slurred speech, unsteady gait or impaired coordination and, eventually, coma.

Support blood pressure and respiration until drug effects subside; monitor vital signs. Mechanical ventilatory assistance via endotracheal tube may be required to maintain a patent airway and support adequate oxygenation. Use I.V. fluids to promote diuresis and vasopressors such as dopamine and phenylephrine to treat hypotension, as needed.

If the patient is conscious, induce emesis with ipecac syrup. Use gastric lavage if ingestion was recent, but only if an endotracheal tube is present to prevent aspiration. After emesis or lavage, administer activated charcoal with a cathartic as a single dose. Dialysis is of limited value. Do not use barbiturates if excitation occurs to avoid exacerbation of excitatory state or potentiation of CNS depressant effects.

▶ Special considerations

Besides those relevant to all *benzodiazepines,* consider the following recommendations.
● Studies have demonstrated a "carryover effect," which causes the drug to be more effective on the second, third, and fourth night of treatment than on the first.
● Long half-life may cause a hangover effect.
● Useful for patients who have trouble falling asleep and who awaken frequently during the night and early in the morning.
● Prolonged use is not recomended, but this drug has proven effective for up to 4 weeks of continuous use.
● Rapid withdrawal after prolonged use can cause withdrawal symptoms.
● Monitor hepatic function, AST (SGOT), ALT (SGPT), bilirubin, and alkaline phosphatase for changes.
● The drug is most effective after 3 or 4 nights of use because of the long half-life. Do not increase dose more frequently than every 5 days.
● Lower doses are effective in patients with renal or hepatic dysfunction.
● Store in a cool, dry place away from light.

Information for the patient

● Advise patient to avoid alcohol while taking flurazepam.
● Advise female patient not to take the drug if she is pregnant. If she suspects pregnancy, she should contact her physician immediately.
● Warn patient about the potential for excessive CNS depression if this drug is taken with alcohol, even if the drug is taken the evening before drinking alcohol.

Geriatric use

● Elderly patients are more susceptible to the CNS depressant effects of flurazepam. They may require assistance and supervision with walking and daily activities during initiation of therapy or after an increase in dose.
● Lower doses usually are effective in elderly patients because of decreased elimination.

Pediatric use

● Closely observe a neonate for withdrawal symptoms if the mother took flurazepam during

---

pregnancy. Use of flurazepam during labor may cause neonatal flaccidity.
- Not for use in children under age 15.
- Neonates are more sensitive to flurazepam because of slower metabolism, which greatly increases the risk of toxicity.

Breast-feeding
Flurazepam is excreted in breast milk. A breast-fed infant may become sedated, have feeding difficulties, or lose weight. Avoid use in breast-feeding women.

---

glutethimide
Doriden, Doriglute

- Pharmacologic classification: piperidinedione
- Therapeutic classification: sedative-hypnotic
- Controlled substance schedule III
- Pregnancy risk category C

How supplied
Available by prescription only
Tablets: 250 mg, 500 mg
Capsules: 500 mg

Indications, route, and dosage
Insomnia
Adults: 250 to 500 mg P.O. h.s. May be repeated, but not less than 4 hours before intended awakening. Total daily dose should not exceed 1 g.

Pharmacodynamics
Sedative-hypnotic action: Glutethimide's cellular mechanism of action is not known. Like the barbiturates, glutethimide produces a nonspecific depression of the CNS. The mesencephalic activating system is particularly affected, decreasing arousal.

Pharmacokinetics
- *Absorption:* Glutethimide is absorbed erratically after oral administration. Peak serum levels may occur at any point from 1 to 6 hours. Action may begin in 30 minutes.
- *Distribution:* Distributed throughout the body, with large concentrations found in fat tissue. Slightly more than 50% of the drug is protein-bound.
- *Metabolism:* Metabolized in the liver to inactive metabolites.
- *Excretion:* Inactive metabolites are excreted primarily in urine, with minor excretion in feces. Less than 2% of the drug is excreted unchanged.

Half-life of glutethimide is 10 to 12 hours; duration of action is 4 to 8 hours.

Contraindications and precautions
Glutethimide is contraindicated in patients with known hypersensitivity to the drug and in those with porphyria, severe renal failure, or uncontrolled pain.

Glutethimide should be used cautiously in patients with conditions such as prostatic hypertrophy, bladder neck obstruction, narrow-angle glaucoma, or stenosing peptic ulcer that may be worsened by the drug's anticholinergic effects.

Because this drug depresses the CNS, avoid use in depressed patients or those with suicidal tendencies and in patients with a history of drug abuse or addiction. The abuse potential, persistence of adverse reactions, and potential lethality of glutethimide overdose mandates the use of other agents in these patients.

Interactions
Glutethimide increases the metabolism of warfarin, decreasing the hypothrombic effect. Glutethimide will add to or potentiate the effects of alcohol, barbiturates, benzodiazepines, narcotics, antihistamines, tranquilizers, and other CNS depressants. Use of glutethimide with tricyclic antidepressants increases anticholinergic effects.

Effects on diagnostic tests
Glutethimide may cause a false-positive phentolamine test. It may interfere with urinary 17-hydroxycorticosteroids (as determined by the Glenn-Nelson technique).

Adverse reactions
- CNS: residual sedation, hangover, headache, vertigo, paradoxical excitation, dizziness, ataxia, confusion.
- DERM: purpuric or urticarial rash, *exfoliative dermatitis* (rarely).
- EENT: dry mouth, blurred vision.
- GI: gastric irritation, nausea, diarrhea, hiccups, dry mouth.
- GU: urine retention, bladder atony.
- Other: hypersensitivity (thrombocytopenic purpura, leukopenia, *aplastic anemia*, jaundice), nocturnal diaphoresis.
  Note: Drug should be discontinued if hypersensitivity, paradoxical excitation, or skin rash occurs.

Overdose and treatment
Clinical manifestations of overdose include prolonged coma, hypotension, hypothermia fol-

lowed by fever, and inadequate ventilation even without significant respiratory depression. Absence of pupillary reflexes, dilated pupils, loss of deep tendon reflexes, tonic muscle spasms, and apnea may occur.

Treatment of overdose involves support of respiration and CV function; mechanical ventilation may be necessary. Maintain adequate urine output with adequate hydration while avoiding pulmonary edema. Empty gastric contents by emesis or by lavage with a 1:1 mixture of water and castor oil. Charcoal and resin hemoperfusion are effective in removing the drug; hemodialysis and peritoneal dialysis are of minimal value. Because of the significant storage of glutethimide in fat tissue, blood levels can often show large fluctuations with worsening of symptoms.

▶ Special considerations
● Assess level of consciousness and vital signs frequently to prevent possible adverse reactions.
● Monitor prothrombin time in patients taking anticoagulants; anticoagulant dosage may need adjusting.
● Drug is effective for short-term use only.
● Abrupt discontinuation may cause withdrawal symptoms. Discontinue gradually.

Information for the patient
● Advise patient to avoid alcohol, barbiturates, benzodiazepines, and other CNS depressants unless prescribed. Tell patient to call for instructions before taking any OTC cold or allergy preparations to prevent possibility of increased CNS depressant activity.
● Warn patient not to increase the dose or frequency unless prescribed.
● Tell patient not to attempt tasks requiring mental alertness or physical coordination until the drug's CNS effects are known.
● Advise patient that abrupt discontinuation of the drug may cause withdrawal symptoms.
● Tell patient to report skin rash or increased excitability.
● Advise patient of potential for physical and psychological dependence with chronic use.
● Advise safety precaution measures (for example, supervised walking and raised bed rails), especially for elderly patients.
● Tell patient to store medicine in a cool, dry, dark place out of the reach of children.
● Warn patient about the danger of combining this drug with alcohol. An additive effect is possible even if the drug is taken the evening before drinking alcohol.

Geriatric use
Elderly patients, especially those with decreased renal function, will have increased effects. Use with caution in lowest possible effective dose.

Pediatric use
Drug is not recommended for use in children.

Breast-feeding
Glutethimide is excreted in breast milk. It may cause sedation in the infants of breast-feeding women and should be used only when benefits far outweigh the risks.

_____

methyprylon
Noludar

● Pharmacologic classification: piperidinedione (glutethimide) derivative
● Therapeutic classification: hypnotic
● Controlled substance schedule III
● Pregnancy risk category B

How supplied
Tablets: 50 mg, 200 mg
Capsules: 300 mg

Indications, route, and dosage
Insomnia
Adults: 200 to 400 mg P.O. 15 minutes before bedtime.

Pharmacodynamics
Hypnotic action: Mechanism is unknown but drug is considered similar to the barbiturates. Methyprylon is structurally related to glutethimide, another hypnotic agent.

Pharmacokinetics
● *Absorption:* Methyprylon is rapidly absorbed after oral administration. Peak plasma levels occur in 1 to 2 hours. Plasma levels for the hypnotic effects are not known.
● *Distribution:* Not well described; the drug is 60% bound to plasma proteins.
● *Metabolism:* Hepatic; enterohepatic recycling occurs.
● *Excretion:* Primarily in the urine; less than 3% of a dose is excreted unchanged.

Contraindications and precautions
Contraindicated in patients hypersensitive to the drug and in patients with acute intermittent

_____

porphyria. Use cautiously in patients with renal or hepatic impairment and in patients with a history of mental depression, suicidal ideation, or drug abuse. Prolonged use may cause psychological or physical dependence.

Interactions
Concomitant use with alcohol or other CNS depressant may result in excessive CNS depression.

Effects on diagnostic tests
May interfere with in vitro determination of 17-ketosteroids using the Holtorff Koch modification of the Zimmerman reaction and 17-hydroxycorticosteroids using the modified Glenn-Nelson technique and the Porter-Silber reaction.

Adverse reactions
- CNS: morning drowsiness, dizziness, headache, paradoxical excitation.
- CV: hypotension, syncope.
- DERM: rash, pruritus.
- GI: nausea, vomiting, diarrhea, esophagitis.
- HEMA: thrombocytopenic purpura, neutropenia, aplastic anemia.
- Other: physical or psychological dependence.

Overdose and treatment
Signs and symptoms of overdose are similar to those following barbiturate overdose: CNS depression, lethargy, coma, circulatory collapse, and respiratory failure.

Treat supportively. Maintain adequate airway and circulation; intubate if necessary. Perform gastric lavage to remove residual drug in the stomach. Hemodialysis may be useful.

▶ Special considerations
- Periodic blood tests are recommended during prolonged use.
- As with many other hypnotic agents, prolonged use is associated with diminished effectiveness. Treatment for longer than 7 days is not recommended.
- Especially in elderly patients, walking should be supervised during treatment.

Information for the patient
- Warn patient that prolonged use is associated with physical or psychological dependence.
- The patient should avoid driving and other hazardous tasks that require alertness until the adverse and residual CNS effects of the drug are known.
- Warn patient about the dangers of combining the drug with alcohol. An additive effect is possible even if the drug is taken the evening before drinking alcohol.

Geriatric use
Use cautiously in elderly patients.

Pediatric use
Not recommended for use in children under age 12.

Breast-feeding
It is unknown if the drug is excreted in breast milk. Use with caution in breast-feeding women.

pentobarbital sodium
Nembutal

- Pharmacologic classification: barbiturate
- Therapeutic classification: sedative-hypnotic, anticonvulsant
- Controlled substance schedule II (suppositories schedule III)
- Pregnancy risk category D

How supplied
Available by prescription only
Capsules: 50 mg, 100 mg
Elixir: 20 mg/5 ml
Injection: 50 mg/ml, 1-ml and 2-ml disposable syringes; 2-ml, 20-ml, and 50-ml vials
Suppositories: 30 mg, 60 mg, 120 mg, 200 mg

Indications, route, and dosage
Sedation
Adults: 20 to 40 mg P.O. b.i.d., t.i.d., or q.i.d.
Children: 2 to 6 mg/kg P.O. daily in divided doses to a maximum of 100 mg/dose.
Insomnia
Adults: 100 to 200 mg P.O. h.s. or 150 to 200 mg deep I.M.; 120 to 200 mg rectally.
Children: 2 to 6 mg/kg I.M., up to a maximum of 100 mg/dose. Or 30 mg rectally (ages 2 months to 1 year), 30 to 60 mg rectally (ages 1 to 4), 60 mg rectally (ages 5 to 12), 60 to 120 mg rectally (ages 12 to 14).
Preanesthetic medication
Adults: 150 to 200 mg I.M. or P.O. in two divided doses.
Seizures
Adults: Initially, 100 mg I.V.; after 1 minute, additional doses may be given. Maximum dosage is 500 mg.
Children: Initially, 50 mg I.M. or I.V.; after 1 minute, additional doses may be given.

† *Treatment of cerebral ischemia or cerebral edema after stroke, head trauma, or Reye's syndrome (barbiturate coma)*
Adults: 1 to 3 mg/kg/hour by I.V. infusion after an initial loading dose sufficient to produce burst suppression of the EEG (5 to 34 mg/kg).

Pharmacodynamics

• *Sedative-hypnotic action:* The exact cellular site and mechanism(s) of action are unknown. Pentobarbital acts throughout the CNS as a non-selective depressant with a fast onset of action and short duration of action. Particularly sensitive to this drug is the reticular activating system, which controls CNS arousal. Pentobarbital decreases both presynaptic and postsynaptic membrane excitability by facilitating the action of gamma-aminobutyric acid (GABA).
• *Anticonvulsant action:* Pentobarbital suppresses the spread of seizure activity produced by epileptogenic foci in the cortex, thalamus, and limbic systems by enhancing the effect of GABA. Both presynaptic and postsynaptic excitability are decreased, and the seizure threshold is raised.

Pharmacokinetics

• *Absorption:* Pentobarbital is absorbed rapidly after oral or rectal administration, with an onset of action of 10 to 15 minutes. Peak serum concentrations occur between 30 and 60 minutes after oral administration. After I.M. injection, the onset of action occurs within 10 to 25 minutes. After I.V. administration, the onset of action occurs immediately. Serum concentrations needed for sedation and hypnosis are 1 to 5 mcg/ml and 5 to 15 mcg/ml, respectively. After oral or rectal administration, duration of hypnosis is 1 to 4 hours.
• *Distribution:* Pentobarbital is distributed widely throughout the body. It accumulates in fat with prolonged use. Approximately 35% to 45% is protein-bound.
• *Metabolism:* Pentobarbital is metabolized in the liver by penultimate oxidation.
• *Excretion:* 99% of pentobarbital is eliminated as glucuronide conjugates and other metabolites in the urine. Terminal half-life ranges from 35 to 50 hours. Duration of action is 3 to 4 hours.

Contraindications and precautions

Pentobarbital is contraindicated in patients with known hypersensitivity to barbiturates and in patients with bronchopneumonia, status asthmaticus, or severe respiratory distress because of the potential for respiratory depression. Pentobarbital should not be used in patients who are depressed or have suicidal ideation because the drug can worsen depression; in patients with uncontrolled acute or chronic pain because exacerbation of pain and paradoxical excitement can occur; or in patients with porphyria because this drug can trigger symptoms of this disease.

Pentobarbital should be used cautiously in patients who must perform hazardous tasks requiring mental alertness, because the drug causes drowsiness. Administer parenteral pentobarbital slowly and with extreme caution to patients with hypotension or severe pulmonary or CV disease because of potential adverse hemodynamic effects. Because tolerance and physical or psychological dependence may occur, prolonged use of high doses should be avoided. Pentobarbital capsules may contain tartrazine, which may cause an allergic reaction in certain individuals, especially those who are sensitive to aspirin. Prenatal exposure to barbiturates is associated with an increased incidence of fetal abnormalities and, possibly, brain tumors. Use of barbiturates in the third trimester may be associated with physical dependence in neonates. Risk-benefit must be considered.

Interactions

Pentobarbital may potentiate or add to CNS and respiratory depressant effects of other sedative-hypnotics, antihistamines, narcotics, antidepressants, tranquilizers, and alcohol.

Pentobarbital enhances the enzymatic degradation of warfarin and other oral anticoagulants; patients may require increased doses of the anticoagulants. Drug also enhances hepatic metabolism of some drugs, including digitoxin (not digoxin), corticosteroids, oral contraceptives and other estrogens, theophylline and other xanthines, and doxycycline. Pentobarbital impairs the effectiveness of griseofulvin by decreasing absorption from the GI tract.

Valproic acid, phenytoin, disulfiram, and MAO inhibitors decrease the metabolism of pentobarbital and can increase its toxicity. Rifampin may decrease pentobarbital levels by increasing hepatic metabolism.

Effects on diagnostic tests

Pentobarbital may cause a false-positive phentolamine test. The drug's physiologic effects may impair the absorption of cyanocobalamin ^{57}Co; it may decrease serum bilirubin concentrations in neonates, patients with seizure disorders, and patients with congenital nonhemolytic unconjugated hyperbilirubinemia. EEG patterns show a change in low-voltage and fast activity;

changes persist for a time after discontinuation of therapy.

Adverse reactions
● CNS: drowsiness, lethargy, vertigo, headache, CNS depression; rebound insomnia, increased dreams or nightmares, and possibly *seizures* (after acute withdrawal or reduction in dosage); mental depression; paradoxical excitement; confusion and agitation (especially in elderly patients).
● CV: hypotension (after rapid I.V. administration), bradycardia, *circulatory collapse.*
● DERM: urticaria, rash, *exfoliative dermatitis, Stevens-Johnson syndrome.*
● EENT: miosis.
● GI: nausea, vomiting, diarrhea, constipation.
● Local: thrombophlebitis, pain and possible tissue damage at the site of extravascular injection.
● Other: laryngospasm, *bronchospasm, respiratory depression,* angioedema, physical or psychological dependence. Vitamin K deficiency and bleeding have occurred in neonates of mothers treated during pregnancy. Hyperalgesia occurs in low doses or in patients with chronic pain.
  Note: Drug should be discontinued if hypersensitivity reaction, profound CNS or respiratory depression, or skin eruptions occur.

Overdose and treatment
Clinical manifestations of overdose include unsteady gait, slurred speech, sustained nystagmus, somnolence, confusion, respiratory depression, pulmonary edema, areflexia, and coma. Typical shock syndrome with tachycardia and hypotension may occur. Jaundice, hypothermia followed by fever, and oliguria also may occur. Serum concentrations greater than 10 mcg/ml may produce profound coma; concentrations greater than 30 mcg/ml may be fatal.
  To treat, maintain and support ventilation and pulmonary function as necessary; support cardiac function and circulation with vasopressors and I.V. fluids, as needed. If patient is conscious and gag reflex is intact, induce emesis (if ingestion was recent) by administering ipecac syrup. If emesis is contraindicated, perform gastric lavage while a cuffed endotracheal tube is in place, to prevent aspiration. Follow with administration of activated charcoal or saline cathartic. Measure intake and output, vital signs, and laboratory parameters. Maintain body temperature.
  Alkalinization of urine may be helpful in removing drug from the body. Hemodialysis may be useful in severe overdose.

▶ Special considerations
Besides those relevant to all *barbiturates,* consider the following recommendations.
● As with many other hypnotic agents, pentobarbital loses its effectiveness after 1 to 2 weeks of therapy.
● Abrupt discontinuation may result in insomnia, nightmares, or increased dreaming.
● After prolonged use, abrupt discontinuation may precipitate withdrawal symptoms.
● I.V. injection should be reserved for emergency treatment and should be given under close supervision. Be prepared for emergency resuscitative measures.
● Avoid I.V. administration at a rate greater than 50 mg/minute to prevent hypotension and respiratory depression.
● High-dose therapy for elevated intracranial pressure may require mechanically assisted ventilation.
● Administer I.M. dose deep into large muscle mass. Do not administer more than 5 ml into any one site.
● Discard any solution that is discolored or contains precipitate.
● Administration of full loading doses over short periods to treat status epilepticus will require ventilatory support in adults.
● To ensure accuracy of dosage, do not divide suppositories.
● Drug has no analgesic effect and may cause restlessness or delirium in patients with pain.
● Nembutal tablets contain tartrazine dye, which may cause allergic reactions in susceptible persons.

Information for the patient
● Advise pregnant patient of potential hazard to fetus or neonate when taking pentobarbital late in pregnancy. Withdrawal symptoms can occur.
● Tell patient not to take drug continuously for longer than 2 weeks.
● Warn patient about the dangers of combining this drug with alcohol. An additive effect is possible, even if the drug is taken the evening before drinking alcohol.

Geriatric use
Elderly patients usually require lower doses because of increased susceptibility to CNS depressant effects of pentobarbital. Confusion, disorientation, and excitability may occur in elderly patients. Use with caution.

Pediatric use
Barbiturates may cause paradoxical excitement in children. Use with caution.

Breast-feeding
Pentobarbital passes into breast milk. Do not administer to breast-feeding women.

---

phenobarbital
Barbita, Gardenal∗, Solfoton

phenobarbital sodium
Luminal

- Pharmacologic classification: barbiturate
- Therapeutic classification: anticonvulsant, sedative-hypnotic
- Controlled substance schedule IV
- Pregnancy risk category D

How supplied
Available by prescription only
Tablets: 8 mg, 15 mg, 16 mg, 30 mg, 32 mg, 60 mg, 65 mg, 100 mg
Capsules: 16 mg
Oral solution: 15 mg/5 ml; 20 mg/5 ml
Elixir: 20 mg/5 ml
Injection: 30 mg/ml, 60 mg/ml, 65 mg/ml, 130 mg/ml
Powder for injection: 120 mg/ampule

Indications, route, and dosage
All forms of seizure disorders, febrile seizures in children
Adults: 100 to 200 mg P.O. daily, divided t.i.d. or given as a single dose h.s.
Children: 4 to 6 mg/kg P.O. daily, usually divided q 12 hours. It can, however, be administered once daily.
Status epilepticus
Adults: 10 mg/kg as I.V. infusion no faster than 50 mg/minute. May give up to 20 mg/kg total. Administer in acute care or emergency area only.
Children: 5 to 10 mg/kg I.V. May repeat q 10 to 15 minutes up to total of 20 mg/kg. I.V. injection rate should not exceed 50 mg/minute.
Sedation
Adults: 30 to 120 mg P.O. daily in two or three divided doses.
Children: 6 mg/kg P.O. divided t.i.d.
Insomnia
Adults: 100 to 320 mg P.O. or I.M.
Children: 3 to 6 mg/kg.

Preoperative sedation
Adults: 100 to 200 mg I.M. 60 to 90 minutes before surgery.
Children: 16 to 100 mg I.M. 60 to 90 minutes before surgery.

Pharmacodynamics
- *Anticonvulsant action:* Phenobarbital suppresses the spread of seizure activity produced by epileptogenic foci in the cortex, thalamus, and limbic systems by enhancing the effect of gamma-aminobutyric acid (GABA). Both presynaptic and postsynaptic excitability are decreased; also, phenobarbital raises the seizure threshold.
- *Sedative-hypnotic action:* Phenobarbital acts throughout the CNS as a nonselective depressant with a slow onset of action and a long duration of action. Particularly sensitive to this drug is the reticular activating system, which controls CNS arousal. Phenobarbital decreases both presynaptic and postsynaptic membrane excitability by facilitating the action of GABA. The exact cellular site and mechanism(s) of action are unknown.

Pharmacokinetics
- *Absorption:* Phenobarbital is absorbed well after oral and rectal administration, with 70% to 90% reaching the bloodstream. Absorption after I.M. administration is 100%. After oral administration, peak serum levels are reached in 1 to 2 hours, and peak levels in the CNS are achieved at 1 to 3 hours. Onset of action occurs 1 hour or longer after oral dosing; onset after I.V. administration is about 5 minutes. A serum concentration of 10 mcg/ml is needed to produce sedation; 40 mcg/ml usually produces sleep. Concentrations of 20 to 40 mcg/ml are considered therapeutic for anticonvulsant therapy.
- *Distribution:* Phenobarbital is distributed widely throughout the body. Phenobarbital is approximately 25% to 30% protein-bound.
- *Metabolism:* Phenobarbital is metabolized by the hepatic microsomal enzyme system.
- *Excretion:* 25% to 50% of a phenobarbital dose is eliminated unchanged in urine. The remainder is excreted as metabolites of glucuronic acid. Phenobarbital's half-life is 5 to 7 days.

Contraindications and precautions
Phenobarbital is contraindicated in patients with known hypersensitivity to barbiturates and in patients with bronchopneumonia, status asthmaticus, or other severe respiratory distress because of the potential for respiratory depression.

Phenobarbital should not be used in patients who are depressed or have suicidal ideation because the drug can worsen depression; in patients with uncontrolled acute or chronic pain because exacerbation of pain or paradoxical excitement can occur; or in patients with porphyria because this drug can trigger symptoms of this disease.

Phenobarbital should be used cautiously in patients who must perform hazardous tasks requiring mental alertness because the drug causes drowsiness and in patients with impaired renal function because up to 50% of phenobarbital is excreted in urine. Administer parenteral phenobarbital slowly and with extreme caution to patients with hypotension or severe pulmonary or cardiovascular disease because of potential adverse hemodynamic effects. Because tolerance and physical or psychological dependence may occur, prolonged use of high doses should be avoided.

Prenatal exposure to barbiturates is associated with an increased incidence of fetal abnormalities and, possibly, brain tumors. Use of barbiturates in the third trimester may be associated with physical dependence in neonates. Risk-benefit must be considered.

Interactions

Phenobarbital may add to or potentiate CNS and respiratory depressant effects of other sedative-hypnotics, antihistamines, narcotics, phenothiazines, antidepressants, tranquilizers, and alcohol.

Phenobarbital enhances the enzymatic degradation of warfarin and other oral anticoagulants; patients may require increased doses of the anticoagulant. Drug also enhances hepatic metabolism of some drugs, including digitoxin (not digoxin), corticosteroids, oral contraceptives and other estrogens, theophylline and other xanthines, and doxycycline.

Phenobarbital impairs the effectiveness of griseofulvin by decreasing absorption from the GI tract.

Valproic acid, phenytoin, disulfiram, and MAO inhibitors decrease the metabolism of phenobarbital and can increase its toxicity.

Rifampin may decrease phenobarbital levels by increasing hepatic metabolism.

Effects on diagnostic tests

Phenobarbital may cause a false-positive phentolamine test. The physiologic effects of the drug may impair the absorption of cyanocobalamin ^{57}Co; it may decrease serum bilirubin concentrations in neonates, patients with seizure disorders, and patients with congenital nonhemolytic unconjugated hyperbilirubinemia. Barbiturates may increase sulfobromophthalein retention. EEG patterns show a change in low-voltage and fast activity; changes persist for a time after discontinuation of therapy.

Adverse reactions

● CNS: drowsiness, lethargy, vertigo, headache, CNS depression, paradoxical excitement; confusion and agitation (in elderly patients); hyperexcitability in children; rebound insomnia, increased dreams or nightmares, and possibly seizures (after acute withdrawal or reduction in dosage).
● CV: hypotension (after rapid I.V. administration), bradycardia, *circulatory collapse.*
● DERM: urticaria, rash, *exfoliative dermatitis, Stevens-Johnson syndrome.*
● EENT: miosis.
● GI: epigastric pain, nausea, vomiting, diarrhea, constipation.
● Local: thrombophlebitis, pain and possible tissue damage at site of extravascular injection.
● Other: *respiratory depression,* laryngospasm, *bronchospasm,* physical or psychological dependence. Vitamin K deficiency and bleeding have occurred in neonates of mothers treated during pregnancy. Hyperalgesia may occur in low doses or in patients with chronic pain.

Note: Drug should be discontinued if hypersensitivity reaction, profound CNS or respiratory depression, or skin eruptions occur.

Overdose and treatment

Clinical manifestations of overdose include unsteady gait, slurred speech, sustained nystagmus, somnolence, confusion, respiratory depression, pulmonary edema, areflexia, and coma. Typical shock syndrome with tachycardia and hypotension along with jaundice, oliguria, and chills followed by fever may occur.

Treatment is aimed at the maintenance and support of ventilation and pulmonary function as necessary; support of cardiac function and circulation with vasopressors and I.V. fluids as needed. If patient is conscious and gag reflex is intact, induce emesis (if ingestion is recent) by administering ipecac syrup. If emesis is contraindicated, perform gastric lavage while a cuffed endotracheal tube is in place, to prevent aspiration. Follow with administration of activated charcoal or saline cathartic. Measure intake and output, vital signs, and laboratory parameters. Maintain body temperature.

Alkalinization of urine may be helpful in removing drug from the body; hemodialysis may be useful in severe overdose. Oral activated charcoal may enhance phenobarbital elimination regardless of its route of administration.

▶ **Special considerations**
Besides those relevant to all *barbiturates,* consider the following recommendations.
● Considered by many clinicians as the "safest" anticonvulsant.
● Oral solution may be mixed with water or juice to improve taste.
● Reconstitute powder for injection with 2.5 to 5 ml sterile water for injection. Roll vial in hands; do not shake.
● Use a larger vein for I.V. administration to prevent extravasation.
● Avoid I.V. administration at a rate greater than 60 mg/minute to prevent hypotension and respiratory depression. It may take up to 30 minutes after I.V. administration to achieve maximum effect.
● Administer parenteral dose within 30 minutes of reconstitution because phenobarbital hydrolyzes in solution and on exposure to air.
● Keep emergency resuscitation equipment on hand when administering phenobarbital I.V.
● Administer I.M. dose deep into a large muscle mass to prevent tissue injury.
● Only parenteral solutions prepared from powder may be given S.C.; however, this route is not recommended.
● Do not use injectable solution if it contains a precipitate.
● Administration of full loading doses over short periods of time to treat status epilepticus will require ventilatory support in adults.
● Full therapeutic effects are not seen for 2 to 3 weeks, except when loading dose is used.

Information for the patient
● Advise patient of potential for physical and psychological dependence with prolonged use.
● Warn patient to avoid alcohol and other CNS depressants while taking this drug. An additive effect is possible even if the drug is taken the evening before drinking alcohol.
● Warn patient that sudden discontinuation of the drug can cause a withdrawal reaction.
● The patient should avoid driving and other hazardous activities that require alertness until the adverse CNS effects of the drug are known.

Geriatric use
Elderly patients are more sensitive to the effects of phenobarbital and usually require lower doses. Confusion, disorientation, and excitability may occur in elderly patients.

Pediatric use
Paradoxical hyperexcitability may occur in children. Use with caution.

Breast-feeding
Phenobarbital passes into breast milk; avoid administering to breast-feeding women.

---

quazepam
Doral

● Pharmacologic classification: benzodiazepine
● Therapeutic classification: hypnotic
● Controlled substance schedule IV
● Pregnancy risk category X

How supplied
Available by prescription only
Tablets: 7.5 mg, 15 mg

Indications, route, and dosage
Insomnia
Adults: 15 mg P.O. h.s. Some patients may respond to lower doses. Decrease dosage in elderly patients to 7.5 mg P.O. h.s. after 2 days of therapy.

Pharmacodynamics
Hypnotic action: Quazepam acts on the limbic system and thalamus of the CNS by binding to specific benzodiazepine receptors responsible for inducing sleep.

Pharmacokinetics
● *Absorption:* Quazepam is well absorbed from the GI tract. Peak plasma levels of about 15 ng/ml occur within 2 hours.
● *Distribution:* Steady-state plasma levels of the parent drug appear after 7 days of once-daily administration. The drug is more than 95% bound to plasma proteins.
● *Metabolism:* Hepatic; two active metabolites (2-oxoquazepam and N-desalkyl-2-oxoquazepam) have been identified.
● *Excretion:* 31% appears in the urine and 23% appears in the feces over a 5-day period. Only a trace of unchanged drug appears in the urine. The mean elimination half-life of the parent drug and 2-oxoquazepam, a metabolite, is 39 hours; of N-desalkyl-2-oxoquazepam, 733 hours.

Contraindications and precautions
Quazepam is contraindicated in patients allergic to the drug or other benzodiazepines, in

---

pregnant patients, and in those with suspected or established sleep apnea.

Interactions
Concomitant use with alcohol, CNS depressants including antihistamines, opiate analgesics, and other benzodiazepines causes increased CNS depression.

Effects on diagnostic tests
None reported.

Adverse reactions
• CNS: fatigue, dizziness, daytime drowsiness, headache.

Overdose and treatment
• Although not specifically reported for quazepam, overdose with other benzodiazepines has produced somnolence, confusion, and coma.
• General supportive measures, including gastric lavage and support of respirations, should be employed. Metaraminol or levarterenol may be used to treat hypotension.

▶ **Special considerations**
• Clinical trials have show that patients do not develop tolerance to quazepam for up to 4 weeks of nightly therapy, unlike other hypnotic agents.
• Prevent hoarding or self-overdosing by hospitalized patients who are depressed, suicidal, or known drug abusers.
• Patients who receive prolonged therapy with benzodiazepines may experience withdrawal symptoms if the drug is suddenly discontinued (possibly after 6 weeks of continuous therapy).

Information for the patient
• Warn the patient about the potentially dangerous depressant effects that can occur with ingestion of alcohol. Additive effects can occur if alcohol is consumed on the day after the use of the drug.
• Warn patients to avoid hazardous activities that require alertness, such as driving a car, until the adverse CNS effects of the drug are known.
• Tell patients not to increase dosage on their own and to call their physician if they notice that the drug is no longer effective.

Geriatric use
• The elimination half-life of the parent drug and of the metabolite 2-oxoquazepam are the same in elderly patients. However, the elimination half-life of N-desalkyl-2-oxoquazepam metabolite is twice that of young adults.

• Elderly patients should have assistance with walking and other activities until the adverse CNS effects of the drug are known.

Pediatric use
Safety and efficacy in children under age 18 have not been established.

Breast-feeding
Because the drug and its metabolites are excreted in breast milk, breast-feeding is not recommended during therapy.

▬▬▬▬▬▬▬▬▬▬▬▬▬▬▬▬▬▬

secobarbital sodium
Novosecobarb∗, Seconal

• Pharmacologic classification: barbiturate
• Therapeutic classification: sedative-hypnotic, anticonvulsant
• Controlled substance schedule II (suppositories are schedule III)
• Pregnancy risk category D

How supplied
Available by prescription only
Tablets: 100 mg
Capsules: 50 mg, 100 mg
Injection: 50 mg/ml in 1-ml and 2-ml disposable syringe; 50 mg/ml in 20-ml vial
Rectal suppositories: 200 mg

Indications, route, and dosage
Preoperative sedation
Adults: 200 to 300 mg P.O. 1 to 2 hours before surgery.
Children: 50 to 100 mg P.O. or 4 to 5 mg/kg rectally 1 to 2 hours before surgery.
Insomnia
Adults: 100 to 200 mg P.O. or I.M.
Children: 3 to 5 mg/kg I.M., not to exceed 100 mg, with no more than 5 ml injected in any one site. Or 4 to 5 mg/kg rectally.
Acute tetanus seizure
Adults and children: 5.5 mg/kg I.M. or slow I.V., repeated q 3 to 4 hours, if needed; I.V. injection rate not to exceed 50 mg/15 seconds.
Acute psychotic agitation
Adults: Initially, 50 mg/minute I.V. up to 250 mg I.V.; additional doses given cautiously after 5 minutes if desired response is not obtained. Not to exceed 500 mg total.
Status epilepticus
Adults and children: 250 to 350 mg I.M. or I.V.

Pharmacodynamics

Sedative-hypnotic action: Secobarbital acts throughout the CNS as a nonselective depressant with a rapid onset of action and short duration of action. Particularly sensitive to this drug is the reticular activating system, which controls CNS arousal. Secobarbital decreases both presynaptic and postsynaptic membrane excitability by facilitating the action of gamma-aminobutyric acid (GABA). The exact cellular site and mechanism(s) of action are unknown.

Anticonvulsant action: Secobarbital suppresses the spread of seizure activity produced by epileptogenic loci in the cortex, thalamus, and limbic systems by enhancing the effects of GABA. Both presynaptic and postsynaptic excitability are decreased and seizure threshold is raised.

Pharmacokinetics

● *Absorption:* After oral administration, 90% of secobarbital is absorbed rapidly. After rectal administration, secobarbital is nearly 100% absorbed. Peak serum concentration after oral or rectal administration occurs between 2 and 4 hours. The onset of action is rapid, occurring within 15 minutes when administered orally. Peak effects are seen 15 to 30 minutes after oral and rectal administration, 7 to 10 minutes after I.M. administration, and 1 to 3 minutes after I.V. administration. Concentrations of 1 to 5 mcg/ml are needed to produce sedation; 5 to 15 mcg/ml are needed for hypnosis. Hypnosis lasts for 1 to 4 hours after oral doses of 100 to 150 mg.

● *Distribution:* Secobarbital is distributed rapidly throughout body tissues and fluids; approximately 30% to 45% is protein-bound.

● *Metabolism:* Secobarbital is oxidized in the liver to inactive metabolites. Duration of action is 3 to 4 hours.

● *Excretion:* 95% of a secobarbital dose is eliminated as glucuronide conjugates and other metabolites in urine.

Contraindications and precautions

Secobarbital is contraindicated in patients with known hypersensitivity to barbiturates and in patients with bronchopneumonia, status asthmaticus, or other severe respiratory distress because of the potential for respiratory depression. Secobarbital has a high potential for abuse and dependence. Secobarbital should not be used in patients who are depressed or have suicidal ideation because the drug can worsen depression; in patients with uncontrolled acute or chronic pain because exacerbation of pain and paradoxical excitement can occur; and in patients with porphyria because this drug can trigger symptoms of this disease.

Secobarbital should be used cautiously in patients who must perform hazardous tasks requiring mental alertness because the drug causes drowsiness. Administer parenteral phenobarbital slowly and with extreme caution to patients with hypotension or severe pulmonary or CV disease because of potential adverse hemodynamic effects. Because tolerance and physical or psychological dependence may occur, prolonged use of high doses should be avoided.

Prenatal exposure to barbiturates is associated with an increased incidence of fetal abnormalities and possibly brain tumors. Use of barbiturates in the third trimester may be associated with physical dependence in neonates. Risk-benefit must be considered.

Interactions

Secobarbital may add to or potentiate CNS and respiratory depressant effects of other sedative-hypnotics, antihistamines, narcotics, antidepressants, tranquilizers, and alcohol.

Secobarbital enhances the enzymatic degradation of warfarin and other oral anticoagulants; patients may require increased doses of the anticoagulant. Drug also enhances hepatic metabolism of some drugs, including digitoxin (not digoxin), corticosteroids, oral contraceptives and other estrogens, theophylline and other xanthines, and doxycycline. Secobarbital impairs the effectiveness of griseofulvin by decreasing absorption from the GI tract.

Valproic acid, phenytoin, disulfiram, and MAO inhibitors decrease the metabolism of secobarbital and can increase its toxicity. Rifampin may decrease secobarbital levels by increasing metabolism.

Effects on diagnostic tests

Secobarbital may cause a false-positive phentolamine test. The physiologic effects of the drug may impair the absorption of cyanocobalamin [57]Co; it may decrease serum bilirubin concentrations in neonates, patients with seizure disorders, and patients with congenital nonhemolytic unconjugated hyperbilirubinemia. EEG patterns show a change in low-voltage and fast activity; changes persist for a time after discontinuation of therapy.

Adverse reactions

● CNS: drowsiness, lethargy, vertigo, headache, CNS depression, paradoxical excitement; confusion and agitation (especially in elderly pa-

tients); rebound insomnia, increased dreams or nightmares, and possibly seizures (after acute withdrawal or reduction in dosage).
- CV: hypotension (after rapid I.V. administration), bradycardia, *circulatory collapse.*
- DERM: urticaria, rash, *exfoliative dermatitis, Stevens-Johnson syndrome.*
- EENT: miosis.
- GI: nausea, vomiting, diarrhea, constipation.
- Local: thrombophlebitis, pain and possible tissue damage at site of extravascular injection.
- Other: *respiratory depression,* laryngospasm, *bronchospasm,* physical or psychological dependence. Reported vitamin K deficiency and bleeding have occurred in neonates of mothers treated during pregnancy. Hyperalgesia may occur with low doses or in patients with chronic pain.

Note: Drug should be discontinued if hypersensitivity reaction, profound CNS or respiratory depression, or skin eruption occurs.

Overdose and treatment
Clinical manifestations of overdose include unsteady gait, slurred speech, sustained nystagmus, somnolence, confusion, respiratory depression, pulmonary edema, areflexia, and coma. Typical shock syndrome with tachycardia and hypotension, jaundice, hypothermia followed by fever, and oliguria may occur.

Maintain and support ventilation and pulmonary function as necessary; support cardiac function and circulation with vasopressors and I.V. fluids as needed. If patient is conscious and gag reflex is intact, induce emesis (if ingestion was recent) by administering ipecac syrup. If emesis is contraindicated, perform gastric lavage while a cuffed endotracheal tube is in place, to prevent aspiration. Follow with administration of activated charcoal or saline cathartic. Measure intake and output, vital signs, and laboratory parameters; maintain body temperature. Patient should be rolled from side to side every 30 minutes to avoid pulmonary congestion.

Alkalinization of urine may be helpful in removing drug from the body; hemodialysis may be useful in severe overdose.

▶ Special considerations
Besides those relevant to all *barbiturates,* consider the following recommendations.
- Generally, barbiturates have been replaced by benzodiazepines and other safer alternatives for the treatment of insomnia.
- Use I.V. route of administration only in emergencies or when other routes are unavailable.

- Dilute secobarbital injection with sterile water for injection solution, 0.9% sodium chloride injection, or Ringer's injection solution. Do not use if solution is discolored or if a precipitate forms.
- Avoid I.V. administration at a rate greater than 50 mg/15 seconds to prevent hypotension and respiratory depression. Have emergency resuscitative equipment on hand.
- Administer I.M. dose deep into large muscle mass to prevent tissue injury.
- Store rectal suppositories in refrigerator. To ensure accurate dosage, do not divide suppository.
- Secobarbital sodium injection, diluted with lukewarm tap water to a concentration of 10 to 15 mg/ml, may be administered rectally in children. A cleansing enema should be administered before secobarbital enema.
- Monitor hepatic and renal studies frequently to prevent possible toxicity.

Information for the patient
- The patient should avoid driving and other hazardous activities that require alertness until the adverse CNS effects of the drug are known.
- Warn patient to avoid alcohol and other CNS depressants while taking this drug. A dangerous additive effect is possible even if the drug is taken the evening before drinking alcohol.
- Warn patient that prolonged use may cause physical or psychological dependence.

Geriatric use
Elderly patients are more susceptible to effects of secobarbital and usually require lower doses. Confusion, disorientation, and excitability may occur in elderly patients.

Pediatric use
Secobarbital may cause paradoxical excitement in children; use cautiously.

Breast-feeding
Secobarbital passes into breast milk; do not administer to breast-feeding women.

temazepam
Razepam, Restoril, Temaz

- Pharmacologic classification: benzodiazepine
- Therapeutic classification: sedative-hypnotic
- Controlled substance schedule IV
- Pregnancy risk category X

How supplied
Available by prescription only
Capsules: 15 mg, 30 mg

Indications, route, and dosage
Insomnia
Adults: 15 to 30 mg P.O. before bedtime.
Adults over age 65: 15 mg P.O. h.s.

Pharmacodynamics
Sedative-hypnotic action: Temazepam depresses the CNS at the limbic and subcortical levels of the brain. It produces a sedative-hypnotic effect by potentiating the effect of the neurotransmitter gamma-aminobutyric acid on its receptor in the ascending reticular activating system, which increases inhibition and blocks both cortical and limbic arousal.

Pharmacokinetics
- *Absorption:* When administered orally, temazepam is well absorbed through the GI tract. Peak levels occur in 1 to 3 hours. Onset of action occurs at 30 to 60 minutes.
- *Distribution:* Temazepam is distributed widely throughout the body. Drug is 98% protein-bound.
- *Metabolism:* Temazepam is metabolized in the liver primarily to inactive metabolites.
- *Excretion:* The metabolites of temazepam are excreted in urine as glucuronide conjugates. The half-life of temazepam ranges from 10 to 17 hours.

Contraindications and precautions
Temazepam is contraindicated in patients with known hypersensitivity to the drug; in patients with acute narrow-angle glaucoma or untreated open-angle glaucoma because of the drug's possible anticholinergic effect; in patients in coma because the drug's hypnotic or hypotensive effect may be prolonged or intensified; in patients with acute alcohol intoxication who have depressed vital signs because the drug will worsen CNS depression; and in pregnant patients. Do

not use in patients with a history of drug abuse or suicidal tendencies.

Temazepam should be used cautiously in patients with psychoses because the drug is rarely beneficial in such patients and may induce paradoxical reactions; in patients with myasthenia gravis, Parkinson's disease, or chronic obstructive pulmonary disease because it may exacerbate these disorders; in patients with impaired hepatic or renal function, which prolongs elimination of the drug; in elderly or debilitated patients, who are usually more sensitive to the drug's CNS effects; and in individuals prone to addiction or drug abuse. Evaluate the patient for the cause of the insomnia, which is frequently a symptom of an underlying disorder, such as depression.

Interactions
Temazepam potentiates the CNS depressant effects of phenothiazines, narcotics, antihistamines, MAO inhibitors, barbiturates, alcohol, general anesthetics, and tricyclic antidepressants.

Concomitant use with cimetidine and possibly disulfiram causes diminished hepatic metabolism of temazepam, which increases its plasma concentration.

Heavy smoking accelerates temazepam metabolism, thus lowering clinical effectiveness.

Benzodiazepines block the therapeutic effects of levodopa.

Temazepam may decrease plasma levels of haloperidol.

Effects on diagnostic tests
Temazepam therapy may increase liver function test results. Minor changes in EEG patterns, usually low-voltage and fast activity, may occur during and after temazepam therapy.

Adverse reactions
- CNS: confusion, depression, drowsiness, lethargy, hangover effect, ataxia, dizziness, syncope, nightmares, fatigue, slurred speech, tremor, vertigo, nervousness, irritability, daytime sedation, headache.
- CV: palpitations, tachycardia, hypotension (rare).
- DERM: rash, urticaria.
- EENT: diplopia, blurred vision, nystagmus.
- GI: constipation, dry mouth, taste alterations, nausea, vomiting, abdominal discomfort, anorexia, diarrhea.
- GU: urinary incontinence, urine retention.
- Other: *respiratory depression,* dysarthria, he-

---

patic dysfunction, changes in libido, physical or psychological dependence.

Note: Drug should be discontinued if hypersensitivity or the following paradoxical reactions occur: acute hyperexcited state, anxiety, hallucinations, increased muscle spasticity, insomnia, or rage.

Overdose and treatment
Clinical manifestations of overdose include somnolence, confusion, hypoactive or absent reflexes, dyspnea, labored breathing, hypotension, bradycardia, slurred speech, unsteady gait or impaired coordination, and, ultimately, coma.

Support blood pressure and respiration until drug effects subside; monitor vital signs. Mechanical ventilatory assistance via endotracheal tube may be required to maintain a patent airway and support adequate oxygenation. Use I.V. fluids and vasopressors such as dopamine and phenylephrine to treat hypotension as needed. If patient is conscious, induce emesis with ipecac syrup. Use gastric lavage if ingestion was recent, but only if an endotracheal tube is present to prevent aspiration. After emesis or lavage, administer activated charcoal with a cathartic as a single dose. Do not use barbiturates if excitation occurs. Dialysis is of limited value.

▶ Special considerations
Besides those relevant to all *benzodiazepines,* consider the following recommendations.
• Useful for patients who have difficulty falling asleep or who awaken frequently during the night and early in the morning.
• Prolonged use is not recommended, although studies have demonstrated effectiveness for up to 4 weeks.
• Remove all potential safety hazards, such as cigarettes, from patient's reach.
• Impose safety measures, such as call bell within reach and side rails raised, to prevent possible injury.
• Monitor hepatic function studies to prevent toxicity; lower doses are indicated in patients with hepatic dysfunction.
• After prolonged use, withdraw the drug slowly (over 6 to 12 weeks).
• Store in a cool, dry place away from light.

Information for the patient
• Instruct patient to seek medical approval before making any changes in medication regimen.
• As necessary, teach patient safety measures to prevent injury, such as gradual position changes and supervised ambulation.

• Advise patient of the potential for physical and psychological dependence with chronic use.
• Do not discontinue the drug abruptly after prolonged use.
• Warn patient about the dangers of combining this drug with alcohol. A dangerous additive effect is possible even if the drug is taken the evening before drinking alcohol.

Geriatric use
• Elderly patients are more susceptible to the CNS depressant effects of temazepam. Use with caution.
• Lower doses are usually effective in elderly patients because of decreased elimination.
• Elderly patients who receive this drug require supervision with ambulation and activities of daily living during initiation of therapy or after an increase in dose.

Pediatric use
Safe use in patients under age 18 has not been established.

Breast-feeding
Temazepam is excreted in breast milk. A breast-fed infant may become sedated, have feeding difficulties, or lose weight. Avoid use in breast-feeding women.

---

triazolam
Halcion

• Pharmacologic classification: benzodiazepine
• Therapeutic classification: sedative-hypnotic
• Controlled substance schedule IV
• Pregnancy risk category X

How supplied
Available by prescription only
Tablets: 0.125 mg, 0.25 mg

Indications, route, and dosage
Insomnia
Adults: 0.125 to 0.25 mg P.O. h.s.
Adults over age 65: 0.125 mg P.O. h.s. May give up to 0.25 mg.

Pharmacodynamics
Sedative-hypnotic action: Triazolam depresses the CNS at the limbic and subcortical levels of the brain. It produces a sedative-hypnotic effect by potentiating the effect of the neurotransmitter gamma-aminobutyric acid on its recep-

tor in the ascending reticular activating system, which increases inhibition and blocks both cortical and limbic arousal.

Pharmacokinetics

• *Absorption:* When administered orally, triazolam is well absorbed through the GI tract. Peak levels occur in 1 to 2 hours. Onset of action occurs at 15 to 30 minutes.

• *Distribution:* Triazolam is distributed widely throughout the body. Drug is 90% protein-bound.

• *Metabolism:* Triazolam is metabolized in the liver primarily to inactive metabolites.

• *Excretion:* The metabolites of triazolam are excreted in urine. The half-life of triazolam ranges from approximately 1½ to 5½ hours.

Contraindications and precautions

Triazolam is contraindicated in patients with known hypersensitivity to the drug; in patients with acute narrow-angle glaucoma or untreated open-angle glaucoma because of the drug's possible anticholinergic effect; in patients in coma because the drug's hypnotic or hypotensive effect may be prolonged or intensified; in pregnant patients because it may be fetotoxic; and in patients with acute alcohol intoxication who have depressed vital signs because the drug will worsen CNS depression.

Triazolam should be used cautiously in patients with psychoses because the drug is rarely beneficial in such patients and may induce paradoxical reactions; in patients with myasthenia gravis or Parkinson's disease because it may exacerbate the disorder; in patients with impaired hepatic function, which prolongs elimination of the drug; in elderly or debilitated patients, who are usually more sensitive to the drug's CNS effects; and in individuals prone to addiction or drug abuse.

Interactions

Triazolam potentiates the CNS depressant effects of phenothiazines, narcotics, antihistamines, MAO inhibitors, barbiturates, alcohol, general anesthetics, and tricyclic antidepressants. Enhanced amnesiac effects have been reported when combined with alcohol (even in small amounts).

Concomitant use with cimetidine and possibly disulfiram causes diminished hepatic metabolism of triazolam, which increases its plasma concentration.

Heavy smoking accelerates triazolam metabolism, thus lowering clinical effectiveness.

Benzodiazepines may decrease the therapeutic effects of levodopa.

Triazolam may decrease serum levels of haloperidol.

Effects on diagnostic tests

Triazolam therapy may elevate liver function test results. Minor changes in EEG patterns, usually low-voltage and fast activity, may occur during and after triazolam therapy.

Adverse reactions

• CNS: confusion, depression, drowsiness, lethargy, hangover effect, ataxia, dizziness, syncope, nightmares, fatigue, slurred speech, tremor, vertigo, headache, light-headedness, amnesia.

• CV: palpitations, chest pains, hypotension (rare).

• DERM: rash, pruritus, urticaria.

• EENT: diplopia, blurred vision, nystagmus.

• GI: constipation, salivation changes, alterations in taste, anorexia, nausea, vomiting, abdominal discomfort.

• GU: urinary incontinence, urine retention.

• Other: *respiratory depression,* dysarthria, hepatic dysfunction, changes in libido, physical or psychological dependence.

Note: Drug should be discontinued if hypersensitivity or the following paradoxical reactions occur: acute hyperexcited state, anxiety, hallucinations, increased muscle spasticity, insomnia, or rage.

Overdose and treatment

Clinical manifestations of overdose include somnolence, confusion, hypoactive reflexes, dyspnea, labored breathing, hypotension, bradycardia, slurred speech, unsteady gait or impaired coordination, and, ultimately, coma.

Support blood pressure and respiration until drug effects subside; monitor vital signs. Mechanical ventilatory assistance via endotracheal tube may be required to maintain a patent airway and support adequate oxygenation. Use I.V. fluids and vasopressors such as dopamine and phenylephrine to treat hypotension as needed. If patient is conscious, induce emesis with ipecac syrup. Use gastric lavage if ingestion was recent, but only if an endotracheal tube is present to prevent aspiration. After emesis or lavage, administer activated charcoal with a cathartic as a single dose. Do not use barbiturates if excitation occurs. Dialysis is of limited value.

▶ Special considerations
Besides those relevant to all *benzodiazepines*, consider the following recommendations.
● Monitor hepatic function studies to prevent toxicity.
● Lower doses are effective in patients with hepatic dysfunction.
● Onset of sedation or hypnosis is rapid; patient should be in bed when taking triazolam.
● Store in a cool, dry place away from light.

Information for the patient
● Instruct patient not to take any OTC drugs or to change medication regimen without medical approval.
● As necessary, teach safety measures, such as gradual position changes, to prevent injury.
● Suggest other measures to promote sleep, such as warm drinks and quiet music, not drinking alcohol near bedtime, regular exercise, and maintaining a regular sleep pattern.
● Warn patient against combining this drug with alcohol.
● Advise patient that rebound insomnia may occur after stopping the drug.
● Advise patient of the potential for physical and psychological dependence.

Geriatric use
● Elderly patients are more susceptible to CNS depressant effects of triazolam. Use with caution.
● Lower doses are usually effective in elderly patients because of decreased elimination.
● Elderly patients who receive triazolam require supervision with ambulation and activities of daily living during initiation of therapy or after an increase in dose.

Pediatric use
Safe use in patients under age 18 has not been established.

Breast-feeding
Triazolam is excreted in breast milk. A breast-fed infant may become sedated, have feeding difficulties, or lose weight. Avoid use in breast-feeding women.

Pharmacologic classes

Most of the drugs listed among the generic drug entries in this volume belong to one of the following pharmacologic classes.

---

amphetamines

amphetamine sulfate
benzphetamine hydrochloride
dextroamphetamine sulfate
diethylpropion hydrochloride
fenfluramine hydrochloride
methamphetamine hydrochloride
phendimetrazine tartrate
phenmetrazine hydrochloride
phentermine hydrochloride

Amphetamines were the first drugs widely prescribed as anorexigenics. They are no longer widely used for this purpose because dependence can develop. The FDA has found no advantage to their use as compared with other, safer anorexigenics. Amphetamines now are used chiefly to control narcolepsy in adults and attention deficit disorder in hyperactive children.

Pharmacology
Amphetamines are sympathomimetic amines with CNS stimulant activity; in children with hyperkinesia, they have a paradoxical calming effect. Their mechanisms of action for narcolepsy, attention deficit disorder, and appetite control are unknown; anorexigenic effects are thought to occur in the hypothalamus, where decreased smell and taste acuity decreases appetite.

The cerebral cortex and reticular activating system appear to be the primary sites of activity; amphetamines release nerve terminal stores of norepinephrine, promoting nerve impulse transmission. At high doses, effects are mediated by dopamine.

Peripheral effects include elevated blood pressure, respiratory stimulation, and weak bronchodilation. At therapeutic dosage levels, cardiac output and cerebral blood flow remain unchanged; high doses may cause arrhythmias.

Clinical indications and actions
Narcolepsy; attention deficit disorder
Amphetamines may be used to treat narcolepsy and as adjuncts to psychosocial measures in attention deficit disorder in children.
Adjunct in managing obesity
Amphetamines may be tried for short-term control of refractory obesity, with caloric restriction and behavior modification; anorexigenic effects persist only a few weeks and patient must be encouraged to learn modification of eating habits rapidly.

Overview of adverse reactions
Adverse reactions to the amphetamines reflect excessive sympathomimetic and CNS stimulation and commonly include insomnia, tremor, and restlessness; toxic dosage levels can induce psychosis, mydriasis, hypertension, *arrhythmias, coma, circulatory collapse, and death.*

Tolerance to amphetamines can occur within a few weeks, necessitating increased dosages to produce desired effects; abusers take an average of 1 to 2 g/day. Both physical tolerance and psychological dependence may occur. Symptoms of chronic abuse include mental impairment, loss of appetite, somnolence, social withdrawal, and occupational and emotional problems; prolonged abuse may cause schizoid syndromes and hallucinations.

▶ Special considerations
● Amphetamines are contraindicated in patients with symptomatic CV disease, hyperthyroidism, nephritis, angina pectoris, any degree of hypertension, arteriosclerosis-induced parkinsonism, certain types of glaucoma, advanced arteriosclerosis, agitated states, or a history of substance abuse.

Amphetamines should be used cautiously in patients with diabetes mellitus; in elderly, debilitated, or hyperexcitable patients; and in children with Gilles de la Tourette's syndrome. Avoid long-term therapy when possible because of the risk of psychic dependence or habituation.
● Patient should receive lowest effective dose

---

with dosage adjusted individually according to response; after long-term use, dosage should be lowered gradually to prevent acute rebound depression.

● Amphetamines may impair ability to perform tasks requiring mental alertness, such as driving a car.

● Vital signs should be checked regularly for increased blood pressure or other signs of excessive stimulation; avoid late-day or evening dosing, especially of long-acting dosage forms, to minimize insomnia.

● Amphetamines are not recommended as first-line therapy for obesity; be sure patients taking amphetamines for weight reduction are on reduced-calorie diet; also monitor calorie intake.

● Amphetamine therapy should be discontinued when tolerance to anorexigenic effects develops; dosage should not be increased.

● Encourage patient to get adequate rest; unusual, compensatory fatigue may result as drug wears off.

● Amphetamine use for analeptic effect is discouraged; CNS stimulation superimposed on CNS depression may cause neuronal instability and seizures.

● Carefully follow manufacturer's directions for reconstitution, storage, and administration of all preparations.

● Prolonged administration of CNS stimulants to children with attention deficit disorders may be associated with temporary decreased growth.

● Amphetamines have a high potential for abuse; they are not recommended to combat the fatigue of exhaustion or the need for sleep but are often abused for this purpose by students, athletes, and truck drivers.

● If overdose occurs, protect patient from excessive noise or stimulation.

Information for the patient

● Explain rationale for therapy and the potential risks and benefits.

● Tell patient to avoid drinks containing caffeine to prevent added CNS stimulation and not to increase dosage.

● Advise narcoleptic patients to take first dose on awakening.

● Advise patients on weight reduction programs to take last dose several hours before bedtime to avoid insomnia.

● Tell patient not to chew or crush sustained-release dosage forms.

● Warn patient not to use drug to mask fatigue, to be sure to obtain adequate rest, and to report excessive CNS stimulation.

● Advise diabetic patients to monitor blood glucose levels carefully, as drug may alter insulin needs.

● Advise patient to avoid tasks that require mental alertness until degree of cognitive impairment is determined.

Geriatric use

Use amphetamines with caution. Elderly patients are usually more sensitive to drugs' effects and may obtain therapeutic effect from lower dosages.

Pediatric use

Amphetamines are not recommended for weight reduction in children under age 12; amphetamine use for hyperactivity is contraindicated in children under age 3.

Breast-feeding

Safety has not been established. An alternate feeding method is recommended during therapy.

anticholinergics

Belladonna alkaloids
atropine sulfate
belladonna leaf
hyoscyamine sulfate
levorotatory alkaloids of belladonna

Semisynthetic belladonna derivative
methscopolamine bromide

Synthetic quaternary anticholinergics
anisotropine methylbromide
clidinium bromide
hexocyclium methylsulfate
isopropamide iodide
mepenzolate bromide
methantheline bromide
oxyphenonium bromide
propantheline bromide

Tertiary synthetic (antispasmodic) derivatives
dicyclomine hydrochloride
oxyphencyclimine hydrochloride

Antiparkinsonian agents
benztropine mesylate
biperiden hydrochloride
biperiden lactate
glycopyrrolate
procyclidine hydrochloride
scopolamine
scopolamine hydrobromide
trihexyphenidyl hydrochloride

Anticholinergics are used to treat various spastic conditions, including acute dystonic reactions, muscle rigidity, parkinsonism, and extrapyramidal disorders. They also are used to reverse neuromuscular blockade, to prevent nausea and vomiting resulting from motion sickness, as adjunctive treatment for peptic ulcer disease and other GI disorders, and preoperatively to decrease secretions and block cardiac reflexes. Belladonna alkaloids are naturally occurring anticholinergics that have been used for centuries. Many semisynthetic alkaloids and synthetic anticholinergic compounds are available; however, most offer few advantages over naturally occurring alkaloids.

Pharmacology
Anticholinergics competitively antagonize the actions of acetylcholine and other cholinergic agonists within the parasympathetic nervous system. Lack of specificity for site of action increases the hazard of adverse effects in association with therapeutic effects.

Antispasmodics are structurally similar to anticholinergics; however, their anticholinergic activity usually occurs only at high doses. They are believed to directly relax smooth muscle.

Clinical indications and actions
Hypersecretory conditions
Many anticholinergics (anisotropine, atropine, belladonna leaf, clidinium, glycopyrrolate, hexocyclium, hyoscyamine, isopropamide, levorotatory alkaloids of belladonna, mepenzolate, and methantheline) are used therapeutically for their antisecretory properties; these properties derive from competitive blockade of cholinergic receptor sites, causing decreased gastric acid secretion, salivation, bronchial secretions, and sweating.

GI tract disorders
Some anticholinergics (atropine, belladonna leaf, glycopyrrolate, hexocyclium, hyoscyamine, isopropamide, levorotatory alkaloids of belladonna, mepenzolate, methantheline, oxyphenonium, propantheline, and methscopolamine),

as well as the antispasmodics dicyclomine and oxyphencyclimine, treat spasms and other GI tract disorders. These drugs competitively block acetylcholine's actions at cholinergic receptor sites. Antispasmodics presumably act by a nonspecific, direct spasmolytic action on smooth muscle. These agents are useful in treating peptic ulcer disease, pylorospasm, ileitis, and irritable bowel syndrome.

Sinus bradycardia
Atropine is used to treat sinus bradycardia caused by drugs, poisons, or sinus node dysfunction. It blocks normal vagal inhibition of the SA node and causes an increase in heart rate.

Dystonia and parkinsonism
Benztropine, biperiden, procyclidine, and trihexyphenidyl are used to treat acute dystonic reactions and drug-induced extrapyramidal adverse effects. They act centrally by blocking cholinergic receptor sites, balancing cholinergic activity.

Perioperative use
Atropine, glycopyrrolate, and hyoscyamine are used postoperatively with anticholinesterase agents to reverse nondepolarizing neuromuscular blockade. These agents block muscarinic effects of anticholinesterase agents by competitively blocking muscarinic receptor sites.

Atropine, glycopyrrolate, and scopolamine are used preoperatively to decrease secretions and block cardiac vagal reflexes. They diminish secretions by competitively inhibiting muscarinic receptor sites; they block cardiac vagal reflexes by preventing normal vagal inhibition of the SA node.

Motion sickness
Scopolamine is effective in preventing nausea and vomiting associated with motion sickness. Its exact mechanism of action is unknown, but it is thought to affect neural pathways originating in the labyrinth of the ear.

Overview of adverse reactions
Dry mouth, decreased sweating or anhidrosis, headache, mydriasis, blurred vision, cycloplegia, urinary hesitancy, urine retention, constipation, palpitations, and tachycardia most commonly occur with therapeutic doses and usually disappear once the drug is discontinued. Signs of drug toxicity include CNS signs resembling psychosis (disorientation, confusion, hallucinations, delusions, anxiety, agitation, and restlessness) and such peripheral effects as dilated, nonreactive pupils; blurred vision; hot, dry, flushed skin; dry mucous membranes; dysphagia; decreased or absent bowel sounds; urine

---

retention; hyperthermia; tachycardia; hypertension; and increased respiration.

▶ **Special considerations**
● Give medication 30 minutes to 1 hour before meals and at bedtime to maximize therapeutic effects. In some instances, drugs should be administered with meals; always follow dosage recommendations.
● Monitor patient's vital signs and urine output and watch for visual changes and signs of impending toxicity.
● Give ice chips, cool drinks, or hard candy to relieve dry mouth.
● Constipation may be relieved by stool softeners or bulk laxatives.
● The safety of anticholinergic therapy during pregnancy has not been determined. Use by pregnant women is indicated only when the drug's benefits outweigh potential risks to the fetus.

Information for the patient
● Teach patient how and when to take drug for his particular condition; caution patient to take drug only as prescribed and not to take other medications with drug except as prescribed.
● Warn patient to avoid driving and other hazardous tasks if he experiences dizziness, drowsiness, or blurred vision.
● Advise patient to avoid alcoholic beverages, because they may cause additive CNS effects.
● Advise patient to consume plenty of fluids and dietary fiber to help avoid constipation.
● Tell patient to promptly report dry mouth, blurred vision, skin rash, eye pain, or any significant change in urine volume or pain or difficulty on urination.
● Warn patient that drug may cause increased sensitivity or intolerance to high temperatures, resulting in dizziness.
● Instruct patient to report confusion and rapid or pounding heartbeat.
● Advise women patients to report pregnancy or the intent to conceive.

Geriatric use
Administer anticholinergics cautiously to elderly patients. Lower doses are usually indicated. Patients over age 40 may be more sensitive to the effects of these drugs.

Pediatric use
Safety and effectiveness have not been established.

Breast-feeding
Some anticholinergics may be excreted in breast milk, possibly resulting in infant toxicity. Breast-feeding women should avoid these drugs. Anticholinergics may decrease milk production.

---

antihistamines

astemizole
azatadine maleate
brompheniramine maleate
buclizine hydrochloride
carbinoxamine maleate
chlorpheniramine maleate
clemastine fumarate
cyclizine hydrochloride
cyclizine lactate
cyproheptadine hydrochloride
dexchlorpheniramine maleate
dimenhydrinate
diphenhydramine hydrochloride
hydroxyzine hydrochloride
hydroxyzine pamoate
meclizine hydrochloride
methdilazine
methdilazine hydrochloride
promethazine hydrochloride
pyrilamine maleate
terfenadine
trimeprazine tartrate
tripelennamine citrate
tripelennamine hydrochloride
triprolidine hydrochloride

Antihistamines, synthetically produced histamine₁- (H_1) receptor antagonists, were discovered in the late 1930s and proliferated rapidly during the next decade. They have many applications related specifically to chemical structure, their widespread use testifying to their versatility and relative safety. Some antihistamines are used primarily to treat rhinitis or pruritus, whereas others are used more often for their antiemetic and antivertigo effects; still others are used as sedative-hypnotics, local anesthetics, and antitussives.

Pharmacology
Antihistamines are structurally related chemicals that compete with histamine for histamine H_1-receptor sites on the smooth muscle of the bronchi, GI tract, uterus, and large blood vessels, binding to the cellular receptors and preventing access and subsequent activity of his-

tamine. They do not directly alter histamine or prevent its release.

Clinical indications and actions
Allergy
Most antihistamines (azatadine, brompheniramine, carbinoxamine, chlorpheniramine, clemastine, cyproheptadine, dexchorpheniramine, diphenhydramine, promethazine, terfenadine, tripelennamine, and triprolidine) are used to treat allergic symptoms, such as rhinitis and urticaria. By preventing access of histamine to H_1-receptor sites, they suppress histamine-induced allergic symptoms.

Pruritus
Cyproheptadine, hydroxyzine, methdilazine, tripelennamine, and trimeprazine are used systemically. It is believed that these drugs counteract histamine-induced pruritus by a combination of peripheral effects on nerve endings and local anesthetic and sedative activity.

Tripelennamine and diphenhydramine are used topically to relieve itching associated with minor skin irritation. Structurally related to local anesthetics, these compounds prevent initiation and transmission of nerve impulses.

Vertigo; nausea and vomiting
Buclizine, cyclizine, dimenhydrinate, and meclizine are used only as antiemetic and antivertigo agents; their antihistaminic activity has not been evaluated. Diphenhydramine and promethazine are used as antiallergic and antivertigo agents and as antiemetics and antinauseants. Although the mechanisms are not fully understood, antiemetic and antivertigo effects probably result from central antimuscarinic activity.

Sedation
Diphenhydramine and promethazine are used for their sedative action; hydroxyzine is used as a sedative and an anxiolytic. The mechanism of antihistamine-induced CNS depression is unknown.

Suppression of cough
Diphenhydramine syrup is used as an antitussive. The cough reflex is suppressed by a direct effect on the medullary cough center.

Dyskinesia
The central antimuscarinic action of diphenhydramine reduces drug-induced dyskinesias and parkinsonism via inhibition of acetylcholine (anticholinergic effect).

Overview of adverse reactions
At therapeutic dosage levels, all antihistamines except terfenadine are likely to cause drowsiness and impaired motor function during initial therapy. Also, their anticholinergic action usually causes dry mouth and throat, blurred vision, and constipation. Antihistamines that are also phenothiazines, such as promethazine, may cause other adverse effects, including cholestatic jaundice (thought to be a hypersensitivity reaction) and may predispose patients to photosensitivity; patients taking such drugs should avoid prolonged exposure to sunlight.

Toxic doses elicit a combination of CNS depression and excitation as well as atropine-like symptoms, including sedation, reduced mental alertness, apnea, CV collapse, hallucinations, tremor, seizures, dry mouth, flushed skin, and fixed, dilated pupils. Toxic effects reverse when medication is discontinued. Used appropriately, in correct dosages, antihistamines are safe for prolonged use.

▶ Special considerations
● Antihistamines are contraindicated during an acute asthma attack, because they may not alleviate the symptoms and antimuscarinic effects can cause thickening of secretions.
● Use antihistamines with caution in elderly patients and in those with increased intraocular pressure, hyperthyroidism, CV or renal disease, diabetes, hypertension, bronchial asthma, urine retention, prostatic hypertrophy, bladder neck obstruction, or stenosing peptic ulcers.
● Monitor blood counts during long-term therapy; watch for signs of blood dyscrasias.
● Reduce GI distress by giving antihistamines with food; give sugarless gum, sour hard candy, or ice chips to relieve dry mouth; increase fluid intake (if allowed) or humidify air to decrease adverse effect of thickened secretions.
● If tolerance develops to one antihistamine, another may be substituted.
● Some antihistamines may mask ototoxicity from high doses of aspirin and other salicylates.

Information for the patient
● Advise patient to take drug with meals or snacks to prevent gastric upset and to use any of the following measures to relieve dry mouth: warm water rinses, artificial saliva, ice chips, or sugarless gum or candy. Patient should avoid overusing mouthwash, which may add to dryness (alcohol content) and destroy normal flora.
● Warn patient to avoid hazardous activities, such as driving a car or operating machinery, until extent of CNS effects are known and to seek medical approval before using alcoholic beverages, tranquilizers, sedatives, pain relievers, or sleeping medications.
● Warn patient to stop taking antihistamines 4

days before diagnostic skin tests, to preserve accuracy of tests. In the case of terfenadine, discontinue drug at least 2 days before the test.

Geriatric use
Elderly patients are usually more sensitive to adverse effects of antihistamines and are especially likely to experience a greater degree of dizziness, sedation, hypotension, and urine retention than younger patients.

Pediatric use
Children, especially those under age 6, may experience paradoxical hyperexcitability with restlessness, insomnia, nervousness, euphoria, tremor, and seizures.

Breast-feeding
Antihistamines should not be used during breast-feeding; many of these drugs are excreted in breast milk, exposing the infant to hazards of unusual excitability; neonates, especially premature infants, may experience seizures.

---

barbiturates

amobarbital
amobarbital sodium
aprobarbital
butabarbital sodium
mephobarbital
metharbital
pentobarbital sodium
phenobarbital
phenobarbital sodium
primidone
secobarbital sodium

Barbituric acid was compounded over 100 years ago in 1864. The first hypnotic barbiturate, barbital, was introduced into medicine in 1903. Although barbiturates have been used extensively as sedative-hypnotics and anxiolytics, benzodiazepines are the current drugs of choice for sedative-hypnotic effects. Phenobarbital remains a cornerstone of anticonvulsant therapy. A few short-acting barbiturates are used as general anesthetics.

Pharmacology
Barbiturates are structurally related compounds that act throughout the central CNS, particularly in the mesencephalic reticular ac-

tivating system, which controls the CNS arousal mechanism. Barbiturates decrease both presynaptic and postsynaptic membrane excitability.

The exact mechanism(s) of action of barbiturates at these sites is unknown, nor is it clear which cellular and synaptic actions result in sedative-hypnotic effects. Barbiturates can produce all levels of CNS depression, from mild sedation to coma to death. Barbiturates exert their effects by facilitating the actions of gamma-aminobutyric acid (GABA). Barbiturates also exert a central effect, which depresses respiration and GI motility. The principal anticonvulsant mechanism of action is reduction of nerve transmission and decreased excitability of the nerve cell. Barbiturates also raise the seizure threshold. After oral or rectal administration, all barbiturates act within 20 to 60 minutes.

Clinical indications and actions
Seizure disorders
Phenobarbital is used in the prophylactic treatment of seizure disorders. It is used mainly in tonic-clonic and partial seizures. At anesthetic doses, all barbiturates have anticonvulsant activity.

Barbiturates suppress the spread of seizure activity produced by epileptogenic foci in the cortex, thalamus, and limbic systems by enhancing the effects of GABA.

Sedation; hypnosis
All currently available barbiturates are used as sedative-hypnotics for short-term (up to 2 weeks) treatment of insomnia because of their nonspecific CNS effects.

Barbiturates are not used as routinely as sedatives because of excess sedation, short-term efficacy, and the potential for severe adverse reactions upon withdrawal or overdose; they have been replaced for such use by benzodiazepines and nonspecific sedatives. Barbiturate-induced sleep differs from physiologic sleep by decreasing the rapid-eye-movement (REM) sleep cycles.

Overview of adverse reactions
Drowsiness, lethargy, vertigo, headache, and CNS depression are common with barbiturates. After hypnotic doses, a hangover effect, subtle distortion of mood, and impairment of judgment or motor skills may continue for many hours. After a decrease in dosage or discontinuation of barbiturates used for hypnosis, rebound insomnia or increased dreaming or nightmares may occur. Barbiturates cause hyperalgesia in

---

subhypnotic doses. Hypersensitivity reactions (rash, fever, serum sickness) are not common and are more likely to occur in patients with a history of asthma or allergies to other drugs; reactions include urticaria, rash, angioedema, and Stevens-Johnson syndrome. Barbiturates can cause paradoxical excitement at low doses, confusion in elderly patients, and hyperactivity in children. High fever, severe headache, stomatitis, conjunctivitis, or rhinitis may precede skin eruptions. Because of the potential for fatal consequences, discontinue barbiturates if dermatologic reactions occur.

Withdrawal symptoms may occur after as little as 2 weeks of uninterrupted therapy. Symptoms of abstinence usually occur within 8 to 12 hours after the last dose, but may be delayed up to 5 days. They include weakness, anxiety, nausea, vomiting, insomnia, hallucinations, and possibly seizures.

▶ **Special considerations**
● Dosage of barbiturates must be individualized for each patient, because different rates of metabolism and enzyme induction occur.
● Parenteral solutions are highly alkaline; avoid extravasation, which may cause local tissue damage and tissue necrosis; inject I.V. or deep I.M. only. Do not exceed 5 ml per I.M. injection site to avoid tissue damage.
● Too-rapid I.V. administration of barbiturates may cause respiratory depression, apnea, laryngospasm, or hypotension. Have resuscitative measures available. Assess I.V. site for signs of infiltration or phlebitis.
● May be given rectally if oral or parenteral route is inappropriate.
● Assess level of consciousness before and frequently during therapy to evaluate effectiveness of drug. Monitor neurologic status for possible alterations or deteriorations. Monitor seizure character, frequency, and duration for changes. Institute seizure precautions, as necessary.
● Vital signs should be checked frequently, especially during I.V. administration.
● Assess patient's sleeping patterns before and during therapy to ensure effectiveness of drug.
● Institute safety measures — side rails, assistance when out of bed, call light within reach — to prevent falls and injury.
● Anticipate possible rebound confusion and excitatory reactions in patient.
● Assess bowel elimination patterns; monitor for complaints of constipation. Advise diet high in fiber, if indicated.
● Monitor prothrombin time carefully in patients taking anticoagulants; dosage of anti-

coagulant may require adjustment to counteract possible interaction.
● Observe patient to prevent hoarding or self-dosing, especially in depressed or suicidal patients or those who are or have a history of being drug-dependent.
● Abrupt discontinuation may cause withdrawal symptoms; discontinue slowly.
● Death is common with an overdose of 2 to 10 g; it may occur at much smaller doses if alcohol is also ingested.
● Avoid administering barbiturates to patients with status asthmaticus.

Information for the patient
● Warn patient to avoid concurrent use of other drugs with CNS depressant effects, such as antihistamines, analgesics, and alcohol, because they will have additive effects and result in increased drowsiness. Instruct patient to seek medical approval before taking any OTC cold or allergy preparations.
● Caution patient not to increase or decrease dose or frequency without medical approval; abrupt discontinuation of medication may trigger rebound insomnia, with increased dreaming, nightmares, or seizures.
● Advise patient against driving and other hazardous tasks that require alertness while taking barbiturates. Instruct patient in safety measures to prevent injury.
● Be sure patient understands that barbiturates are capable of causing physical or psychological dependence (addiction), and that these effects may be transmitted to the fetus; withdrawal symptoms can occur in neonates whose mothers took barbiturates in the third trimester.
● Instruct patient to report any skin eruption or other marked adverse effect.
● Explain that a morning hangover is common after therapeutic use of barbiturates.

Geriatric use
Elderly patients and patients receiving subhypnotic doses may experience hyperactivity, excitement, or hyperalgesia. Use with caution.

Pediatric use
Premature infants are more susceptible to the depressant effects of barbiturates because of immature hepatic metabolism. Children receiving barbiturates may experience hyperactivity, excitement, or hyperalgia.

Breast-feeding

Barbiturates are excreted in breast milk and may result in infant CNS depression. Use with caution.

---

benzodiazepines

alprazolam
chlordiazepoxide hydrochloride
clonazepam
clorazepate dipotassium
chlordiazepoxide
diazepam
estazolam
flurazepam hydrochloride
halazepam
lorazepam
midazolam
oxazepam
prazepam
quazepam
temazepam
triazolam

Benzodiazepines, synthetically produced sedative-hypnotics, gained popularity in the early 1960s, replacing barbiturates as the treatment of choice for anxiety, seizure disorders, and sedation. These drugs are preferred over barbiturates because therapeutic doses produce less drowsiness and impairment of motor function and toxic doses are less likely to be fatal.

Pharmacology

Benzodiazepines are a group of structurally related chemicals that selectively act on polysynaptic neuronal pathways throughout the CNS. Their precise sites and mechanisms of action are not completely known. However, the benzodiazepines are thought to enhance or facilitate the action of gamma-aminobutyric acid (GABA), an inhibitory neurotransmitter in the CNS. All of the benzodiazepines have CNS-depressant activities; however, individual derivatives act more selectively at specific sites, allowing them to be subclassified into five categories based on their predominant clinical use.

Clinical indications and actions
Seizure disorders

Four of the benzodiazepines (diazepam, clonazepam, clorazepate, and parenteral lorazepam) are used as anticonvulsants. Their anticonvulsant properties are derived from an ability to suppress the spread of seizure activity produced by epileptogenic foci in the cortex, thalamus, and limbic systems by enhancing presynaptic inhibition. Clonazepam is particularly useful in the adjunctive treatment of petit mal variant (Lennox-Gastaut syndrome), myoclonic, or akinetic seizures. Parenteral diazepam is indicated to treat status epilepticus.

Anxiety, tension, and insomnia

Most benzodiazepines (alprazolam, chlordiazepoxide, clorazepate, diazepam, estazolam, flurazepam, halazepam, lorazepam, oxazepam, prazepam, quazepam, temazepam, and triazolam) are useful as anxiolytics or sedative-hypnotics. They have a similar mechanism of action: they are believed to facilitate the effects of GABA in the ascending reticular activating system, increasing inhibition and blocking both cortical and limbic arousal.

They are used to treat anxiety and tension that occur alone or as an adverse reaction of a primary disorder. They are not recommended for tension associated with everyday stress. The choice of a specific benzodiazepine depends on individual metabolic characteristics of the drug. For instance, in patients with depressed renal or hepatic function, alprazolam, lorazepam, or oxazepam may be selected because they have a relatively short duration of action and have no active metabolites. The sedative-hypnotic properties of chlordiazepoxide, clorazepate, diazepam, lorazepam, and oxazepam make these the drugs of choice as preoperative medication and as an adjunct in the rehabilitation of alcoholics.

Surgical adjuncts for conscious sedation or amnesia

Diazepam, midazolam, and lorazepam have amnesic effects. The mechanism of such action is not known. Parenteral administration before such procedures as endoscopy or elective cardioversion causes impairment of recent memory and interferes with the establishment of memory trace, producing anterograde amnesia.

Skeletal muscle spasm; tremor

Because oral forms of diazepam and chlordiazepoxide have skeletal muscle relaxant properties, they are often used to treat neurologic conditions involving muscle spasms and tetanus. The mechanism of such action is unknown, but they are believed to inhibit spinal polysynaptic and monosynaptic afferent pathways.

Overview of adverse reactions

Therapeutic dosage of the benzodiazepines usually causes drowsiness and impaired motor function, which should be monitored early in

---

treatment. GI discomfort, such as constipation, diarrhea, vomiting, and changes in appetite, with urinary alterations also have been reported. Visual disturbances and CV irregularities also are common. Continuing confusion, severe depression, shakiness, vertigo, slurred speech, staggering, bradycardia, shortness of breath or difficulty breathing, and severe weakness usually indicate a toxic dose level. Prolonged or frequent use of benzodiazepines can cause physical dependency and withdrawal syndrome when use is discontinued.

▶ Special considerations
● Administer with milk or immediately after meals to prevent GI upset. Give antacid, if needed, at least 1 hour before or after dose to prevent interaction and ensure maximum drug absorption and effectiveness.
● Crush tablet or empty capsule and mix with food if patient has difficulty swallowing.
● Assess level of consciousness and neurologic status before and frequently during therapy for changes. Monitor for paradoxical reactions, especially early in therapy.
● Assess sleep patterns and quality. Institute seizure precautions. Assess for changes in seizure character, frequency, or duration.
● Assess vital signs frequently during therapy. Significant changes in blood pressure and heart rate may indicate impending toxicity.
● Monitor renal and hepatic function periodically to ensure adequate drug removal and prevent cumulative effects.
● Comfort measures – such as back rubs and relaxation techniques – may enhance drug effectiveness.
● As needed, institute safety measures – raised side rails and ambulatory assistance – to prevent injury. Anticipate possible rebound excitement reactions.
● Patient should be observed to prevent drug hoarding or self-dosing, especially in depressed or suicidal patients or those who are, or who have a history of being, drug-dependent. Patient's mouth should be checked to be sure tablet or capsule was swallowed.
● After prolonged use, abrupt discontinuation may cause withdrawal symptoms; discontinue gradually.

Information for the patient
● Warn patient to avoid use of alcohol or other CNS depressants, such as antihistamines, analgesics, MAO inhibitors, antidepressants, and barbiturates, while taking benzodiazepines to prevent additive depressant effects.

● Caution patient not to take the drug except as prescribed and not to give medication to others. Tell patient not to increase the dose or frequency and to call before taking any OTC cold or allergy preparations that may potentiate CNS depressant effects.
● Warn patient to avoid activities requiring alertness and good psychomotor coordination until the CNS response to the drug is determined. Instruct patient in safety measures to prevent injury.
● Tell patient to avoid using antacids, which may delay drug absorption, unless prescribed.
● Be sure patient understands that benzodiazepines are capable of causing physical and psychological dependence with prolonged use.
● Warn patient not to stop taking the drug abruptly to prevent withdrawal symptoms after prolonged therapy.
● Tell patient that smoking decreases the drug's effectiveness. Encourage patient to stop smoking during therapy.
● Tell patient to report any adverse effects. These are often dose-related and can be relieved by dosage adjustments.
● Inform women who are taking the drug to report if they suspect they are pregnant or intend to become pregnant.

Geriatric use
● Because they are sensitive to its CNS effects, elderly patients receiving benzodiazepines require lower doses. Use with caution.
● Parenteral administration of these drugs is more likely to cause apnea, hypotension, bradycardia, and cardiac arrest in elderly patients.
● Geriatric patients may show prolonged elimination of benzodiazepines, except possibly of oxazepam, lorazepam, temazapam, and triazolam.

Pediatric use
● Because children, particularly very young ones, are sensitive to the CNS depressant effects of benzodiazepines, caution must be exercised. A neonate whose mother took a benzodiazepine during pregnancy may exhibit withdrawal symptoms.
● Use of benzodiazepines during labor may cause neonatal flaccidity.

Breast-feeding
The breast-fed infant of a mother who uses a benzodiazepine drug may show sedation, feeding difficulties, and weight loss. Safe use has not been established.

■

beta-adrenergic blockers

beta₁ blockers
acebutolol
atenolol
metoprolol tartrate

beta₁ and beta₂ blockers
betaxolol hydrochloride
carteolol hydrochloride
esmolol
labetalol
levobunolol
nadolol
penbutolol sulfate
pindolol
propranolol hydrochloride
timolol maleate

Beta-adrenergic blockers were first used clinically in the early 1960s; they are now widely used in the management of hypertension, angina pectoris, and arrhythmias.

Beta blockers have been used in the treatment of genrealized anxiety, adjustment disorders, and acute stress reactions. They appear particularly useful for treating anxiety accompanied by somatic symptoms (sweating, tremor, palpitations). Although they are not FDA-approved for these uses, these drugs are widely used and are well tolerated by most patients.

Pharmacology
Beta blockers are chemicals that compete with beta agonists for available beta-receptor sites; individual agents differ in their ability to affect beta receptors. Most available agents are considered nonselective; that is, they block both beta₁ receptors in cardiac muscle and beta₂ receptors in bronchial and vascular smooth muscle. Several agents are cardioselective and in lower doses primarily inhibit beta₁ receptors. Some beta blockers have intrinsic sympathomimetic activity and simultaneously stimulate and block beta receptors, decreasing cardiac output; still others also have membrane-stabilizing activity, which affects cardiac action potential.

Clinical indications and actions
Hypertension
All currently available beta blockers are used to treat hypertension. Although the exact mechanism of their antihypertensive effect is un-

known, the action is thought to result from decreased cardiac output, decreased sympathetic outflow from the CNS, and suppression of renin release.
Angina
Propranolol and nadolol are used to treat angina pectoris; they decrease myocardial oxygen requirements via blockade of catecholamine-induced increases in heart rate, blood pressure, and the extent of myocardial contraction.
Arrhythmia
Propranolol, acebutolol, and esmolol are used to treat arrhythmias; they prolong the refractory period of the AV node and slow AV conduction.
Glaucoma
The mechanism by which betaxolol, levobunolol, and timolol reduce intraocular pressure is unknown, but the drug effect is at least partially caused by decreased production of aqueous humor.
MI
Timolol, propranolol, and metoprolol are used to prevent MI in susceptible patients; the mechanism of this protective effect is unknown.
Migraine prophylaxis
Propranolol is used to prevent recurrent attacks of migraine and other vascular headaches. The exact mechanism by which propranolol decreases the incidence of migraine headache attacks is unknown, but it is thought to result from inhibition of vasodilation of cerebral vessels.
Other uses
Beta blockers have been used as anxiolytics, as adjunctive therapy of bleeding esophageal varices, and to treat portal hypertension.

Overview of adverse reactions
Therapeutic doses of beta-adrenergic blockers usually cause bradycardia, fatigue, and dizziness; some may cause other CNS disturbances such as nightmares, depression, memory loss, and hallucinations. Impotence, cold extremities, and elevated serum cholesterol levels have been reported. *Severe hypotension, bradycardia, heart failure, or bronchospasm* usually indicates toxic dosage levels.

▶ Special considerations
● Check apical pulse rate daily; discontinue and reevaluate therapy if extremes occur (for example, a pulse rate below 60 beats/minute).
● Monitor blood pressure, ECG, and heart rate and rhythm frequently; be alert for progression of AV block or severe bradycardia.
● Weigh patients with CHF regularly; watch for gains of more than 5 lb (2.25 kg) per week.

• Signs of hypoglycemic shock are masked; watch diabetic patients for sweating, fatigue, and hunger.

• *Do not discontinue these drugs before surgery for pheochromocytoma;* before any surgical procedure, notify anesthesiologist that patient is taking a beta-adrenergic blocker.

• Glucagon may be prescribed to reverse signs and symptoms of beta blocker overdose.

Information for the patient
• Explain rationale for therapy, and emphasize importance of taking drugs as prescribed, even when patient is feeling well.

• Warn patient not to discontinue these drugs suddenly; abrupt discontinuation can exacerbate angina or precipitate MI.

• Explain potential adverse reactions and importance of reporting any unusual effects.

• Teach patient to minimize dizziness from orthostatic hypotension by taking dose at bedtime and by rising slowly and avoiding sudden position changes.

• Advise patient to seek medical approval before taking OTC cold preparations.

Geriatric use
Elderly patients may require lower maintenance doses of beta-adrenergic blockers because of increased bioavailability or delayed metabolism; they also may experience enhanced adverse reactions.

Pediatric use
Safety and efficacy of beta-adrenergic blocking agents in children have not been established; they should be used only if potential benefit outweighs risk.

Breast-feeding
Beta-adrenergic blockers are distributed into breast milk. Recommendations for breast-feeding vary with individual drugs.

---

carbonic anhydrase inhibitors

acetazolamide
dichlorphenamide
methazolamide

The carbonic anhydrase inhibitors were developed in the 1940s during research aimed at synthesizing sulfonamide compounds with the carbonic anhydrase inhibitory properties of sulfanilamide. Most studies have been conducted with acetazolamide, the prototype for this class of drugs. Carbonic anhydrase inhibitors have been largely replaced by thiazides and are seldom used as diuretics because their propensity for causing metabolic acidosis makes patients refractory to their diuretic effects, requiring intermittent therapy to restore effective diuresis.

Pharmacology
As their name implies, carbonic anhydrase inhibitors act by noncompetitive reversible inhibition of the enzyme carbonic anhydrase, which is responsible for formation of hydrogen and bicarbonate ions from carbon dioxide and water. This inhibition results in decreased hydrogen levels in the renal tubules, promoting excretion of bicarbonate, sodium, potassium, and water; because carbon dioxide is not eliminated as rapidly, systemic acidosis may occur.

Clinical indications and actions
Open-angle glaucoma and angle-closure glaucoma
Because carbonic anhydrase inhibitors reduce the formation of aqueous humor, lowering intraocular pressure, they are useful as adjunctive therapy in patients with glaucoma.
Seizure disorders
Acetazolamide is used with other anticonvulsants in various types of seizures, particularly absence. It acts to inhibit seizures by an unknown mechanism; it may act by inducing metabolic acidosis or by increasing carbon dioxide tension within the CNS.
Diuresis
Acetazolamide, a carbonic anhydrase inhibitor, reversibly blocks the enzyme responsible for formation of hydrogen and bicarbonate ions from carbon dioxide and water. This decreases hydrogen concentration in the renal tubules, promoting excretion of bicarbonate, sodium, potassium, and water.
Mountain sickness
Acetazolamide shortens the period of high-altitude acclimatization; by inhibiting conversion of carbon dioxide to bicarbonate, it may increase carbon dioxide tension in tissues and decrease it in the lungs; the resultant metabolic acidosis may also increase oxygenation during hypoxia.

Overview of adverse reactions
Many adverse reactions associated with carbonic anhydrase inhibitors are dose-related and respond to lowered dosage; each drug has a

---

slightly different adverse reaction profile, and patients who cannot tolerate one of the drugs may be able to tolerate another. Serious adverse reactions are infrequent, because drugs are primarily given for short-term use. Some of the more common adverse reactions include generalized weakness, tiredness, or discomfort; nausea; vomiting; diarrhea; loss of appetite; metallic taste in the mouth; peripheral numbness or tingling in hands, fingers, toes, or tongue.

▶ **Special considerations**

● Drug use in glaucoma may be limited because of the propensity for causing metabolic acidosis; signs and symptoms include weakness, malaise, headache, abdominal pain, nausea, vomiting, and poor skin turgor.

● In treating edema, intermittent dosage schedules may minimize tendency to cause metabolic acidosis and permit diuresis.

● Because they alkalize urine, these drugs may cause false-positive results on test for proteinuria.

● Establish baseline values before therapy, and monitor blood pressure and pulse rate for changes. Impose safety measures until patient's response to the diuretic is known.

● Establish baseline and periodically review laboratory tests: CBC, including WBC count; serum electrolyte, carbon dioxide, BUN, and creatinine levels; and, especially, liver function tests. Patients with liver disease are especially susceptible to diuretic-induced electrolyte imbalance; in extreme cases, stupor, coma, and death can result.

● Administer diuretics in the morning so that major diuresis occurs before bedtime. To prevent nocturia, diuretics should not be administered after 6 p.m.

● Consider possible dosage adjustment: reduced dosage for patients with hepatic dysfunction and those taking other antihypertensive agents; increased dosage for patients with renal impairment, oliguria, or decreased diuresis (inadequate urine output may result in circulatory overload, causing water intoxication, pulmonary edema, and CHF); and increased doses of insulin or oral hypoglycemics in diabetic patients.

● Monitor for signs of toxicity: postural hypotension; muscle weakness and cardiac arrhythmia (signs of hypokalemia); leg cramps, nausea, muscle weakness, dry mouth, and dizziness (hyponatremia); lethargy, confusion, stupor, muscle twitching, increased reflexes, and seizures (water intoxication); severe weakness, headache, abdominal pain, malaise, nausea, and vomiting (metabolic acidosis); sore throat, rash, or jaundice (blood dyscrasia from hypersensitivity); and joint swelling, redness, and pain (hyperuricemia).

● Monitor patient for edema. Observe lower extremities of ambulatory patients and the sacral area of patients on bed rest. Check abdominal girth with tape measure to detect ascites. Dosage adjustment may be indicated. Patient's weight should be recorded each morning immediately after voiding and before breakfast; the patient should be weighed in the same type of clothing and on the same scale. Weight provides an index for dosage adjustments.

● Consult with dietitian on possible need for high-potassium diet or supplement.

● Patient should have urinal or commode readily available.

Information for the patient

● Explain rationale for therapy and diuretic effect of these drugs (increased volume and frequency of urination).

● Teach patient signs of adverse reactions, especially hypokalemia (weakness, fatigue, muscle cramps, paresthesia, confusion, nausea, vomiting, diarrhea, headache, dizziness, or palpitations), and importance of reporting these symptoms promptly.

● Advise patient to eat potassium-rich foods, such as citrus fruits, potatoes, dates, raisins, and bananas; to avoid high-sodium foods, such as lunch meat, smoked meats, and processed cheeses; and not to add salt to other foods. Recommend salt substitutes.

● Counsel patient to avoid smoking because nicotine increases blood pressure.

● Tell patient to seek medical approval before taking OTC drugs; many contain sodium and potassium and can cause electrolyte imbalance.

● Warn patient of photosensitivity reactions. Explain that this reaction is a photoallergy in which ultraviolet radiation alters drug structure, causing allergic reactions in some persons; reactions occur 10 days to 2 weeks after initial sun exposure.

● Emphasize importance of keeping follow-up appointments to monitor effectiveness of diuretic therapy.

● Tell patient to report increased edema or weight or excess diuresis (more than 2-lb weight loss/day) and to record weight each morning after voiding and before breakfast, using the same scale and wearing the same type of clothing.

● Caution patient to change position slowly, es-

pecially when rising from lying or sitting position, to prevent dizziness from orthostatic hypotension.
• Instruct patient to immediately report chest, back, or leg pain; shortness of breath; or dyspnea.
• Tell patient to take drugs only as prescribed and at the same time each day, to prevent night diuresis and interrupted sleep.

Geriatric use
Elderly and debilitated patients require close observation, because they are more susceptible to drug-induced diuresis. In elderly patients excessive diuresis can quickly lead to rapid dehydration, hypovolemia, hypokalemia, and hyponatremia and may cause circulatory collapse. Reduced dosages may be indicated.

Pediatric use
Guidelines for safe use vary with each drug.

Breast-feeding
Safety has not been established.

---

hydantoin derivatives

ethotoin
mephenytoin
phenacemide
phenytoin
phenytoin sodium

Hydantoins, of which phenytoin is the prototype, are used primarily to control generalized tonic-clonic and partial seizures. Ethotoin and mephenytoin are used to treat partial seizures refractory to less toxic agents; because of its extreme toxicity, phenacemide usually is reserved for refractory seizures. Ethotoin is less toxic than phenytoin but also less effective. Mephenytoin is more likely to produce fatal blood dyscrasias than either ethotoin or phenytoin but is less likely to cause ataxia, gingival hyperplasia, hypertrichosis, or GI distress.

Pharmacology
The hydantoins exert their anticonvulsant effects by inhibiting the spread of seizure activity in the motor cortex; they stabilize seizure threshold against hyperexcitability produced by excessive stimulation and decrease post-tetanic potentiation that accompanies abnormal focal discharge.

Phenytoin's antiarrhythmic effects are similar to those produced by quinidine or procainamide; it improves atrioventricular conduction, especially that depressed by digitalis, and prolongs the effective refractory period.

Clinical indications and actions
Seizure disorders
Hydantoins are used to control generalized tonic-clonic and psychomotor seizures; phenytoin, the only parenteral hydantoin, is used to control status epilepticus and seizures occurring during neurosurgery and in patients who cannot receive oral therapy. Mephenytoin is used only for focal, jacksonian, and psychomotor seizures and in patients with refractory seizures.
Arrhythmias
Phenytoin is also used to counteract arrhythmias, especially those produced by digitalis. However, this is an unlabeled use.

Overview of adverse reactions
The most common adverse reactions to hydantoins involve the CNS and are dose-related, especially drowsiness, headache, ataxia, and dizziness. Other adverse reactions include GI irritation, severe dermatologic and hematopoietic reactions, lymphadenopathy, gingival hyperplasia, and hepatotoxicity.

▶ Special considerations
• Monitor baseline liver function and hematologic laboratory studies and repeat at monthly intervals.
• Observe patient closely during therapy for possible adverse reactions, especially at start of therapy. Hydantoins may cause gingival hyperplasia; good oral hygiene and gum care are essential to minimize effects.
• The hydantoin anticonvulsants should not be discontinued abruptly, but rather slowly over 6 weeks; abrupt discontinuation may cause status epilepticus.
• Drug interactions are frequently a problem, primarily with hepatically cleared drugs, such as chloramphenicol, digitoxin, isoniazid, and griseofulvin; be especially alert for toxic symptoms or breakthrough seizures in patients taking any of these drugs.
• Carefully follow manufacturer's directions for reconstitution, storage, and administration of all preparations.

Information for the patient

- Tell patient not to use alcohol while taking drug, as it may decrease drug's effectiveness and may increase CNS adverse reactions.
- Advise patient to avoid hazardous tasks that require mental alertness until degree of CNS sedative effect is determined.
- Tell patient to take oral drug with food if GI distress occurs.
- Teach patient signs and symptoms of hypersensitivity, liver dysfunction, and blood dyscrasias and to call at once if any of the following occurs: sore throat, fever, bleeding, easy bruising, lymphadenopathy, or rash.
- Tell patient to notify physician immediately if pregnancy occurs.
- Warn patient never to discontinue drug suddenly or without medical supervision.
- Encourage patient to wear medical alert identification listing medication and seizure disorders while taking anticonvulsants.
- Caution patient to consult pharmacist before changing brand or using generic drug; therapeutic effect may change.
- Explain that drug may increase gum growth and sensitivity (gingival hyperplasia); teach proper oral hygiene and urge patient or parent to establish good mouth care.
- Assure patient that pink or reddish brown discoloration of urine is normal and harmless.

Geriatric use

Use anticonvulsants with caution. Elderly patients metabolize and excrete all drugs more slowly and may obtain therapeutic effect from lower dosages.

Pediatric use

Be sure to administer only dosage forms prepared for pediatric use.

Breast-feeding

Hydantoin anticonvulsants are excreted in breast milk; women should discontinue breast-feeding while taking these drugs.

monoamine oxidase inhibitors

isocarboxazid
pargyline hydrochloride
phenelzine sulfate
selegiline hydrochloride
tranylcypromine sulfate

Antidepressant effects of MAO inhibitors were first noted in 1952 during studies with iproniazid, a hydrazine derivative of the antitubercular agent isoniazid. Because of excessive hepatotoxicity, iproniazid was never used clinically. Currently available MAO inhibitors include two hydrazine derivatives, isocarboxazid and phenelzine sulfate, and a nonhydrazine derivative, tranylcypromine sulfate, all of which are less hepatotoxic than iproniazid. All four have antihypertensive activity and antidepressant effects; only pargyline is used (rarely) to treat severe hypertension.

MAO inhibitors can cause serious adverse reactions and interact adversely with many foods and drugs. They are useful drugs for treating dysthymic disorders (particulary depression with hypersomnia, hyperphagia, or severe anxiety) or depression unresponsive to TCAs. They are also used for panic disorders.

Pharmacology

Some forms of depression are thought to result from low CNS levels of neurotransmitters, including norepinephrine and serotonin. MAO inhibitors, as their name implies, depress the effects of MAO, an enzyme that is present principally in the CNS and inactivates amine-containing substances, including the neurotransmitters. Many adverse effects from MAO inhibitors are attributed to gradual buildup and increased activity of neurotransmitters after enzyme inhibition.

Selegiline specifically inhibits MAO type B, which is found only in the CNS.

Clinical indications and actions
Depression

MAO inhibitors are used to treat severe, atypical neurotic depression refractory to TCAs. Data suggest that depressed patients with coexisting obsessive-compulsive behavior, hysteria, or phobia respond more favorably to MAO inhibitors than to TCAs.

Parkinson's disease

Selegiline is used as an adjunct to carbidopa-levodopa in the treatment of Parkinson's disease.

Overview of adverse reactions

MAO inhibitors' most serious adverse effects involve blood pressure. Hypotensive reactions appear to follow gradual accumulation of false neurotransmitters (phenylethylamines) in adrenergic nerve terminals; normal breakdown of these agents is also inhibited by MAO. Severe hypertension may result from interaction with drugs with sympathomimetic activity, such as pseudoephedrine, phenylephrine, and phenylpropanolamine, other false neurotransmitters, and other drugs with vasoconstrictive effects.

Ingestion of food or beverages containing tyramine may provoke hypertensive crisis—a rapid and severe increase in blood pressure. Hypertensive crisis is attributed to displacement of norepinephrine by false neurotransmitters; prodromal symptoms include severe occipital headache, tachycardia, sweating, and visual disturbances.

All MAO inhibitors cause CNS adverse effects, including restlessness, hyperexcitability, insomnia, and headache. Over time, tolerance develops to most adverse reactions.

▶ Special considerations

● Implement all precautions for use of MAO inhibitors, given alone or with other drugs, for 14 days after discontinuation of drug. Check for potential interactions with other drugs patient may be taking, and especially avoid concomitant use of MAO inhibitors with alcohol or alcohol-containing drugs, phenothiazines, other CNS stimulants, and food and beverages containing tyramine.
● MAO inhibitors impair ability to perform tasks requiring mental alertness, such as driving a car.
● Check vital signs regularly for increased blood pressure or other signs of excessive CNS stimulation.
● Patient should be observed to be sure each dose of drug is swallowed; as depressed patients begin to improve, they may hoard pills for suicide attempt.
● MAO inhibitors may be used with electroconvulsive therapy.

Information for the patient

● Explain rationale for therapy and the risks and benefits that may be anticipated; also explain that full therapeutic effect of drug may not occur for several weeks.
● Advise patient to promptly report any unusual reactions, especially severe headache, rash, dark urine, pale stools, or jaundice.
● Tell patient to avoid beverages and drugs containing alcohol and not to take any other drug (including OTC products) unless prescribed.
● Give patient a list of tyramine-containing foods and beverages and explain why patient should avoid these.
● Tell patient during initial therapy to rise slowly from recumbent position (take at least 2 minutes when getting out of bed) to avoid dizziness from orthostatic hypotension.
● Teach patient how and when to take drug, not to increase dosage unless prescribed, and never to discontinue drug abruptly.
● Advise diabetic patient to monitor serum glucose levels, as drug may alter insulin needs.
● Advise patient to avoid hazardous tasks that require mental alertness until full effect of drug is determined.
● Urge patient to obtain medical alert identification listing therapy with MAO inhibitors.

Geriatric use

MAO inhibitors are not recommended for use in patients over age 60.

Pediatric use

MAO inhibitors are not recommended for children under age 16.

Breast-feeding

Safety has not been established.

■■■■■■■■■■

oxazolidinedione derivatives

paramethadione
trimethadione

Oxazolidinediones, which are similar in structure to hydantoins, are used primarily to control absence seizures; because of their greater toxicity, they usually are reserved for seizures refractory to other anticonvulsants. This class has been replaced largely by the less toxic succinimides.

Pharmacology

Oxazolidinediones elevate the seizure threshold in the cerebral cortex and basal ganglia; they are less effective than either hydantoins or barbiturates. They cause CNS sedation, which may lead to ataxia at high doses; paramethadione has the least sedative effect.

Clinical indications and actions
Seizure disorders
Oxazolidinediones are used to control absence seizures refractory to anticonvulsants, especially in patients with mixed seizures. They have no value in generalized tonic-clonic seizures and may precipitate a first tonic-clonic seizure.

Overview of adverse reactions
The most common adverse reactions from oxazolidinediones include blurred vision, drowsiness, and such GI disturbances as nausea and vomiting. Toxic effects include fatal hematologic and renal reactions, lupuslike syndromes, and lymphadenopathy resembling malignant lymphoma. Strict medical supervision is necessary during the first year of treatment. Because of their potential teratogenicity and toxic adverse reactions, these drugs should be reserved for severely refractory seizure disorders.

▶ Special considerations
● Oxazolidinediones are contraindicated during pregnancy because of their potential to cause fetal malformations and in patients with known hypersensitivity to oxazolidinediones. These drugs should be used with caution in patients with renal or hepatic dysfunction, severe blood dyscrasias, and retinal or optic nerve disease because of their potential to cause severe toxicities in these organs and systems.
● Monitor baseline liver and renal function and CBC at beginning of therapy and monthly during therapy.
● Drug should be discontinued if neutrophil count falls below 2,500/mm³ or if any of the following occur: hypersensitivity, scotomata, hepatitis, systemic lupus erythematosus, lymphadenopathy, rash, nephrosis, alopecia, or generalized tonic-clonic seizures.
● Anticonvulsants should not be discontinued abruptly.

Information for the patient
● Explain rationale for treatment and the need for close medical supervision.
● Teach patient signs and symptoms of hypersensitivity, liver dysfunction, and blood dyscrasias and to report any of the following: sore throat, fever, malaise, bleeding, easy bruising, petechiae, lymphadenopathy, scotomata, or rash.

● Tell patient to notify physician immediately if pregnancy occurs.
● Warn patient never to discontinue drug without medical supervision.
● Advise patient not to use alcohol while taking drug, as it may decrease drug's effectiveness and increase CNS adverse effects.
● Advise patient to avoid tasks that require mental alertness, such as driving a car, until degree of sedative effect is determined. Drug may cause dizziness, drowsiness, or blurred vision.
● Tell patient to take drug with food if GI distress occurs.
● Encourage patient to wear medical alert identification listing medication and seizure disorders while taking anticonvulsants.
● Advise patient to wear dark glasses if photophobia occurs and to use a sunscreen if photosensitivity develops.

Geriatric use
Use anticonvulsant drugs with caution. Elderly patients metabolize and excrete all drugs slowly and may obtain therapeutic effect from lower doses.

Pediatric use
Be sure to administer only dosage forms prepared for pediatric use; these drugs are not recommended for children under age 2.

Breast-feeding
It is unknown if oxazolidinediones are excreted in breast milk. Alternate feeding method is recommended during therapy.

---

phenothiazines

Aliphatic derivatives
chlorpromazine hydrochloride
promazine hydrochloride
promethazine hydrochloride

Piperazine derivatives
acetophenazine maleate
fluphenazine decanoate
fluphenazine enanthate
fluphenazine hydrochloride
perphenazine
prochlorperazine
prochlorperazine edisylate
prochlorperazine maleate
trifluoperazine hydrochloride

Piperidine derivatives
mesoridazine besylate
thioridazine
thioridazine hydrochloride

Pyrollidine derivative
methdilazine

Thioxanthenes
chlorprothixene
chlorprothixene hydrochloride
thiothixene
thiothixene hydrochloride

The phenothiazines were originally synthesized by European scientists seeking aniline-like dyes in the late 1800s. Several decades later, in the 1930s, promethazine was identified and found to have sedative, antihistaminic, and narcotic-potentiating effects. Chlorpromazine was synthesized in the 1950s; this drug proved to have many effects, among them strong antipsychotic activity.

Pharmacology
Phenothiazines are classified in terms of chemical structure: the aliphatic agents (chlorpromazine, promazine, and promethazine) have a greater sedative, hypotensive, allergic, and convulsant activity; the piperazines (acetophenazine, perphenazine, prochlorperazine, fluphenazine, and trifluoperazine) are more likely to produce extrapyramidal symptoms; the piperidines (thioridazine and mesoridazine) have intermediate effects. Thioxanthenes are chemically similar to phenothiazines, and pharma-cologically similar to piperazine phenothiazines.

All antipsychotics have fundamentally similar mechanisms of action; they are believed to function as dopamine antagonists, blocking postsynaptic dopamine receptors in various parts of the CNS; their antiemetic effects result from blockage of the chemoreceptor trigger zone. They also produce varying degrees of anticholinergic and alpha-adrenergic receptor blocking actions. The drugs are structurally similar to TCAs and share many adverse reactions.

All antipsychotics have comparable clinical efficacy when given in equivalent doses; choice of specific therapy is determined primarily by the individual patient's response and adverse reaction profile. A patient who does not respond to one drug may respond to another.

Onset of full therapeutic effects requires 6 weeks to 6 months of therapy; therefore, dosage adjustment is recommended at not less than weekly intervals.

Clinical indications and actions
Psychoses
The phenothiazines and thioxanthenes are indicated to treat agitated psychotic states. They are especially effective in controlling hallucinations in schizophrenic patients, the manic phase of manic-depressive illness, and excessive motor and autonomic activity.
†Anxiety
Chlorpromazine, mesoridazine, promethazine, prochlorperazine, and trifluoperazine may be used for short-term treatment of moderate anxiety in selected nonpsychotic patients, for example, to control anxiety before surgery.
Severe behavior problems
Chlorpromazine and thioridazine are indicated to control combativeness and hyperexcitability in children with severe behavior problems. They also are used in hyperactive children for short-term treatment of excessive motor activity with labile moods, impulsive behavior, aggressiveness, attention deficit, and poor tolerance of frustration. Mesoridazine is used to manage hypersensitivity and to promote cooperative behavior in patients with mental deficiency and chronic brain syndrome.
Anxiety and depression
Thioridazine is effective in adults with moderate to severe anxiety and depression and in elderly patients with multiple mental and emotional symptoms such as agitation, depression, anxiety, apprehension, and insomnia. Thiothixine also has been used as an antidepressant.

Nausea and vomiting

Chlorpromazine, perphenazine, prochlorperazine, and triflupromazine are effective in controlling severe nausea and vomiting induced by CNS disturbances. They do not prevent motion sickness or vertigo.

Tetanus

Chlorpromazine is an effective adjunct in treating tetanus.

Porphyria

Because of its effects on the autonomic nervous system, chlorpromazine is effective in controlling abdominal pain in patients with acute intermittent porphyria.

Intractable hiccups

Chlorpromazine has been used to treat patients with intractable hiccups. The mechanism is unknown.

Neurogenic pain

Fluphenazine is a useful adjunct managing selected chronic pain states (such as narcotic withdrawal).

Allergies and pruritus

Because of their potent antihistaminic effects, many of these drugs (including methdilazine and promethazine) are used to relieve itching or symptomatic rhinitis.

Overview of adverse reactions

Phenothiazines may produce extrapyramidal symptoms (dystonic movements, torticollis, oculogyric crises, parkinsonian symptoms) from akathisia during early treatment to tardive dyskinesia after prolonged use. In some cases, such symptoms can be alleviated by dosage reduction or treatment with diphenhydramine, trihexyphenidyl, or benztropine. Dystonia usually occurs on initial therapy or at increased dosage in children and younger adults; parkinsonian symptoms and tardive dyskinesia more often affect older patients, especially women.

A neuroleptic malignant syndrome resembling severe parkinsonism may occur (most often in young men taking fluphenazine); it consists of rapid onset of hyperthermia, muscular hyperreflexia, marked extrapyramidal and autonomic dysfunction, arrhythmias, sweating, and several other unpleasant reactions. Although rare, this condition carries a 10% mortality and requires immediate treatment, including cooling blankets, neuromuscular blocking agents, dantrolene, and supportive measures.

Other adverse reactions are similar to those seen with TCAs, including varying degrees of sedative and anticholinergic effects, orthostatic hypotension with reflex tachycardia, fainting and dizziness, and arrhythmias; GI reactions including anorexia, nausea, vomiting, abdominal pain and local gastric irritation; seizures; endocrine effects; hematologic disorders; ocular changes and other visual disturbances; skin eruptions; and photosensitivity. Allergic manifestations are usually marked by elevation of liver enzymes progressing to obstructive jaundice.

Generally, piperidine derivatives, mesoridazine, and thioridazine have the most pronounced CV effects, while piperazine derivatives have the least. As might be anticipated, parenteral administration is more often associated with CV effects because of more rapid absorption. Seizures are most common with aliphatic derivatives.

▶ Special considerations

● Phenothiazines are contraindicated in patients with known hypersensitivity to phenothiazines and related compounds, including allergic reactions involving hepatic function; with blood dyscrasias and bone marrow depression; with coma, brain damage, CNS depression, circulatory collapse, or cerebrovascular disease, since additive CNS depression and accompanying blood pressure alteration may seriously worsen these states; and in conjunction with adrenergic blocking agents or spinal or epidural anesthesia because of the potential for excessive postural hypotension.

● Phenothiazines should be used cautiously in patients with cardiac disease (arrhythmias, CHF, angina pectoris, valvular disease, or heart block) to avoid further compromise of cardiac function from alpha blockade; such reactions are particularly likely in patients with preexisting cardiac compromise or a history of arrhythmias.

● Phenothiazines should be used cautiously in patients with encephalitis, Reye's syndrome, or head injury because these drugs' antiemetic and CNS depressant effects may mask signs and symptoms and obscure diagnosis; in patients with respiratory disease because of hazard of respiratory depression and suppression of cough reflex subsequent to additive CNS depression; and in patients with seizure disorders because these drugs lower seizure threshold and may require additional dosage of anticonvulsants.

● Phenothiazines should be used cautiously in patients with glaucoma, prostatic hypertrophy, paralytic ileus, and urine retention because drugs have significant antimuscarinic effects that may exacerbate these conditions; in patients with hepatic or renal dysfunction because of the hazard of drug accumulation; in patients with Parkinson's disease because drugs may aggravate tremor and other symptoms; in patients with pheochromocytoma because of possible adverse CV effects; and in patients with hypocalcemia because of increased risk of extrapyramidal symptoms.

• Check vital signs regularly for decreased blood pressure (especially before and after parenteral therapy) or tachycardia; observe patient carefully for other adverse reactions.

• Check intake and output for urine retention or constipation, which may require dosage reduction.

• Monitor bilirubin levels weekly for first 4 weeks; monitor CBC, ECG (for quinidine-like effects), liver and renal function studies, electrolyte levels (especially potassium), and eye examinations at baseline and periodically thereafter, especially in patients on long-term therapy.

• Observe patient for mood changes to monitor progress; benefits may not be apparent for several weeks.

• Monitor for involuntary movements. Check patient receiving prolonged treatment at least once every 6 months.

• Do not withdraw drug abruptly; although physical dependence does not occur with antipsychotic drugs, rebound exacerbation of psychotic symptoms may occur and many drug effects persist.

• Carefully follow manufacturer's instructions for reconstitution, dilution, administration, and storage of drugs; slightly discolored liquids may or may not be all right to use. Check with pharmacist.

Information for the patient

• Explain rationale and anticipated risks and benefits of therapy and that full therapeutic effect may not occur for several weeks.

• Teach signs and symptoms of adverse reactions and importance of reporting *any* unusual effects, especially involuntary movements.

• Tell patient to avoid beverages and drugs containing alcohol and not to take any other drug (especially CNS depressants) including OTC products without medical approval.

• Instruct diabetic patients to monitor blood sugar, as drug may alter insulin needs.

• Teach patient how and when to take drug, not to increase dose without medical approval, and never to discontinue drug abruptly; suggest taking full dose at bedtime if daytime sedation is troublesome.

• Advise patient to lie down for 30 minutes after first dose (1 hour if I.M.) and to rise slowly from sitting or supine position to prevent orthostatic hypotension.

• Warn patient to avoid tasks requiring mental alertness and psychomotor coordination, such as driving, until full effects of drug are established; emphasize that sedative effects will lessen after several weeks.

• Drugs are locally irritating; advise taking with milk or food to minimize GI distress. Warn that oral concentrates and solutions will irritate skin and tell patient not to crush or open sustained-release products, but rather to swallow them whole.

• Warn patient that excessive exposure to sunlight, heat lamps, or tanning beds may cause photosensitivity reactions (burn and abnormal hyperpigmentation).

• Tell patient to avoid exposure to extremes of heat or cold because of risk of hypothermia or hyperthermia induced by alteration in thermoregulatory function.

• Recommend sugarless gum, hard candy, or ice chips to relieve dry mouth.

• Explain that phenothiazines may cause pink to brown discoloration of urine.

Geriatric use

Lower doses are indicated in geriatric patients, who are more sensitive to therapeutic and adverse reactions, especially cardiac toxicity, tardive dyskinesia, and other extrapyramidal effects. Titrate dosage to patient response.

Pediatric use

Unless otherwise specified, antipsychotics are not recommended for children under age 12; be very careful when using phenothiazines for nausea and vomiting, as acutely ill children (chicken pox, measles, CNS infections, dehydration) are at greatly increased risk of dystonic reactions.

Breast-feeding

If feasible, patient should not breast-feed while taking antipsychotics; most phenothiazines are excreted in breast milk and have a direct effect on prolactin levels. Benefit to mother must outweigh hazard to infant.

succinimide derivatives

ethosuximide
methsuximide
phensuximide

Succinimides, of which ethosuximide is the prototype, are similar in ring structure to hydantoins. They evolved from an attempt to synthesize less toxic oxazolidinedione derivatives.

Pharmacology
Like the oxazolidinediones, succinimides elevate the seizure threshold in the basal ganglia and cerebral cortex and attenuate the synaptic response to repetitive stimulation. They do not affect post-tetanic potentiation. These drugs suppress the characteristic spike-and-wave pattern of the EEG seen with absence seizures.

Clinical indications and actions
Seizure disorders
Succinimides are used primarily to control absence seizures; they are used with other anticonvulsants when absence seizures are accompanied by other forms of seizure disorders. Ethosuximide is the drug of choice; phensuximide is both the least effective and least toxic of this class. Methsuximide is used to control absence seizures refractory to other anticonvulsants. A beneficial therapeutic effect has been noted in patients with myoclonus and partial seizures with complex symptomatology.

Overview of adverse reactions
Most common adverse reactions from succinimides involve the CNS and include drowsiness, headache, and blurred vision. Other adverse reactions include acute dermatologic reactions (Stevens-Johnson syndrome), blood dyscrasias, renal dysfunction, and systemic lupus erythematosus. Drug should be used with caution in patients with acute intermittent porphyria.

▶ Special considerations
● Succinimides are contraindicated in patients with known hypersensitivity to succinimides; they should be used with caution in patients with hepatic or renal dysfunction.
● Monitor baseline liver and renal function studies and blood studies; repeat CBCs every 3 months and urinalysis and liver function tests every 6 months.
● Observe patient closely for dermatologic reactions at initiation of therapy.
● Monitor closely for signs of hypersensitivity or adverse reactions: skin rash, sore throat, joint pain, unexplained fever, or unusual bleeding or bruising.
● Succinimide anticonvulsants should not be discontinued abruptly.
● Succinimides add to CNS depressant effects of alcohol, narcotics, anxiolytics, antidepressants, and tranquilizers.
● Carefully follow manufacturer's directions for reconstitution, storage, and administration of all preparations.

Information for the patient
● Tell patient not to use alcohol while taking drug; it may decrease drug's effectiveness and increase CNS adverse effects.
● Advise patient to avoid hazardous tasks that require mental alertness until degree of sedative effect is determined.
● Tell patient to take oral drug with food if GI distress occurs.
● Teach patient signs and symptoms of hypersensitivity, liver dysfunction, and blood dyscrasias and advise patient to report them promptly. Also tell patient to notify physician immediately if pregnancy occurs.
● Warn patient never to discontinue drug or to change dosage without medical approval.
● Encourage patient to wear medical alert identification listing medication and seizure disorder while taking anticonvulsants.
● Inform patient to protect capsules from excessive heat, such as in a closed car or near a heat source.

Geriatric use
Use anticonvulsant drugs with caution. Elderly patients metabolize and excrete all drugs slowly and may obtain therapeutic effect from lower doses.

Pediatric use
Use with caution in children.

Breast-feeding
It is unknown whether succinimide anticonvulsants are excreted in breast milk; women should discontinue breast-feeding while taking these drugs.

---

tricyclic antidepressants

amitriptyline hydrochloride
amoxapine
clomipramine hydrochloride
desipramine hydrochloride
doxepin hydrochloride
imipramine hydrochloride
imipramine pamoate
maprotiline hydrochloride
nortriptyline hydrochloride
protriptyline hydrochloride
trimipramine maleate

The inherent mood-elevating activity of TCAs was discovered during research with iminodibenzyl, a compound originally investigated for sedative, analgesic, antihistaminic, and anti-parkinsonian effects. Clinical trials in 1958 with the class prototype, imipramine, found no antipsychotic activity, but clearly demonstrated marked mood-elevating effects.

Pharmacology
Although the precise mechanism of their CNS effects is not established, TCAs may exert their effects by inhibiting reuptake of the neurotransmitters norepinephrine and serotonin in CNS nerve terminals (presynaptic neurons), resulting in increased concentration and enhanced activity of neurotransmitters in the synaptic cleft. TCAs also have antihistaminic, sedative, anticholinergic, vasodilatory, and quinidine-like effects; the drugs are structurally similar to phenothiazines and share similar adverse reactions.

Individual TCAs differ somewhat in their degree of CNS inhibitory effect. The tertiary amines (amitriptyline, doxepin, imipramine, and trimipramine) exert greater sedative effects; tertiary amines and protriptyline have more profound effects on cardiac conduction, whereas desipramine has the least anticholinergic activity. All of the currently available TCAs have equal clinical efficacy when given in equivalent therapeutic doses; choice of specific therapy is determined primarily by pharmacokinetic properties and the patient's adverse reaction profile. Patients may respond to some TCAs and not others; if a patient does not respond to one drug, another should be tried.

Clinical indications and actions
Depression
TCAs are used to treat major depression. Depressed patients who are also anxious are helped most by the more sedating agents—doxepin, imipramine, and trimipramine. Protriptyline has a stimulant effect that evokes a favorable response in withdrawn depressed patients; only maprotiline has FDA approval for use in depression mixed with anxiety. Some studies suggest that amoxapine may have a more rapid onset of antidepressant effects, but this has not been substantiated.

Obsessive-compulsive disorder (OCD)
Clomipramine is used in the treatment of OCD.

Enuresis
Imipramine is used to treat enuresis in children over age 6.

Severe, chronic pain
TCAs, especially amitriptyline, desipramine, doxepin, imipramine, and nortriptyline, are useful in the management of severe chronic pain.

Overview of adverse reactions
Adverse reactions to TCAs are similar to those seen with phenothiazine antipsychotic agents, including varying degrees of sedation, anticholinergic effects, and orthostatic hypotension. The tertiary amines have the strongest sedative effects; tolerance to these effects usually develops in a few weeks. Protriptyline has the least sedative effect (and may be stimulatory), but shares with the tertiary amines the most pronounced effects on blood pressure and cardiac tissue. Maprotiline and amoxapine are most likely to cause seizures, especially in overdose situations. Desipramine has a greater margin of safety in patients with prostatic hypertrophy, paralytic ileus, glaucoma, and urine retention because of its relatively low level of anticholinergic activity.

▶ Special considerations
● TCAs impair ability to perform tasks requiring mental alertness, such as driving a car.
● Check vital signs regularly for decreased blood pressure or tachycardia; observe patient carefully for other adverse reactions and report changes. Check ECG in patients over age 40. Consider having patient take the first dose in the office to allow close observation for adverse reactions.
● Check for anticholinergic adverse reactions (urine retention or constipation), which may require dosage reduction.
● Caregiver should be sure patient swallows each dose of drug when given; as depressed

---

patients begin to improve, they may hoard pills for suicide attempt.

● Observe patients for mood changes to monitor progress; benefits may not be apparent for several (3 to 6) weeks.

● Do not withdraw full dose of drug abruptly; gradually reduce dosage over a period of weeks to avoid rebound effect or other adverse reactions.

● Carefully follow manufacturer's instructions for reconstitution, dilution, and storage of drugs.

● Investigational uses include treating peptic ulcer, migraine prophylaxis, and allergy. Potential toxicity has, to date, outweighed most advantages.

Information for the patient

● Explain rationale for therapy and anticipated risks and benefits; also explain that full therapeutic effect may not occur for several weeks.

● Teach signs and symptoms of adverse reactions and the importance of reporting any that occur.

● Tell patient to avoid beverages and drugs containing alcohol and not to take any other drug (including OTC products) without medical approval.

● Teach patient how and when to take drug, not to increase dosage without medical approval, and never to discontinue drug abruptly.

● Advise patient to lie down for 30 minutes after first dose and to rise slowly to prevent orthostatic hypotension.

● Advise taking drug with milk or food to minimize GI distress; suggest taking full dose at bedtime if daytime sedation is troublesome.

● Urge diabetic patients to monitor blood sugar, as drug may alter insulin needs.

● Advise patient to avoid tasks that require mental alertness until full effect of drug is determined.

● Warn patient that excessive exposure to sunlight, heat lamps, or tanning beds may cause burn and abnormal hyperpigmentation.

● Recommend sugarless gum or hard candy, artificial saliva, or ice chips to relieve dry mouth.

● Advise patient that unpleasant adverse reactions (except dry mouth) generally diminish over time.

Geriatric use

Lower doses are indicated in geriatric patients, because they are more sensitive to both therapeutic and adverse effects of TCAs. Recommended starting dosage is 25 mg P.O. t.i.d.

Pediatric use

TCAs are not recommended for children under age 12.

Breast-feeding

Safety in breast-feeding has not been established.

Selected references

American Hospital Formulary Service (AHFS) Drug Information. Bethesda, Md.: American Society of Hospital Pharmacists, 1991.

Bleck, T.P., and Klawans, H.L. "Convulsive Disorders: Mechanisms of Epilepsy and Anticonvulsant Action," Clinical Neuropharmacology 13(2):121-28, April 1990.

Brodie, M.J. "Established Anticonvulsants and Treatment of Refractory Epilepsy," Lancet 336(8711):350-54, August 11, 1990.

Bryant, S.G., et al. "Long-term vs. Short-term Amitriptyline Side Effects as Measured by a Postmarketing Surveillance System," Journal of Clinical Psychopharmacology 7(2):78-82, April 1987.

Campanella, G., et al. "Drugs Affecting Movement Disorders" Annual Review of Pharmacology and Toxicology 276:113-36, 1987.

Carpenter, W.T., Jr., et al. "A Comparative Trial of Pharmacologic Strategies in Schizophrenia," American Journal of Psychiatry 144(11):1466-70, November 1987.

Chan, C.H., et al. "Response of Psychotic and Nonpsychotic Depressed Patients to Tricyclic Antidepressants," Journal of Clinical Psychiatry 48(5):197-200, May 1987.

Drug Information for the Health Care Professional. Rockville, Md.: United States Pharmacopeial Convention, Inc., 1991.

Dubin, W.R., and Feld, J.A. "Tranquilization of the Violent Patient," American Journal of Emergency Medicine 7(3):313-20, May 1989.

Dubin, W.R., et al. "Pharmacotherapy of Psychiatric Emergencies," Journal of Clinical Psychopharmacology 6(4):210-22, August 1986.

Facts and Comparisons. St. Louis: J.B. Lippincott Co., Facts and Comparisons Division, 1991.

Gilman, A., et al., eds. Goodman and Gillman's The Pharmacological Basis of Therapeutics, 8th ed. New York: Pergamon Press, 1990.

Goa, K.L., and Ward, A. "Buspirone: A Preliminary Review of its Pharmacological Properties and Therapeutic Efficacy as an Anxiolytic," Drugs 32(2):114-29, August 1986.

Lader, M. "Rational Use of Anxiolytic Drugs," Rational Drug Therapy 21(9):1-5, September 1987.

Mikati, M.A., and Browne, T.R. "Comparative Efficacy of Antiepileptic Drugs," Clinical Neuropharmacology 11(2):130-40, April 1988.

Physician's 1991 Drug Handbook. Springhouse, Pa.: Springhouse Corp., 1991.

Shorvon, S.D. "Medical Assessment and Treatment of Chronic Epilepsy," British Medical Journal 302(6773):363-66, February 16, 1991.

Theodore, W.H., et al. "Carbamazepine and its Epoxide: Relation of Plasma Levels to Toxicity and Seizure Control," Annals of Neurology 25(2):194-96, February 1989.

Yaari, Y., et al. "Phenytoin: Mechanisms of its Anticonvulsant Action," Annals of Neurology 20(2):171-84, August 1986.

Appendices and Index

DSM-III-R DIAGNOSES AND *ICD-9-CM* CODES: DIAGNOSIS LIST

V62.30	Academic problem
	Adjustment disorder
309.24	with anxious mood
309.00	with depressed mood
309.30	with disturbance of conduct
309.40	with mixed disturbance of emotions and conduct
309.28	with mixed emotional features
309.82	with physical complaints
309.83	with withdrawal
309.23	with work (or academic) inhibition
309.90	Adjustment disorder NOS
V71.01	Adult antisocial behavior
300.22	Agoraphobia without history of panic disorder
	Alcohol
305.00	abuse
291.10	amnestic disorder
303.90	dependence
291.30	hallucinosis
291.40	idiosyncratic intoxication
303.00	intoxication
291.00	withdrawal delirium
294.00	Amnestic disorder (etiology noted on Axis III or is unknown)
	Amphetamine or similarly acting sympathomimetic
305.70	abuse
292.81	delirium
292.11	delusional disorder
304.40	dependence
305.70	intoxication
292.00	withdrawal
307.10	Anorexia nervosa
301.70	Antisocial personality disorder
300.00	Anxiety disorder NOS
314.01	Attention-deficit hyperactivity disorder
299.00	Autistic disorder
313.21	Avoidant disorder of childhood or adolescence
301.82	Avoidant personality disorder
	Bipolar disorder, depressed
296.56	in full remission
296.51	mild
296.52	moderate
296.55	in partial remission
296.54	with psychotic features
296.53	severe, without psychotic features
296.50	unspecified
	Bipolar disorder, manic
296.46	in full remission
296.41	mild
296.42	moderate
296.45	in partial remission
296.44	with psychotic features
296.43	severe, without psychotic features
296.40	unspecified
	Bipolar disorder, mixed
296.66	in full remission
296.61	mild
296.62	moderate
296.65	in partial remission

(continued)

NOS = not otherwise specified

***DSM-III-R* DIAGNOSES AND *ICD-9-CM* CODES: DIAGNOSIS LIST** *(continued)*

	Bipolar disorder, mixed *(continued)*
296.64	with psychotic features
296.63	severe, without psychotic features
296.60	unspecified
296.70	Bipolar disorder NOS
300.70	Body dysmorphic disorder
V40.00	Borderline intellectual functioning
301.83	Borderline personality disorder
298.80	Brief reactive psychosis
307.51	Bulimia nervosa
305.90	Caffeine intoxication
	Cannabis
305.20	abuse
292.11	delusional disorder
304.30	dependence
305.20	intoxication
V71.02	Childhood or adolescent antisocial behavior
307.22	Chronic motor or vocal tic disorder
307.00	Cluttering
	Cocaine
305.60	abuse
292.81	delirium
292.11	delusional disorder
304.20	dependence
305.60	intoxication
292.00	withdrawal
	Conduct disorder
312.20	group type
312.00	solitary aggressive type
312.90	undifferentiated type
300.11	Conversion disorder
301.13	Cyclothymia
293.00	Delirium (etiology noted on Axis III or is unknown)
297.10	Delusional disorder
294.10	Dementia (etiology noted on Axis III or is unknown)
291.20	Dementia associated with alcoholism
301.60	Dependent personality disorder
300.60	Depersonalization disorder
311.00	Depressive disorder NOS
	Developmental
315.10	arithmetic disorder
315.39	articulation disorder
315.40	coordination disorder
315.90	disorder NOS
315.31	expressive language disorder
315.80	expressive writing disorder
315.00	reading disorder
315.31	receptive language disorder
799.90	Diagnosis or condition deferred on Axis I
799.90	Diagnosis or condition deferred on Axis II
300.15	Dissociative disorder NOS
307.47	Dream anxiety disorder (Nightmare disorder)
302.76	Dyspareunia
307.40	Dyssomnia NOS
300.40	Dysthymia
307.50	Eating disorder NOS
313.23	Elective mutism
302.40	Exhibitionism

NOS = not otherwise specified

DSM-III-R DIAGNOSES AND ICD-9-CM CODES: DIAGNOSIS LIST (continued)

	Factitious disorder
	Factitious disorder
301.51	with physical symptoms
300.16	with psychological symptoms
300.19	Factitious disorder NOS
302.72	Female sexual arousal disorder
302.81	Fetishism
302.89	Frotteurism
307.70	Functional encopresis
307.60	Functional enuresis
	Gender identity disorder
302.85	of adolescence or adulthood, nontranssexual type
302.60	of childhood
302.85	NOS
300.02	Generalized anxiety disorder
	Hallucinogen
305.30	abuse
292.11	delusional disorder
304.50	dependence
305.30	hallucinosis
292.84	mood disorder
301.50	Histrionic personality disorder
780.50	Hypersomnia related to a known organic factor
307.44	Hypersomnia related to another mental disorder (nonorganic)
302.71	Hypoactive sexual desire disorder
300.70	Hypochondriasis
313.82	Identity disorder
312.39	Impulse control disorder NOS
297.30	Induced psychotic disorder
	Inhalant
305.90	abuse
304.60	dependence
305.90	intoxication
302.73	Inhibited female orgasm
302.74	Inhibited male orgasm
780.50	Insomnia related to a known organic factor
307.42	Insomnia related to another mental disorder (nonorganic)
312.34	Intermittent explosive disorder
312.32	Kleptomania
307.90	Late luteal phase dysphoric disorder
	Major depression, recurrent
296.36	in full remission
296.31	mild
296.32	moderate
296.35	in partial remission
296.34	with psychotic features
296.33	severe, without psychotic features
296.30	unspecified
	Major depression, single episode
296.26	in full remission
296.21	mild
296.22	moderate
296.25	in partial remission
296.24	with psychotic features
296.23	severe, without psychotic features
296.20	unspecified
302.72	Male erectile disorder
V65.20	Malingering

(continued)

NOS = not otherwise specified

DSM-III-R DIAGNOSES AND *ICD-9-CM* CODES: DIAGNOSIS LIST *(continued)*

V61.10	Marital problem
317.00	Mild mental retardation
318.00	Moderate mental retardation
	Multi-infarct dementia
290.41	with delirium
290.42	with delusions
290.43	with depression
290.40	uncomplicated
300.14	Multiple personality disorder
301.81	Narcissistic personality disorder
	Nicotine
305.10	dependence
292.00	withdrawal
V71.09	No diagnosis or condition on Axls I
V71.09	No diagnosis or condition on Axis II
V15.81	Noncompliance with medical treatment
300.30	Obsessive-compulsive disorder
301.40	Obsessive-compulsive personality disorder
V62.20	Occupational problem
	Opioid
305.50	abuse
304.00	dependence
305.50	intoxication
292.00	withdrawal
313.81	Oppositional defiant disorder
294.80	Organic anxiety disorder (etiology noted on Axis III or is unknown)
293.81	Organic delusional disorder (etiology noted on Axis III or is unknown)
293.82	Organic hallucinosis (etiology noted on Axis III or is unknown)
294.80	Organic mental disorder NOS (etiology noted on Axis III or is unknown)
293.83	Organic mood disorder (etiology noted on Axis III or is unknown)
310.10	Organic personality disorder (etiology noted on Axis III or is unknown)
	Other or unspecified psychoactive substance
292.83	amnestic disorder
292.89	anxiety disorder
292.81	delirium
292.11	delusional disorder
292.82	dementia
292.12	hallucinosis
305.90	intoxication
292.84	mood disorder
292.90	organic mental disorder NOS
292.89	personality disorder
292.00	withdrawal
V62.81	Other interpersonal problem
V61.80	Other specified family circumstances
313.00	Overanxious disorder
	Panic disorder
300.21	with agoraphobia
300.01	without agoraphobia
301.00	Paranoid personality disorder
302.90	Paraphilia NOS
307.40	Parasomnia NOS
V61.20	Parent-child problem
301.84	Passive-aggressive personality disorder
312.31	Pathological gambling
302.20	Pedophilia
301.90	Personality disorder NOS
299.80	Pervasive developmental disorder NOS

NOS = not otherwise specified

DSM-III-R DIAGNOSES AND *ICD-9-CM* CODES: DIAGNOSIS LIST *(continued)*

V62.89	Phase of life problem or other life circumstance problem
	Phencyclidine (PCP) or similarly acting arylcyclohexylamine
305.90	abuse
292.81	delirium
292.11	delusional disorder
304.50	dependence
305.90	intoxication
292.84	mood disorder
292.90	organic mental disorder NOS
307.52	Pica
305.90	Polysubstance abuse
304.90	Polysubstance dependence
292.89	Posthallucinogen perception disorder
309.89	Post-traumatic stress disorder
302.75	Premature ejaculation
290.10	Presenile dementia NOS
	Primary degenerative dementia of the Alzheimer type
290.11	presenile onset, with delirium
290.12	presenile onset, with delusions
290.13	presenile onset, with depression
290.10	presenile onset, uncomplicated
	Primary degenerative dementia of the Alzheimer type
290.30	senile onset, with delirium
290.20	senile onset, with delusions
290.21	senile onset, with depression
290.00	senile onset, uncomplicated
780.54	Primary hypersomnia
307.42	Primary insomnia
318.20	Profound mental retardation
305.90	Psychoactive substance abuse NOS
304.90	Psychoactive substance dependence NOS
300.12	Psychogenic amnesia
300.13	Psychogenic fugue
316.00	Psychological factors affecting physical condition
298.90	Psychotic disorder NOS
312.33	Pyromania
313.89	Reactive attachment disorder of infancy or early childhood
307.53	Rumination disorder of infancy
295.70	Schizoaffective disorder
301.20	Schizoid personality disorder
	Schizophrenia, catatonic type
295.22	chronic
295.24	chronic with acute exacerbation
295.25	in remisslon
295.21	subchronic
295.23	subchronic with acute exacerbation
295.20	unspecified
	Schizophrenia, disorganized type
295.12	chronic
295.14	chronic with acute exacerbation
295.15	in remission
295.11	subchronic
295.13	subchronic with acute exacerbation
295.10	unspecified
	Schizophrenia, paranoid type
295.32	chronic
295.34	chronic with acute exacerbatlon

(continued)

NOS = not otherwise specified

DSM-III-R DIAGNOSES AND *ICD-9-CM* CODES: DIAGNOSIS LIST *(continued)*

	Schizophrenia, paranoid type *(continued)*
295.35	in remission
295.31	subchronic
295.33	subchronic with acute exacerbation
295.30	unspecified
	Schizophrenia, residual type
295.62	chronic
295.61	subchronic
295.60	unspecified
	Schizophrenia, undifferentiated type
295.92	chronic
295.94	chronic with acute exacerbation
295.95	in remission
295.91	subchronic
295.93	subchronic with acute exacerbation
295.90	unspecified
295.40	Schizophreniform disorder
301.22	Schizotypal personality disorder
	Sedative, hypnotic, or anxiolytic
305.40	abuse
292.83	amnestic disorder
304.10	dependence
305.40	intoxication
292.00	withdrawal delirium
290.00	Senile dementia NOS
309.21	Separation anxiety disorder
318.10	Severe mental retardation
302.79	Sexual aversion disorder
302.90	Sexual disorder NOS
302.70	Sexual dysfunction NOS
302.83	Sexual masochism
302.84	Sexual sadism
300.29	Simple phobia
307.46	Sleep terror disorder
307.45	Sleep-wake schedule disorder
307.46	Sleepwalking disorder
300.23	Social phobia
300.81	Somatization disorder
300.70	Somatoform disorder NOS
307.80	Somatoform pain disorder
315.90	Specific developmental disorder NOS
307.30	Stereotypy/habit disorder
307.00	Stuttering
307.20	Tic disorder NOS
307.23	Tourette's disorder
307.21	Transient tic disorder
302.50	Transsexualism
302.30	Transvestic fetishism
312.39	Trichotillomania
291.80	Uncomplicated alcohol withdrawal
V62.82	Uncomplicated bereavement
292.00	Uncomplicated sedative, hypnotic, or anxiolytic withdrawal
314.00	Undifferentiated attention-deficit disorder
300.70	Undifferentiated somatoform disorder
300.90	Unspecified mental disorder (nonpsychotic)
319.00	Unspecified mental retardation
306.51	Vaginismus
302.82	Voyeurism

NOS = not otherwise specified

DSM-III-R DIAGNOSES AND *ICD-9-CM* CODES: NUMERIC LIST

To maintain compatibility with *ICD-9-CM*, some *DSM-III-R* diagnoses share the same code numbers. In this list, such groups of diagnoses are separated by rules.

290.00	Primary degenerative dementia of the Alzheimer type, senile onset, uncomplicated
290.00	Senile dementia NOS
290.10	Presenile dementia NOS
290.10	Primary degenerative dementia of the Alzheimer type, presenile onset, uncomplicated
290.11	Primary degenerative dementia of the Alzheimer type, presenile onset, with delirium
290.12	Primary degenerative dementia of the Alzheimer type, presenile onset, with delusions
290.13	Primary degenerative dementia of the Alzheimer type, presenile onset, with depression
290.20	Primary degenerative dementia of the Alzheimer type, senile onset, with delusions
290.21	Primary degenerative dementia of the Alzheimer type, senile onset, with depression
290.30	Primary degenerative dementia of the Alzheimer type, senile onset, with delirium
290.40	Multi-infarct dementia, uncomplicated
290.41	Mutli-infarct dementia, with delirium
290.42	Mutli-infarct dementia, with delusions
290.43	Mutli-infarct dementia, with depression
291.00	Alcohol withdrawal delirium
291.10	Alcohol amnestic disorder
291.20	Dementia associated with alcoholism
291.30	Alcohol hallucinosis
291.40	Alcohol idiosyncratic intoxication
291.80	Uncomplicated alcohol withdrawal
292.00	Amphetamine or similarly acting sympathomimetic withdrawal
292.00	Cocaine withdrawal
292.00	Nicotine withdrawal
292.00	Opioid withdrawal
292.00	Other or unspecified psychoactive substance withdrawal
292.00	Sedative, hypnotic, or anxiolytic withdrawal delirium
292.00	Uncomplicated sedative, hypnotic, or anxiolytic withdrawal
292.11	Amphetamine or similarly acting sympathomimetic delusional disorder
292.11	Cannabis delusional disorder
292.11	Cocaine delusional disorder
292.11	Hallucinogen delusional disorder
292.11	Other or unspecified psychoactive substance delusional disorder
292.11	Phencyclidine (PCP) or similarly acting arylcyclohexylamine delusional disorder
292.12	Other or unspecified psychoactive substance hallucinosis
292.81	Amphetamine or similarly acting sympathomimetic delirium
292.81	Cocaine delirium
292.81	Other or unspecified psychoactive substance delirium
292.81	Phencyclidine (PCP) or similarly acting arylcyclohexylamine delirium
292.82	Other or unspecified psychoactive substance dementia
292.83	Other or unspecified psychoactive substance amnestic disorder
292.83	Sedative, hypnotic, or anxiolytic amnestic disorder
292.84	Hallucinogen mood disorder
292.84	Other or unspecified psychoactive substance mood disorder
292.84	Phencyclidine (PCP) or similarly acting arylcyclohexylamine mood disorder

(continued)

DSM-III-R DIAGNOSES AND ICD-9-CM CODES: NUMERIC LIST *(continued)*

292.89	Other or unspecified psychoactive substance anxiety disorder
292.89	Other or unspecified psychoactive substance personality disorder
292.89	Posthallucinogen perception disorder

292.90	Other or unspecified psychoactive substance organic mental disorder NOS
292.90	Phencyclidine (PCP) or similarly acting arylcyclohexylamine organic mental disorder NOS

293.00	Delirium (etiology noted on Axis III or is unknown)
293.81	Organic delusional disorder (etiology noted on Axis III or is unknown)
293.82	Organic hallucinosis (etiology noted on Axis III or is unknown)
293.83	Organic mood disorder (etiology noted on Axis III or is unknown)
294.00	Amnestic disorder (etiology noted on Axis III or is unknown)
294.10	Dementia (etiology noted on Axis III or is unknown)

294.80	Organic anxiety disorder (etiology noted on Axis III or is unknown)
294.80	Organic mental disorder NOS (etiology noted on Axis III or is unknown)

295.10	Schizophrenia, disorganized type, unspecified
295.11	Schizophrenia, disorganized type, subchronic
295.12	Schizophrenia, disorganized type, chronic
295.13	Schizophrenia, disorganized type, subchronic with acute exacerbation
295.14	Schizophrenia, disorganized type, chronic with acute exacerbation
295.15	Schizophrenia, disorganized type, in remission
295.20	Schizophrenia, catatonic type, unspecified
295.21	Schizophrenia, catatonic type, subchronic
295.22	Schizophrenia, catatonic type, chronic
295.23	Schizophrenia, catatonic type, subchronic with acute exacerbation
295.24	Schizophrenia, catatonic type, chronic, with acute exacerbation
295.25	Schizophrenia, catatonic type, in remission
295.30	Schizophrenia, paranoid type, unspecified
295.31	Schizophrenia, paranoid type, subchronic
295.32	Schizophrenia, paranoid type, chronic
295.33	Schizophrenia, paranoid type, subchronic with acute exacerbation
295.34	Schizophrenia, paranoid type, chronic with acute exacerbation
295.35	Schizophrenia, paranoid type, in remission
295.40	Schizophreniform disorder
295.60	Schizophrenia, residual type, unspecified
295.61	Schizophrenia, residual type, subchronic
295.62	Schizophrenia, residual type, chronic
295.70	Schizoaffective disorder
295.90	Schizophrenia, undifferentiated type, unspecified
295.91	Schizophrenia, undifferentiated type, subchronic
295.92	Schizophrenia, undifferentiated type, chronic
295.93	Schizophrenia, undifferentiated type, subchronic with acute exacerbation
295.94	Schizophrenia, undifferentiated type, chronic with acute exacerbation
295.95	Schizophrenia, undifferentiated type, in remission
296.20	Major depression, single episode, unspecified
296.21	Major depression, single episode, mild
296.22	Major depression, single episode, moderate
296.23	Major depression, single episode, severe, without psychotic features
296.24	Major depression, single episode, with psychotic features
296.25	Major depression, single episode, in partial remission
296.26	Major depression, single episode, in full remission
296.30	Major depression, recurrent, unspecified
296.31	Major depression, recurrent, mild
296.32	Major depression, recurrent, moderate
296.33	Major depression, recurrent, severe, without psychotic features
296.34	Major depression, recurrent, with psychotic features
296.35	Major depression, recurrent, in partial remission

NOS = not otherwise specified

DSM-III-R DIAGNOSES AND ICD-9-CM CODES: NUMERIC LIST (continued)

296.36	Major depression, recurrent, in full remission
296.40	Bipolar disorder, manic, unspecified
296.41	Bipolar disorder, manic, mild
296.42	Bipolar disorder, manic, moderate
296.43	Bipolar disorder, manic, severe, without psychotic features
296.44	Bipolar disorder, manic, with psychotic features
296.45	Bipolar disorder, manic, in partial remission
296.46	Bipolar disorder, manic, in full remission
296.50	Bipolar disorder, depressed, unspecified
296.51	Bipolar disorder, depressed, mild
296.52	Bipolar disorder, depressed, moderate
296.53	Bipolar disorder, depressed, severe, without psychotic features
296.54	Bipolar disorder, depressed, with psychotic features
296.55	Bipolar disorder, depressed, in partial remission
296.56	Bipolar disorder, depressed, in full remission
296.60	Bipolar disorder, mixed, unspecified
296.61	Bipolar disorder, mixed, mild
296.62	Bipolar disorder, mixed, moderate
296.63	Bipolar disorder, mixed, severe, without psychotic features
296.64	Bipolar disorder, mixed, with psychotic features
296.65	Bipolar disorder, mixed, in partial remission
296.66	Bipolar disorder, mixed, in full remission
296.70	Bipolar disorder NOS
297.10	Delusional disorder
297.30	Induced psychotic disorder
298.80	Brief reactive psychosis
298.90	Psychotic disorder NOS
299.00	Autistic disorder
299.80	Pervasive developmental disorder NOS
300.00	Anxiety disorder NOS
300.01	Panic disorder without agoraphobia
300.02	Generalized anxiety disorder
300.11	Conversion disorder
300.12	Psychogenic amnesia
300.13	Psychogenic fugue
300.14	Multiple personality disorder
300.15	Dissociative disorder NOS
300.16	Factitious disorder with psychological symptoms
300.19	Factitious disorder NOS
300.21	Panic disorder with agoraphobia
300.22	Agoraphobia without history of panic disorder
300.23	Social phobia
300.29	Simple phobia
300.30	Obsessive-compulsive disorder
300.40	Dysthymia
300.60	Depersonalization disorder
300.70	Body dysmorphic disorder
300.70	Hypochondriasis
300.70	Somatoform disorder NOS
300.70	Undifferentiated somatoform disorder
300.81	Somatization disorder
300.90	Unspecified mental disorder (nonpsychotic)
301.00	Paranoid personality disorder
301.13	Cyclothymia
301.20	Schizoid personality disorder
301.22	Schizotypal personality disorder

(continued)

NOS = not otherwise specified

DSM-III-R DIAGNOSES AND *ICD-9-CM* CODES: NUMERIC LIST *(continued)*

301.40	Obsessive-compulsive personality disorder
301.50	Histrionic personality disorder
301.51	Factitious disorder with physical symptoms
301.60	Dependent personality disorder
301.70	Antisocial personality disorder
301.81	Narcissistic personality disorder
301.82	Avoidant personality disorder
301.83	Borderline personality disorder
301.84	Passive-aggressive personality disorder
301.90	Personality disorder NOS
302.20	Pedophilia
302.30	Transvestic fetishism
302.40	Exhibitionism
302.50	Transsexualism
302.60	Gender identity disorder of childhood
302.70	Sexual dysfunction NOS
302.71	Hypoactive sexual desire disorder

302.72	Female sexual arousal disorder
302.72	Male erectile disorder

302.73	Inhibited female orgasm
302.74	Inhibited male orgasm
302.75	Premature ejaculation
302.76	Dyspareunia
302.79	Sexual aversion disorder
302.81	Fetishism
302.82	Voyeurism
302.83	Sexual masochism
302.84	Sexual sadism

302.85	Gender identity disorder NOS
302.85	Gender identity disorder of adolescence or adulthood, nontranssexual type

302.89	Frotteurism

302.90	Sexual disorder NOS
302.90	Paraphilia NOS

303.00	Alcohol intoxication
303.90	Alcohol dependence
304.00	Opioid dependence
304.10	Sedative, hypnotic, or anxiolytic dependence
304.20	Cocaine dependence
304.30	Cannabis dependence
304.40	Amphetamine or similarly acting sympathomimetic dependence

304.50	Hallucinogen dependence
304.50	Phencyclidine (PCP) or similarly acting arylcyclohexylamine dependence

304.60	Inhalant dependence

304.90	Polysubstance dependence
304.90	Psychoactive substance dependence NOS

305.00	Alcohol abuse
305.10	Nicotine dependence

305.20	Cannabis abuse
305.20	Cannabis intoxication

NOS = not otherwise specified

DSM-III-R DIAGNOSES AND *ICD-9-CM* CODES: NUMERIC LIST *(continued)*

305.30	Hallucinogen abuse
305.30	Hallucinogen hallucinosis
305.40	Sedative, hypnotic, or anxiolytic abuse
305.40	Sedative, hypnotlc, or anxiolytic intoxication
305.50	Opioid abuse
305.50	Opioid intoxication
305.60	Cocaine abuse
305.60	Cocaine intoxication
305.70	Amphetamine or similarly acting sympathomimetic abuse
305.70	Amphetamine or similarly acting sympathomimetic intoxication
305.90	Caffeine intoxication
305.90	Inhalant abuse
305.90	Inhalant intoxication
305.90	Other or unspecified psychoactive substance intoxication
305.90	Phencyclidine (PCP) or similarly acting arylcyclohexylamine abuse
305.90	Phencyclidine (PCP) or similarly acting arylcyclohexylamine intoxication
305.90	Polysubstance abuse
305.90	Psychoactive substance abuse NOS
306.51	Vaginismus
307.00	Cluttering
307.00	Stuttering
307.10	Anorexia nervosa
307.20	Tic disorder NOS
307.21	Transient tic disorder
307.22	Chronic motor or vocal tic disorder
307.23	Tourette's disorder
307.30	Stereotypy/habit disorder
307.40	Dyssomnia NOS
307.40	Parasomnia NOS
307.42	Insomnia related to another mental disorder (nonorganic)
307.42	Primary insomnia
307.44	Hypersomnia related to another mental disorder (nonorganic)
307.45	Sleep-wake schedule disorder
307.46	Sleep terror disorder
307.46	Sleepwalking disorder
307.47	Dream anxiety disorder (Nightmare disorder)
307.50	Eating disorder NOS
307.51	Bulimia nervosa
307.52	Pica
307.53	Rumination disorder of infancy
307.60	Functional enuresis
307.70	Functional encopresis
307.80	Somatoform pain disorder
307.90	Late luteal phase dysphoric disorder
309.00	Adjustment disorder with depressed mood
309.21	Separation anxiety disorder

(continued)

NOS = not otherwise specified

DSM-III-R DIAGNOSES AND ICD-9-CM CODES: NUMERIC LIST *(continued)*

309.23	Adjustment disorder with work (or academic) inhibition
309.24	Adjustment disorder with anxious mood
309.28	Adjustment disorder with mixed emotional features
309.30	Adjustment disorder with disturbance of conduct
309.40	Adjustment disorder with mixed disturbance of emotions and conduct
309.82	Adjustment disorder with physical complaints
309.83	Adjustment disorder with withdrawal
309.89	Post-traumatic stress disorder
309.90	Adjustment disorder NOS
310.10	Organic personality disorder (etiology noted on Axis III or is unknown)
311.00	Depressive disorder NOS
312.00	Conduct disorder, solitary aggressive type
312.20	Conduct disorder, group type
312.31	Pathological gambling
312.32	Kleptomania
312.33	Pyromania
312.34	Intermittent explosive disorder
312.39	Impulse control disorder NOS
312.39	Trichotillomania
312.90	Conduct disorder, undifferentiated type
313.00	Overanxious disorder
313.21	Avoidant disorder of childhood or adolescence
313.23	Elective mutism
313.81	Oppositional defiant disorder
313.82	Identity disorder
313.89	Reactive attachment disorder of infancy or early childhood
314.00	Undifferentiated attention-deficit disorder
314.01	Attention-deficit hyperactivity disorder
315.00	Developmental reading disorder
315.10	Developmental arithmetic disorder
315.31	Developmental expressive language disorder
315.31	Developmental receptive language disorder
315.39	Developmental articulation disorder
315.40	Developmental coordination disorder
315.80	Developmental expressive writing disorder
315.90	Developmental disorder NOS
315.90	Specific developmental disorder NOS
316.00	Psychological factors affecting physical condition
317.00	Mild mental retardation
318.00	Moderate mental retardation
318.10	Severe mental retardation
318.20	Profound mental retardation
319.00	Unspecified mental retardation
780.50	Hypersomnia related to a known organic factor
780.50	Insomnia related to a known organic factor
780.54	Primary hypersomnia
799.90	Diagnosis or condition deferred on Axis I
799.90	Diagnosis or condition deferred on Axis II

NOS = not otherwise specified

DSM-III-R DIAGNOSES AND *ICD-9-CM* CODES: NUMERIC LIST *(continued)*

V15.81	Noncompliance with medical treatment
V40.00	Borderline intellectual functioning
V61.10	Marital problem
V61.20	Parent-child problem
V61.80	Other specified family circumstances
V62.20	Occupational problem
V62.30	Academic problem
V62.81	Other interpersonal problem
V62.82	Uncomplicated bereavement
V62.89	Phase of life problem or other life circumstance problem
V65.20	Malingering
V71.01	Adult antisocial behavior
V71.02	Childhood or adolescent antisocial behavior
V71.09	No diagnosis or condition on Axis I
V71.09	No diagnosis or condition on Axis II

NOS = not otherwise specified

RECOMMENDED LABORATORY TESTS IN CHRONIC DRUG THERAPY

Long-term use of drugs can cause physiologic abnormalities best detected by laboratory tests. This chart lists recommended laboratory tests during therapy with drugs listed in this volume. The drugs are grouped below, as in preceding chapters, according to primary therapeutic use.

DRUG	LABORATORY TESTS	RATIONALE	SPECIAL CONSIDERATIONS
Anticonvulsants			
acetazolamide	CBC, platelet count	To detect aplastic anemia	Perform at least every 3 months.
	Urine calcium	To detect hypercalcuria	Perform before initiating therapy; avoid renal calculi formation in predisposed patients.
	Serum electrolytes (Na, K)	To detect excess electrolyte loss	Especially important in patients receiving digitalis glycosides.
	Serum uric acid	To detect hyperuricemia	Levels return to pretreatment values when drug is discontinued.
carbamazepine	CBC, platelet count	To detect aplastic anemia or agranulocytosis	Establish baseline and monitor routinely; incidence of aplastic anemia is low. Transient decreases in platelet and leukocyte counts are common and usually don't signal impending problem.
	Liver function tests	To detect hepatotoxicity	Establish baseline and repeat periodically. Hepatotoxicity may occur after prolonged use.
	Urinalysis, BUN	To detect nephrotoxicity	Establish baseline and repeat periodically.
	Ophthalmologic examinations (fundoscopy, slit-lamp, and tonometry)	To detect adverse ophthalmologic effects, including glaucoma	Drug has mild anticholinergic effects and may elevate intraocular pressure.
clonazepam	Liver function tests	To detect hepatotoxicity	Transient elevations of serum aminotransferase and alkaline phosphatase may occur.
	Ophthalmologic tests	To detect glaucoma	Contraindicated in acute angle-closure glaucoma; establish baseline screening to identify undiagnosed glaucoma.
	Renal function tests	To detect nephrotoxicity	Renal problems are relatively rare with prolonged use.
	Blood counts	To detect blood dyscrasias	A few cases of leukopenia and aplastic anemia reported with other benzodiazepines.
clorazepate	CBC, platelet count	To detect blood dyscrasias	Relatively rare; establish baseline and repeat periodically.
	Liver function tests	To detect hepatotoxicity	Establish baseline and repeat periodically; elevated AST (SGOT), ALT (SGPT), lactate dehydrogenase, and total and direct bilirubin has occurred with benzodiazepines.

RECOMMENDED LABORATORY TESTS IN CHRONIC DRUG THERAPY *(continued)*

DRUG	LABORATORY TESTS	RATIONALE	SPECIAL CONSIDERATIONS
Anticonvulsants			
clorazepate *(continued)*	Kidney function tests	To detect nephrotoxicity	Establish baseline and repeat periodically.
ethosuximide	CBC, platelet count	To detect blood dyscrasias	May produce direct positive Coomb's test or systemic lupus erythematosus.
	Urinalysis	To detect nephrotoxicity	Establish baseline and repeat periodically.
	Liver function tests	To detect hepatotoxicity	Establish baseline and repeat periodically. Hepatotoxicity may occur after prolonged use.
ethotoin	CBC, platelet count	To detect blood dyscrasias	Reversible lymphadenopathy has been reported.
	Liver function tests	To detect hepatotoxicity	Establish baseline and repeat periodically. Hepatotoxicity may occur after prolonged use.
mephenytoin	CBC, platelet count	To detect blood dyscrasias	Higher incidence than some other anticonvulsants; establish baseline, repeat after 2 weeks of initial therapy, then after 2 weeks of maintainance. Repeat monthly for first year then at 3-month intervals.
	Liver function tests	To detect hepatotoxicity	Establish baseline and repeat periodically. Hepatotoxicity may occur after prolonged use.
mephobarbital	CBC, platelet count	To detect blood dyscrasias	Establish baseline and repeat periodically.
methsuximide	CBC, platelet count	To detect blood dyscrasias	Establish baseline and repeat periodically.
	Liver function tests	To detect hepatotoxicity	Establish baseline and repeat periodically. Hepatotoxicity may occur after prolonged use.
	Urinalysis	To detect nephrotoxicity	Establish baseline and repeat periodically.
paraldehyde	Liver function tests	To detect hepatotoxicity	Establish baseline and repeat periodically. Toxic hepatitis reported after chronic use.
	Renal function tests	To detect nephrotoxicity	Nephrosis reported after chronic use.
paramethadione	CBC, platelet count	To detect blood dyscrasias	Higher incidence of blood dyscrasias than some other anticonvulsants; establish baseline and repeat monthly for the first year.

(continued)

RECOMMENDED LABORATORY TESTS IN CHRONIC DRUG THERAPY (continued)

DRUG	LABORATORY TESTS	RATIONALE	SPECIAL CONSIDERATIONS
Anticonvulsants			
paramethadione (continued)	Urinalysis	To detect nephrotoxicity	Establish baseline and repeat monthly for the first year.
	Liver function tests	To detect hepatotoxicity	Establish baseline and repeat monthly for the first year.
phenacemide	CBC, platelet count	To detect blood dyscrasias	Establish baseline then repeat monthly for first year; reduce frequency if no problems detected after 1 year.
	Urinalysis	To detect nephrotoxicity	Establish baseline and repeat periodically.
	Liver function tests	To detect hepatotoxicity	Establish baseline and repeat monthly.
phenobarbital	CBC, platelet count	To detect blood dyscrasias	Establish baseline and repeat periodically.
phensuximide	CBC, platelet count	To detect blood dyscrasias	Establish baseline and repeat periodically.
	Urinalysis	To detect nephrotoxicity	Establish baseline and repeat periodically.
	Liver function tests	To detect hepatotoxicity	Establish baseline and repeat periodically. Hepatotoxicity may occur after prolonged use.
phenytoin	CBC, platelet count	To detect blood dyscrasias	Macrocytosis and megaloblastic anemia may respond to folic acid therapy. May be associated with lymphoma.
	Liver function tests	To detect hepatotoxicity	Establish baseline and repeat periodically. Hepatotoxicity may occur after prolonged use.
	Renal function studies	To prevent toxicity	Higher incidence of glycosuria and hyperglycemia in patients with renal impairment.
primidone	CBC, platelet count	To detect blood dyscrasias	Establish CBC and SMA 12 every 6 months.
	Liver function tests	To detect hepatotoxocity	Establish baseline and repeat periodically. Hepatotoxicity may occur after prolonged use.
trimethadione	CBC, platelet count	To detect blood dyscrasias	Higher incidence than some other anticonvulsants; establish baseline and repeat monthly for the first year.
	Urinalysis	To detect nephrotoxicity	Establish baseline and repeat monthly for the first year.

RECOMMENDED LABORATORY TESTS IN CHRONIC DRUG THERAPY *(continued)*

DRUG	LABORATORY TESTS	RATIONALE	SPECIAL CONSIDERATIONS
Anticonvulsants			
trimethadione *(continued)*	Liver function tests	To detect hepatotoxicity	Establish baseline and repeat monthly for the first year.
	Ophthalmologic examinations	To detect hemeralopia or other visual disturbances	Discontinue if scotomata is detected.
valproic acid	Liver function tests	To detect hepatotoxicity	Establish baseline and repeat frequently, especially during first 6 months. May be dose-related. Higher incidence of fatal hepatotoxicity in children under age 2. Hepatotoxic effects not always preceded by abnormal liver function tests.
	Platelet count, bleeding time, coagulation studies	To detect clotting abnormalities	Some clinicians recommend thromboelastograpy as the most reliable assessment of drug effects on coagulation.
	Liver function tests	To detect hepatotoxicity	Establish baseline and repeat periodically. Hepatotoxicity may occur after prolonged use.
Antidepressants			
amitriptyline	Liver function tests	To detect hepatotoxicity	Establish baseline and repeat periodically; asymptomatic elevations of transaminase and alkaline phosphatase levels, which can progress to signs of hepatic failure, have occurred in patients receiving TCAs.
	Blood counts	To detect blood dyscrasias	Establish baseline and repeat periodically, especially in symptomatic patients.
	ECG	To detect cardiotoxicity	Establish baseline and repeat periodically, especially in patients receiving high doses.
	Ophthalmologic examinations, including tonometry	To detect glaucoma	Anticholinergic effects may exacerbate glaucoma.
amoxapine	Liver function tests	To detect hepatotoxicity	Establish baseline and repeat periodically; asymptomatic elevations of transaminase and alkaline phosphatase levels, which can progress to signs of hepatic failure, have occurred in patients receiving TCAs.
	Blood counts	To detect blood dyscrasias	Establish baseline and repeat periodically, especially in symptomatic patients.

(continued)

RECOMMENDED LABORATORY TESTS IN CHRONIC DRUG THERAPY *(continued)*

DRUG	LABORATORY TESTS	RATIONALE	SPECIAL CONSIDERATIONS
Antidepressants			
amoxapine *(continued)*	ECG	To detect cardiotoxicity	Establish baseline and repeat periodically, especially in patients receiving high doses.
	Ophthalmologic examinations, including tonometry	To detect glaucoma	Anticholinergic effects may exacerbate glaucoma.
bupropion	Blood counts	To detect blood dyscrasias	Establish baseline and repeat periodically, especially in symptomatic patients.
	ECG	To detect cardiotoxicity	Establish baseline and repeat periodically; bupropion has minimal effects on ECG.
	Body weight	To detect excessive weight loss	Anorectic action noted with short-term use.
clomipramine	Liver function tests	To detect hepatotoxicity	Establish baseline and repeat periodically; asymptomatic elevations of transaminase and alkaline phosphatase levels, which can progress to signs of hepatic failure, have occurred in patients receiving TCAs.
	Blood counts	To detect blood dyscrasias	Establish baseline and repeat periodically, especially in symptomatic patients.
	ECG	To detect cardiotoxicity	Establish baseline and repeat periodically, especially in patients receiving high doses.
	Ophthalmologic examinations, including tonometry	To detect glaucoma	Anticholinergic effects may exacerbate glaucoma.
desipramine	Liver function tests	To detect hepatotoxicity	Establish baseline and repeat periodically; asymptomatic elevations of transaminase and alkaline phosphatase levels, which can progress to signs of hepatic failure, have occurred in patients receiving TCAs.
	Blood counts	To detect blood dyscrasias	Establish baseline and repeat periodically, especially in symptomatic patients.
	ECG	To detect cardiotoxicity	Establish baseline and repeat periodically, especially in patients receiving high doses.
	Ophthalmologic examinations, including tonometry	To detect glaucoma	Anticholinergic effects may exacerbate glaucoma.

RECOMMENDED LABORATORY TESTS IN CHRONIC DRUG THERAPY *(continued)*

DRUG	LABORATORY TESTS	RATIONALE	SPECIAL CONSIDERATIONS
Antidepressants			
doxepin	Liver function tests	To detect hepato-toxicity	Establish baseline and repeat periodically; asymptomatic elevations of transaminase and alkaline phosphatase levels, which can progress to signs of hepatic failure, have occurred in patients receiving TCAs.
	Blood counts	To detect blood dyscrasias	Establish baseline and repeat periodically, especially in symptomatic patients.
	ECG	To detect cardio-toxicity	Establish baseline and repeat periodically, especially in patients receiving high doses.
	Ophthalmologic examinations, including tonometry	To detect glaucoma	Anticholinergic effects may exacerbate glaucoma.
fluoxetine	Blood counts	To detect blood dyscrasias	Establish baseline and repeat periodically, especially in symptomatic patients.
	ECG	To detect cardio-toxicity	Establish baseline and repeat periodically; fluoxetine has minimal effects on ECG
	Ophthalmologic examinations, including tonometry	To detect glaucoma	Anticholinergic effects may exacerbate glaucoma.
	Body weight	To detect excessive weight loss	Anorectic action noted with short-term use.
imipramine	Liver function tests	To detect hepato-toxicity	Establish baseline and repeat periodically; asymptomatic elevations of transaminase and alkaline phosphatase levels, which can progress to signs of hepatic failure, have occurred in patients receiving TCAs.
	Blood counts	To detect blood dyscrasias	Establish baseline and repeat periodically, especially in symptomatic patients.
	ECG	To detect cardio-toxicity	Establish baseline and repeat periodically, especially in patients receiving high doses.
	Ophthalmologic examinations, including tonometry	To detect glaucoma	Anticholinergic effects may exacerbate glaucoma.
isocarboxazid	Blood pressure	To detect toxicity	May cause orthostatic hypotension, especially in hypertensive patients.

(continued)

RECOMMENDED LABORATORY TESTS IN CHRONIC DRUG THERAPY *(continued)*

DRUG	LABORATORY TESTS	RATIONALE	SPECIAL CONSIDERATIONS
Antidepressants			
isocarboxazid *(continued)*	Ophthamologic examinations	To detect toxicity	Prolonged use may be associated rarely with amblyopia, visual disturbances, or glaucoma.
	Blood counts	To detect blood dyscrasias	Establish baseline and repeat periodically; normocytic and normochromic anemia, leukocytosis, agranulocytosis, and thrombocytopenia have been reported with MAO inhibitors.
	Liver function studies	To detect hepatotoxicity	Prevalent in patients on prolonged, high-dose therapy.
maprotiline	Liver function tests	To detect hepatotoxicity	Establish baseline and repeat periodically; asymptomatic elevations of transaminase and alkaline phosphatase levels, which can progress to signs of hepatic failure, have occurred in patients receiving TCAs.
	Blood counts	To detect blood dyscrasias	Establish baseline and repeat periodically, especially in symptomatic patients.
	ECG	To detect cardiotoxicity	Establish baseline and repeat periodically, especially in patients receiving high doses.
	Ophthalmologic examinations, including tonometry	To detect glaucoma	Anticholinergic effects may exacerbate glaucoma.
nortriptyline	Liver function tests	To detect hepatotoxicity	Establish baseline and repeat periodically; asymptomatic elevations of transaminase and alkaline phosphatase levels, which can progress to signs of hepatic failure, have occurred in patients receiving TCAs.
	Blood counts	To detect blood dyscrasias	Establish baseline and repeat periodically, especially in symptomatic patients.
	ECG	To detect cardiotoxicity	Establish baseline and repeat periodically, especially in patients receiving high doses.
	Ophthalmologic examinations, including tonometry	To detect glaucoma	Anticholinergic effects may exacerbate glaucoma.
phenelzine	Blood pressure	To detect toxicity	May cause orthostatic hypotension, especially in hypertensive patients.
	Ophthamologic examinations	To detect toxicity	Prolonged use may be associated rarely with amblyopia, visual disturbances, or glaucoma.

RECOMMENDED LABORATORY TESTS IN CHRONIC DRUG THERAPY *(continued)*

DRUG	LABORATORY TESTS	RATIONALE	SPECIAL CONSIDERATIONS
Antidepressants			
phenelzine *(continued)*	Blood counts	To detect blood dyscrasias	Establish baseline and repeat periodically; normocytic and normochromic anemia, leukocytosis, agranulocytosis, and thrombocytopenia have been reported with MAO inhibitors.
	Liver function studies	To detect hepatotoxicity	Prevalent in patients on prolonged, high-dose therapy.
protriptyline	Liver function tests	To detect hepatotoxicity	Establish baseline and repeat periodically; asymptomatic elevations of transaminase and alkaline phosphatase levels, which can progress to signs of hepatic failure, have occurred in patients receiving TCAs.
	Blood counts	To detect blood dyscrasias	Establish baseline and repeat periodically, especially in symptomatic patients.
	ECG	To detect cardiotoxicity	Establish baseline and repeat periodically, especially in patients receiving high doses.
	Ophthalmologic examinations, including tonometry	To detect glaucoma	Anticholinergic effects may exacerbate glaucoma.
tranylcypromine	Blood pressure	To detect toxicity	May cause orthostatic hypotension, especially in hypertensive patients.
	Ophthalmologic examinations	To detect toxicity	Prolonged use may be associated rarely with amblyopia, visual disturbances, or glaucoma.
	Blood counts	To detect blood dyscrasias	Establish baseline and repeat periodically; normocytic and normochromic anemia, leukocytosis, agranulocytosis, and thrombocytopenia have been reported with MAO inhibitors.
	Liver function studies	To detect hepatotoxicity	Prevalent in patients on prolonged, high-dose therapy
trazodone	Blood counts	To detect blood dyscrasias	Establish baseline and repeat periodically, especially in symptomatic patients.
	ECG	To detect cardiotoxicity	Establish baseline and repeat periodically, especially in patients receiving high doses.

RECOMMENDED LABORATORY TESTS IN CHRONIC DRUG THERAPY *(continued)*

DRUG	LABORATORY TESTS	RATIONALE	SPECIAL CONSIDERATIONS
Antidepressants			
trimipramine	Liver function tests	To detect hepatotoxicity	Establish baseline and repeat periodically; asymptomatic elevations of transaminase and alkaline phosphatase levels, which can progress to signs of hepatic failure, have occurred in patients receiving TCAs.
	Blood counts	To detect blood dyscrasias	Establish baseline and check periodically, especially in symptomatic patients.
	ECG	To detect cardiotoxicity	Establish baseline and repeat periodically, especially in patients receiving high doses.
	Ophthalmologic examinations, including tonometry	To detect glaucoma	Anticholinergic effects may exacerbate glaucoma.
Antiparkinsonian agents			
amantadine	Liver function studies	To detect toxicity	Establish baseline and repeat periodically; reversible elevations in liver enzymes seen occasionally.
benztropine	Ophthalmologic examinations, especially tonometry	To detect toxic effect	Anticholinergic effect may unmask glaucoma in predisposed patients.
biperiden	Ophthalmologic examinations, especially tonometry	To detect toxic effect	Anticholinergic effect may unmask glaucoma in predisposed patients.
bromocriptine	Blood pressure	To detect hypotension	Orthostatic hypotension is common when therapy is initiated; however, a persistent hypotensive effect usually accompanies therapy.
	Hematologic studies	To detect chronic toxicity	Recommended by most clinicians for patients on prolonged therapy; establish baseline and repeat periodically.
	Liver function studies	To detect and prevent toxicity	Transient elevations of AST (SGOT), ALT (SGPT), CPK, and alkaline phosphatase levels and of some transaminases have been noted.
	Renal function studies	To detect and prevent toxicity	Transient elevations of BUN and uric acid levels have been noted.
carbidopa-levodopa	Liver function studies	To detect toxic effects	Establish baseline and repeat periodically.
	Hematologic tests	To detect toxic effects	Establish baseline and repeat periodically; check clotting studies before any surgical procedures.

RECOMMENDED LABORATORY TESTS IN CHRONIC DRUG THERAPY *(continued)*

DRUG	LABORATORY TESTS	RATIONALE	SPECIAL CONSIDERATIONS
Antiparkinsonian agents			
carbidopa-levodopa *(continued)*	CV studies (ECG, blood pressure)	To detect toxicity	Establish baseline and repeat periodically; orthostatic hypotension is common, especially at initiation of therapy and during dosage increases.
	Renal function	To detect toxicity	Establish baseline and repeat periodically.
diphenhydramine	Blood counts	To detect toxicity	Establish baseline and repeat periodically; pancytopenia, agranulocytosis, and thrombocytopenia reported rarely with prolonged use.
levodopa	Liver function studies	To detect toxic effects	Establish baseline and repeat periodically.
	Hematologic tests	To detect toxic effects	Establish baseline and repeat periodically; check clotting studies before any surgical procedures.
	CV studies (ECG, blood pressure)	To detect toxicity	Check baseline and repeat periodically; orthostatic hypotension is common, especially at initiation of therapy and during dosage increases.
	Renal function	To detect toxicity	Establish baseline and repeat periodically.
orphenadrine	Ophthalmologic examinations, especially tonometry	To detect toxic effect	Anticholinergic effect may unmask glaucoma in predisposed patients.
pergolide	Ophthalmologic examinations, especially tonometry	To detect toxic effect	Anticholinergic effect may unmask glaucoma in predisposed patients.
procyclidine	Ophthalmologic examinations, especially tonometry	To detect toxic effect	Anticholinergic effect may unmask glaucoma in predisposed patients.
trihexyphenidyl	Ophthalmologic examinations, especially tonometry	To detect toxic effect	Anticholinergic effect may unmask glaucoma in predisposed patients.
Antimanic agent			
lithium	Blood counts	To detect blood dyscrasias	Establish baseline and repeat periodically.
	Serum electrolytes (particularly sodium)	To prevent toxicity	Sodium depletion can decrease lithium clearance and increase risk of toxicity.
	Serum lithium levels	To prevent toxicity	Toxic effects associated with levels above 1.5 mEq/liter.

(continued)

RECOMMENDED LABORATORY TESTS IN CHRONIC DRUG THERAPY *(continued)*

DRUG	LABORATORY TESTS	RATIONALE	SPECIAL CONSIDERATIONS
Antimanic agent			
lithium *(continued)*	Thyroid function studies	To evaluate decreased thyroid function	About 5% of all patients develop goiters; evaluate triiodothyronine, thyroxine, and thyroid-stimulating hormone concentrations.
	Kidney function tests	To detect nephron atrophy	Establish baseline renal function (serum creatinine, urinalysis) every 1 to 2 months for the first 6 months then every 6 months thereafter.
	Urine specific gravity	To detect diabetes insipidus	Specific gravity should be above 1.015.
Antipsychotic agents			
acetophenazine	Blood counts	To detect blood dyscrasias	Phenothiazines can cause mild leukopenia; agranulocytosis is more frequently seen in females after 4 to 10 weeks of therapy. Incidence of blood dyscrasias is low but mortality is high; check blood studies promptly in symptomatic patients.
	Ophthalmologic examinations	To detect adverse drug effect	Corneal opacities and retinopathy have been reported after prolonged, high-dose therapy.
	ECG	To detect toxicity	Establish baseline and check periodically.
	Blood pressure	To detect adverse drug effects	Orthostatic hypotension may be problematic at initiation of therapy.
chlorpromazine	Blood counts	To detect blood dyscrasias	Phenothiazines can cause mild leukopenia; agranulocytosis is more frequently seen in females after 4 to 10 weeks of therapy. Incidence of blood dyscrasias is low but mortality is high. Check blood studies promptly in symptomatic patients.
	Ophthalmologic examinations	To detect adverse drug effect	Corneal opacities and retinopathy have been reported after prolonged, high-dose therapy.
	ECG	To detect toxicity	Establish baseline and check periodically.
	Blood pressure	To detect adverse drug effects	Orthostatic hypotension may be problematic at initiation of therapy.
chlorprothixene	Blood counts	To detect blood dyscrasias	Drug can cause mild leukopenia or agranulocytosis. Incidence of blood dyscrasias is low. Check blood studies promptly in symptomatic patients.

RECOMMENDED LABORATORY TESTS IN CHRONIC DRUG THERAPY *(continued)*

DRUG	LABORATORY TESTS	RATIONALE	SPECIAL CONSIDERATIONS
Antipsychotic agents			
chlorprothixene *(continued)*	Ophthalmologic examinations	To detect adverse drug effect	Corneal opacities and retinopathy may occur after prolonged, high-dose therapy.
	ECG	To detect toxicity	Establish baseline and repeat periodically.
	Blood pressure	To detect adverse drug effects	Orthostatic hypotension may be problematic at initiation of therapy.
clozapine	Blood counts	To detect adverse drug effects	Drug can cause granulocytopenia or fatal agranulocytosis; baseline WBC count and differential required before therapy, and weekly WBC and granulocyte counts are mandatory during therapy and for at least 4 weeks after drug is discontinued.
droperidol	Blood counts	To detect blood dyscrasias	Drug can cause mild leukopenia or agranulocytosis. Incidence of blood dyscrasias is low. Check blood studies promptly in symptomatic patients.
	ECG	To detect toxicity	Establish baseline and repeat periodically.
	Blood pressure	To detect adverse drug effects	Orthostatic hypotension may be problematic at initiation of therapy; hypertension can occur with prolonged use.
fluphenazine	Blood counts	To detect blood dyscrasias	Phenothiazines can cause mild leukopenia; agranulocytosis is more frequently seen in females after 4 to 10 weeks of therapy. Incidence of blood dyscrasias is low but mortality is high. Check blood studies promptly in symptomatic patients.
	Ophthalmologic examinations	To detect adverse drug effects	Corneal opacities and retinopathy have been reported after prolonged, high-dose therapy.
	ECG	To detect toxicity	Establish baseline and repeat periodically.
	Blood pressure	To detect adverse drug effects	Orthostatic hypotension may be problematic at initiation of therapy.
haloperidol	Blood counts	To detect blood dyscrasias	Drug can cause mild leukopenia or agranulocytosis (only when combined with other drugs). Incidence of blood dyscrasias is low. Check blood studies promptly in symptomatic patients.

(continued)

RECOMMENDED LABORATORY TESTS IN CHRONIC DRUG THERAPY *(continued)*

DRUG	LABORATORY TESTS	RATIONALE	SPECIAL CONSIDERATIONS
Antipsychotic agents			
haloperidol *(continued)*	ECG	To detect toxicity	Establish baseline and check periodically
	Blood pressure	To detect adverse drug effects	Orthostatic hypotension may be problematic at initiation of therapy; hypertension can occur with prolonged use.
loxapine	Blood counts	To detect blood dyscrasias	Drug can cause mild leukopenia or agranulocytosis. Incidence of blood dyscrasias is low. Check blood studies promptly in symptomatic patients.
	Ophthalmologic examinations	To detect adverse drug effectd	Corneal opacities and retinopathy may occur after prolonged, high-dose therapy. Anticholinergic effects may aggravate glaucoma.
	ECG	To detect toxicity	Establish baseline and repeat periodically.
	Blood pressure	To detect adverse drug effects	Tachycardia or orthostatic hypotension may be problematic, especially at initiation of therapy.
mesoridazine	Blood counts	To detect blood dyscrasias	Phenothiazines can cause mild leukopenia; agranulocytosis is more frequently seen in females after 4 to 10 weeks of therapy. Incidence of blood dyscrasias is low but mortality is high. Check blood studies promptly in symptomatic patients.
	Ophthalmologic examinations	To detect adverse drug effects.	Corneal opacities and retinopathy have been reported after prolonged, high-dose therapy.
	ECG	To detect toxicity	Establish baseline and repeat periodically.
	Blood pressure	To detect adverse drug effects	Orthostatic hypotension may be problematic at initiation of therapy.
molindone	Blood counts	To detect blood dyscrasias	Drug can cause mild leukopenia or agranulocytosis. Incidence of blood dyscrasias is low. Check blood studies promptly in symptomatic patients.
	Ophthalmologic examinations	To detect adverse drug effects	Corneal opacities and retinopathy may occur after prolonged, high-dose therapy. Anticholinergic effects may aggravate glaucoma.
	ECG	To detect toxicity	Establish baseline and repeat periodically.

RECOMMENDED LABORATORY TESTS IN CHRONIC DRUG THERAPY *(continued)*

DRUG	LABORATORY TESTS	RATIONALE	SPECIAL CONSIDERATIONS
Antipsychotic agents			
molindone *(continued)*	Blood pressure	To detect adverse drug effects	Tachycardia or orthostatic hypotension may be problematic, especially at initiation of therapy.
perphenazine	Blood counts	To detect blood dyscrasias	Phenothiazines can cause mild leukopenia; agranulocytosis is more frequently seen in females after 4 to 10 weeks of therapy. Incidence of blood dyscrasias is low but mortality is high. Check blood studies promptly in symptomatic patients.
	Ophthalmologic examinations	To detect adverse drug effects	Corneal opacities and retinopathy have been reported after prolonged, high-dose therapy.
	ECG	To detect toxicity	Establish baseline and repeat periodically.
	Blood pressure	To detect adverse drug effects	Orthostatic hypotension may be problematic at initiation of therapy.
prochlorperazine	Blood counts	To detect blood dyscrasias	Phenothiazines can cause mild leukopenia; agranulocytosis is more frequently seen in females after 4 to 10 weeks of therapy. Incidence of blood dyscrasias is low but mortality is high. Check blood studies promptly in symptomatic patients.
	Ophthalmologic examinations	To detect adverse drug effects	Corneal opacities and retinopathy have been reported after prolonged, high-dose therapy.
	ECG	To detect toxicity	Establish baseline and repeat periodically.
	Blood pressure	To detect adverse drug effects	Orthostatic hypotension may be problematic at initiation of therapy.
promazine	Blood counts	To detect blood dyscrasias	Phenothiazines can cause mild leukopenia; agranulocytosis is more frequently seen in females after 4 to 10 weeks of therapy. Incidence of blood dyscrasias is low but mortality is high. Check blood studies promptly in symptomatic patients.
	Ophthalmologic examinations	To detect adverse drug effects	Corneal opacities and retinopathy have been reported after prolonged, high-dose therapy.
	ECG	To detect toxicity	Establish baseline and repeat periodically.

(continued)

RECOMMENDED LABORATORY TESTS IN CHRONIC DRUG THERAPY *(continued)*

DRUG	LABORATORY TESTS	RATIONALE	SPECIAL CONSIDERATIONS
Antipsychotic agents			
promazine *(continued)*	Blood pressure	To detect adverse drug effects	Orthostatic hypotension may be problematic at initiation of therapy.
thioridazine	Blood counts	To detect blood dyscrasias	Phenothiazines can cause mild leukopenia; agranulocytosis is more frequently seen in females after 4 to 10 weeks of therapy. Incidence of blood dyscrasias is low but mortality is high. Check blood studies promptly in symptomatic patients.
	Ophthalmologic examinations	To detect adverse drug effect	Corneal opacities and retinopathy have been reported after prolonged, high-dose therapy.
	ECG	To detect toxicity	Establish baseline and repeat periodically
	Blood pressure	To detect adverse drug effects	Orthostatic hypotension may be problematic at initiation of therapy.
thiothixene	Blood counts	To detect blood dyscrasias	Drug can cause mild leukopenia or agranulocytosis. Incidence of blood dyscrasias is low. Check blood studies promptly in symptomatic patients.
	Ophthalmologic examinations	To detect adverse drug effects	Corneal opacities and retinopathy may occur after prolonged, high-dose therapy.
	ECG	To detect toxicity	Establish baseline and repeat periodically
	Blood pressure	To detect adverse drug effects	Orthostatic hypotension may be problematic at initiation of therapy.
trifluoperazine	Blood counts	To detect blood dyscrasias	Phenothiazines can cause mild leukopenia; agranulocytosis is more frequently seen in females after 4 to 10 weeks of therapy. Incidence of blood dyscrasias is low but mortality is high. Check blood studies promptly in symptomatic patients.
	Ophthalmologic examinations	To detect adverse drug effects	Corneal opacities and retinopathy have been reported after prolonged, high-dose therapy.
	ECG	To detect toxicity	Establish baseline and repeat periodically.
	Blood pressure	To detect adverse drug effects	Orthostatic hypotension may be problematic at initiation of therapy.

RECOMMENDED LABORATORY TESTS IN CHRONIC DRUG THERAPY *(continued)*

DRUG	LABORATORY TESTS	RATIONALE	SPECIAL CONSIDERATIONS
Anxiolytics			
alprazolam	Blood counts	To detect blood dyscrasias	Establish baseline and repeat periodically during prolonged therapy.
	Liver function tests	To detect hepato-toxicity	Elevated liver function tests reported after prolonged benzodiazepine use.
	Renal function tests	To detect nephro-toxicity	Decreased renal function may occur after prolonged benzodiazepine use.
chlordiaze-poxide	Blood counts	To detect blood dyscrasias	Establish baseline and repeat periodically during prolonged therapy.
	Liver function tests	To detect hepato-toxicity	Elevated liver function tests reported after prolonged benzodiazepine use.
	Renal function tests	To detect nephro-toxicity	Decreased renal function may occur after prolonged benzodiazepine use.
diazepam	Blood counts	To detect blood dyscrasias	Relatively rare; establish baseline and repeat periodically during prolonged therapy.
	Plasma testolactone levels	To detect chronic toxicity	Decreases reported in males with prolonged therapy.
	Liver function tests	To detect hepato-toxicity	Elevated AST (SGOT), ALT (SGPT), lactate dehydrogenase, alkaline phosphatase, and total and direct bilirubin reported occasionally with chronic use.
	Renal function studies	To detect nephro-toxicity	May occur with prolonged use; also transient decreased renal function after parenteral diazepam has been reported.
halazepam	Blood counts	To detect blood dyscrasias	Establish baseline and repeat periodically during prolonged therapy.
	Liver function tests	To detect hepato-toxicity	Elevated liver function tests reported after prolonged benzodiazepine use.
	Renal function tests	To detect nephro-toxicity	Decreased renal function may occur after prolonged benzodiazepine use.
lorazepam	Liver function tests	To detect hepato-toxicity	Elevated liver enzymes reported after prolonged benzodiazepine use.
	Blood counts	To detect blood dyscrasias	Establish baseline and repeat periodically during prolonged use.
	Renal function tests	To detect nephro-toxicity	Nephrotoxicity may occur after prolonged use.

(continued)

RECOMMENDED LABORATORY TESTS IN CHRONIC DRUG THERAPY *(continued)*

DRUG	LABORATORY TESTS	RATIONALE	SPECIAL CONSIDERATIONS
Anxiolytics			
meprobamate	Blood counts	To detect blood dyscrasias	Establish baseline and repeat periodically; blood dyscrasias has been reported rarely.
oxazepam	Blood counts	To detect blood dyscrasias	Establish baseline and repeat periodically.
	Kidney function tests	To detect nephrotoxicity	May occur after prolonged benzodiazepine use.
	Liver function tests	To detect hepatotoxicity	May occur after prolonged benzodiazepine use.
prazepam	Blood counts	To detect blood dyscrasias	Establish baseline and repeat periodically.
	Kidney function tests	To detect nephrotoxicity	May occur after prolonged benzodiazepine use.
	Liver function tests	To detect hepatotoxicity	May occur after prolonged benzodiazepine use.
Sedative-hypnotics			
amobarbital	CBC, platelet count	To detect blood dyscrasias	Establish baseline and repeat periodically.
aprobarbital	CBC, platelet count	To detect blood dyscrasias	Establish baseline and repeat periodically.
butabarbital	CBC, platelet count	To detect blood dyscrasias	Establish baseline and repeat periodically.
chloral hydrate	Blood counts	To detect blood dyscrasias	Leukopenia and eosinophilia reported rarely with prolonged use.
flurazepam	Blood counts	To detect blood dyscrasias	Establish baseline and repeat periodically.
	Liver function tests	To detect hepatotoxicity	Reported with prolonged benzodiazepine use.
	Kidney function tests	To detect nephrotoxicity	Reported with prolonged benzodiazepine use.
glutethimide	Blood counts	To detect blood dyscrasias	May be symptom of an acute hypersensitivity reaction.
pentobarbital	CBC, platelet count	To detect blood dyscrasias	Establish baseline and repeat periodically.
quazepam	Blood counts	To detect blood dyscrasias	Establish baseline and repeat periodically.
	Kidney function tests	To detect nephrotoxicity	Reported with prolonged use of benzodiazepines.
	Liver function tests	To detect hepatotoxicity	Reported with prolonged benzodiazepine use.

RECOMMENDED LABORATORY TESTS IN CHRONIC DRUG THERAPY *(continued)*

DRUG	LABORATORY TESTS	RATIONALE	SPECIAL CONSIDERATIONS
Sedative-hypnotics			
secobarbital	CBC, platelet count	To detect blood dyscrasias	Establish baseline and repeat periodically.
temazepam	Blood counts	To detect blood dyscrasias	Establish baseline and repeat periodically.
	Liver function tests	To detect hepato-toxicity	Reported with prolonged benzodiazepine use.
	Kidney function tests	To detect nephro-toxicity	Reported with prolonged benzodiazepine use.
triazolam	Blood counts	To detect blood dyscrasias	Establish baseline and repeat periodically.
	Liver function tests	To detect hepato-toxicity	Reported with prolonged benzodiazepine use.
	Kidney function tests	To detect nephro-toxicity	Reported with prolonged benzodiazepine use.

PSYCHIATRIC DRUG REACTIONS

The following list reports generic drugs and pharmacologic classes that have been associated with psychiatric symptoms or disorders. If unspecified, reported incidence for individual drugs is less than 1%.

SYMPTOM	GENERIC NAME	TRADE NAME	INCIDENCE
Agitation	alprazolam	Xanax	
	antidepressants		
	atropine		
	bromocriptine	Parlodel	
	clonidine	Catapres	3%
	diazepam	Valium	
	diphenhydramine	Benadryl	
	ephedrine		
	fluoxetine	Prozac	
	indapamide	Lozol	5%
	isoniazid (INH)		
	MAO inhibitors		
	methadone		
	morphine sulfate		
Akathisia	alprazolam	Xanax	
	chlorprothixene	Taractan	common
	phenothiazines		
Amnesia	alprazolam	Xanax	>1%
	benzodiazepines		
	triazolam	Halcion	
Anxiety	amantadine	Symmetrel	1% to 5%
	CNS stimulants		
	diazoxide	Proglycem	frequent
	dronabinol	Marinol	16%
	epinephrine	Adrenalin	
	indapamide	Lozol	5%
	indomethacin	Indocin	
	leuprolide acetate	Lupron	>3%
	maprotiline	Ludiomil	3%
	naltrexone	Trexan	>10%
	oxymetazoline		
	pindolol	Visken	4%
	ritodrine	Yutopar	5% to 6% (I.V.)
	sympathomimetics		
	theophylline		
Apathy	CNS depressants		
	digitalis glycosides		
	halazepam	Paxipam	9%
Behavioral changes	clonazepam	Klonopin	25%
	meperidine	Demerol	
Catatonia	atenolol	Tenormin	
	butyrophenones		
	chlorprothixine	Taractan	

PSYCHIATRIC DRUG REACTIONS *(continued)*

SYMPTOM	GENERIC NAME	TRADE NAME	INCIDENCE
Catatonia *(continued)*	fluphenazine hydrochloride	Permitil Hydrochloride	
	labetalol	Trandate	
	methdilazine hydrochloride	Tacaryl	
	perphenazine	Trilafon	
	perphenazine and amitriptyline	Etrafon, Triavil	
	phenothiazines		
	prochlorperazine	Compazine	
	promethazine	Phenergan	
	propranolol	Inderal	
	propranolol and hydrochlorothiazide	Inderide	
	thioxanthines		
	trifluoperazine	Stelazine	
	trimeprazine	Temaril	
Choreoathetotic movements	chlorprothixene	Taractan	
	levodopa	Larodopa	
	lithium	Cibalith, Eskalith	
	loxapine hydrochloride	Loxitane C	
	methyldopa	Aldomet	
	methyldopa and chlorothiazide	Aldoclor	
	methyldopa and hydrochlorothiazide	Aldoril	
Clonic movements	lithium	Eskalith, Lithane	
Clonus	doxapram	Dopram	
Confusion	alprazolam	Xanax	9.9%
	amantadine	Symmetrel	1% to 5%
	baclofen	Lioresal	1% to 11%
	benzodiazepines		
	carbamazepine	Mazepine, Tegretol	
	clonidine	Catapres	
	CNS depressants		
	cyclosporine	Sandimmune	2%
	diazepam	Valium	
	esmolol	Brevibloc	2%
	guanadrel sulfate	Hylorel	14.8%
	halazepam	Paxipam	9%
	interferon alfa-2a, recombinant	Roferon-A	10%
	isocarboxazid	Marplan	most common
	levodopa	Larodopa	
	MAO inhibitors		
	meperidine	Demerol	
	metoclopramide	Octamide	> 10%
	mexiletine	Mexitil	2.6%
	penicillin		
	pentazocine	Fortral, Talwin	30%
	phenobarbital		

(continued)

PSYCHIATRIC DRUG REACTIONS (continued)

SYMPTOM	GENERIC NAME	TRADE NAME	INCIDENCE
Confusion (continued)	phenytoin	Dilantin	most common
	temazepam	Restoril	2% to 3%
	tocainide	Tonocard	>1%
	valproic acid	Depakene	
Delirium	acyclovir	Zovirax	
	amantadine	Symmetrel	
	amphetamines		
	anticholinergics		
	atropine		
	baclofen	Lioresal	
	chloramphenicol	Chloromycetin	
	cimetidine	Tagamet	
	clonidine	Catapres	
	corticosteroids		
	digitalis glycosides		
	ephedrine		
	famotidine	Pepcid	
	fentanyl citrate with droperidol	Innovar	
	indomethacin	Indocin	
	lithium	Eskalith, Lithane	
	lorazepam	Ativan	
	meperidine	Demerol	
	methohexital sodium	Brevital Sodium	
	methoxyflurane	Penthrane	
	methyldopa	Aldomet	
	mexiletine	Mexitil	
	nizatidine	Axid	
	opium alkaloids	Pentopon	
	pentazocine	Talwin	
	phenelzine	Nardil	
	phenylephrine		
	phenylpropanolamine		
	phenytoin	Dilantin	
	propranolol	Inderal	
	quinidine gluconate	Duraquin	
	ranitidine	Zantac	
	sympathomimetics		
	thiamylal	Surital	
Delusions	amitriptyline	Elavil	
	carbidopa-levodopa	Sinemet	
	chlordiazepoxide hydrochloride	Limbitrol	
	desipramine	Pertofrane	
	imipramine	Tofranil	
	levodopa	Larodopa	frequent
	nortriptyline	Pamelor	
	perphenazine and amitriptyline	Etrafon, Triavil	
	protriptyline	Vivactil	
	trimipramine	Surmontil	

PSYCHIATRIC DRUG REACTIONS *(continued)*

SYMPTOM	GENERIC NAME	TRADE NAME	INCIDENCE
Dementia	carbidopa-levodopa	Sinemet	
	levodopa	Larodopa	
	methotrexate	Mexate	
	quinidine sulfate	Quinidex Extentabs	
Depression	alprazolam	Xanax	
	amantadine	Symmetrel	1% to 5%
	atenolol	Tenormin	12%
	atenolol and chlorthalidone	Tenoretic	12%
	baclofen	Lioresal	
	clonidine	Catapres	
	digitalis glycosides		
	dronabinol	Marinol	7%
	flecainide	Tambocor	1% to 3%
	flunisolide	Aerobid Inhaler	1% to 3%
	guanabenz	Wytensin	3%
	guanadrel	Hylorel	1.9%
	halazepam	Paxipam	9%
	indapamide	Lozol	5%
	indomethacin	Indocin	1% to 3%
	metoclopramide	Octamide	<10%
	metoprolol	Lopressor	5%
	mexiletine	Mexitil	2.4%
	naltrexone	Trexan	<10%
	NSAIDs		
	reserpine	Serpasil	
	tolmetin	Tolectin	<3%
Disorientation	benzodiazepines		
	cimetidine	Tagamet	
	CNS depressants		
	famotidine	Pepcid	
	halazepam	Paxipam	9%
	lidocaine	Xylocaine	
	methadone		
	metronidazole	Flagyl	
	morphine		
	nizatidine	Axid	
	NSAIDs		
	penicillin		
	pentazocine	Talwin	30%
	ranitidine	Zantac	
Dysphoria	metoclopramide	Octamide, Reglan	10%
	opiates		
Emotional disturbances	imipramine	Tofranil	
	primidone	Mysoline	
	ritodrine	Yutopar	5 to 6%
	valproic acid	Depakene	

(continued)

PSYCHIATRIC DRUG REACTIONS (continued)

SYMPTOM	GENERIC NAME	TRADE NAME	INCIDENCE
Euphoria	antidepressants		
	atropine		
	baclofen	Lioresal	
	levodopa	Larodopa	
	methadone		
	morphine sulfate		
	pentazocine	Talwin	
Hallucinations	acyclovir	Zovirax	
	amantadine	Symmetrel	1% to 5%
	atropine		
	baclofen	Lioresal	
	beta-adrenergic blockers		
	bromocriptine	Parlodel	
	carbidopa-levodopa	Sinemet	
	cimetidine	Tagamet	
	corticosteroids		
	diazepam	Valium	
	digitalis glycosides		
	diphenhydramine	Benadryl	
	dronabinol	Marinol	5%
	ephedrine		
	famotidine	Pepcid	
	levodopa	Larodopa	
	lidocaine	Xylocaine	
	methyldopa	Aldomet	
	metronidazole	Flagyl	
	nizatidine	Axid	
	oxymetazoline		
	penicillin		
	pentazocine	Talwin	
	phenylephrine		
	propranolol	Inderal	
	ranitidine	Zantac	
Hyperirritability	dinoprostone	Prostin E^2	
	phenylpropanolamine		
	primidone	Mysoline	
	thiabendazole	Mintezol	
Hysteria	azatidine	Optimine	
	clemastine	Tavist	
	clonazepam	Klonopin	
	codeine and bromodiphenhydramine	Ambenyl	
	cyproheptadine	Periactin	
	dexchlorpheniramine, pseudoephedrine, and guaifenesin	Polaramine	
	ethchlorvynol	Placidyl	
	methdilazine hydrochloride	Tacaryl	

PSYCHIATRIC DRUG REACTIONS *(continued)*

SYMPTOM	GENERIC NAME	TRADE NAME	INCIDENCE
Hysteria *(continued)*	phenylpropanolamine and chlorpheniramine	Ornade, Triaminic	
	promethazine	Phenergan	
	pseudoephedrine		
	trimeprazine	Temaril	
	tripelennamine	PBZ	
	triprolidine, pseudoephedrine, and codeine phosphate	Actifed with codeine	
Insomnia	acebutolol	Sectral	3%
	albuterol	Proventil, Ventolin	2%
	alprazolam	Xanax	>8%
	amantadine	Symmetrel	5% to 10%
	amphetamines		
	antidepressants		
	baclofen	Lioresal	2% to 7%
	clomiphene	Serophene	1.9%
	estramustine	Emcyt	3% to 4%
	fluoxetine	Prozac	
	guanfacine	Tenex	4%
	indapamide	Lozol	<5%
	interferon alfa-2b, recombinant	Intron	5%
	isocarboxazid	Marplan	most frequent
	ketoprofen	Orudis	>3%
	leuprolide acetate	Lupron	<3%
	MAO inhibitors		
	maprotiline	Ludiomil	2%
	metoclopramide	Octamide	10%
	pentoxifylline	Trental	2.3%
	phenylpropanolamine		
	pindolol	Visken	19%
	sympathomimetics		
	theophylline		
Irritability	amantadine	Symmetrel	1% to 5%
	dronabinol	Marinol	7%
	flunisolide	AeroBid Inhaler	3% to 9%
	indapamide	Lozol	5%
	naltrexone	Trexan	>10%
Jitteriness	acyclovir	Zovirax	
	amitriptyline	Elavil	
	amphetamines		
	chlorpromazine	Thorazine	
	diethylpropion	Tenuate	
	isocarboxazid	Marplan	most frequent
	metoclopramide	Octamide	
	nifedipine	Adalat, Procardia	2%
	phenelzine	Nardil	
	prochlorperazine	Compazine	

(continued)

PSYCHIATRIC DRUG REACTIONS (continued)

SYMPTOM	GENERIC NAME	TRADE NAME	INCIDENCE
Jitteriness (continued)	ritodrine	Yutopar	5% to 8%
	sympathomimetics		
	trifluoperazine	Stelazine	
Lethargy	atenolol	Tenormin	3%
	atenolol and chlorthalidone	Tenoretic	3%
	butalbital, aspirin, caffeine and codeine phosphate	Fiorinal with codeine	most common
	butorphanol	Stadol	2%
	clonidine	Catapres	3%
	estramustine	Emcyt	3% to 4%
	etretinate	Tegison	1% to 10%
	immune globulin	RhoGam	25%
	indapamide	Lozol	5%
	interferon alfa-2a, recombinant	Roferon-A	3%
	leuprolide acetate	Lupron	3%
	metoprolol	Lopressor	10%
	pindolol	Visken	3%
	temazepam	Restoril	3%
Manic symptoms	alprazolam	Xanax	
	antidepressants		20% to 30%
	baclofen	Lioresal	
	bromocriptine	Parlodel	
	corticosteroids		
	levodopa	Larodopa	
	metoclopramide	Octamide	
	propranolol	Inderal	
	triazolam	Halcion	
Memory impairment	acebutolol	Sectral	
	alprazolam	Xanax	>1%
	atenolol	Tenormin	
	atenolol and chlorthalidone	Tenoretic	
	benztropine	Cogentin	
	carbamazepine	Tegretol	
	clonazepam	Klonopin	
	diphenhydramine	Benadryl	
	glutethimide	Doriden	
	isocarboxazid	Marplan	most frequent
	isoniazid (INH)		
	labetalol	Trandate	
	leuprolide acetate	Lupron	<3%
	lithium	Eskalith	
	MAO inhibitors		
	maprotiline	Ludiomil	
	metoprolol	Lopressor	
	oxazepam	Serax	
	phenobarbital		
	phenytoin	Dilantin	

PSYCHIATRIC DRUG REACTIONS *(continued)*

SYMPTOM	GENERIC NAME	TRADE NAME	INCIDENCE
Memory impairment *(continued)*	propranolol and hydrochlorothiazide	Inderide	
	timolol	Blocadren, Timoptic	
	tocainide	Tonocard	
	trazodone	Desyrel	>1%
	triazolam	Halcion	
	valproic acid	Depakene	
Memory loss, short term	benzodiazepines		
	mexilitine	Mexitil	
	propranolol	Inderal	
Mood changes	carbidopa-levodopa	Sinemet	
	fenfluramine	Pondimin	
	flunisolide	AeroBid Inhaler	1% to 3%
	hydrocodone and acetaminophen	Co-Gesic, Vicodin	
	hydrocodone, aspirin, and caffeine	Damason P	
	hydrocodone and chlorpheniramine	Hycomine	
	hydromorphone	Dilaudid	
	nifedipine	Adalat, Procardia	
	phenelzine	Nardil	
	piroxicam	Feldene	
	tocainide	Tonocard	>1%
Nervousness	albuterol	Proventil, Ventolin	4% to 20%
	alprazolam	Xanax	4.1%
	bitolterol	Tornalate	5%
	dicyclomine	Bentyl	6%
	flunisolide	AeroBid Inhaler	3% to 9%
	indapamide	Lozol	>5%
	ipratropium bromide	Atrovent	3.1%
	isoetharine hydrochloride	Arm-a-Med Isoetharine	
	ketoprofen	Orudis	>3%
	maprotiline	Ludiomil	6%
	metaproterenol	Alupent	
	mexiletine	Mexitil	5%
	naltrexone	Trexan	>10%
	nifedipine	Adalat, Procardia	7%
	pindolol	Visken	11%
	ritodrine	Yutopar	5% to 6%
	triazolam	Halcion	5.2%
	trihexyphenidyl	Artane	30% to 50%
Neuromuscular reactions, extra-pyramidal	butyrophenones		frequent
	chlorpromazine	Thorazine	frequent
	haloperidol	Haldol	frequent
	phenothiazines		frequent
	pimozide	Orap	frequent

(continued)

PSYCHIATRIC DRUG REACTIONS *(continued)*

SYMPTOM	GENERIC NAME	TRADE NAME	INCIDENCE
Neuromuscular reactions, extra-pyramidal *(continued)*	prochlorperazine	Compazine	frequent
	thioxanthines		
	trifluoperazine	Stelazine	frequent
	vincristine	Vincasar PFS	frequent
Nightmares	amantadine	Symmetrel	
	amoxapine	Asendin	>1%
	atropine		
	baclofen	Lioresal	
	beta-adrenergic blockers		
	bromocriptine	Parlodel	
	levodopa	Larodopa	frequent
	propranolol	Inderal	
Night terrors	ethosuximide	Zarontin	
	penicillin		
Paradoxical anxiety	hydrochlorothiazide and deserpidine	Oreticyl	
	methyclothiazide	Enduron	
	perphenazine	Trilafon	
Paranoia	alprazolam	Xanax	
	amphetamines		
	bromocriptine	Parlodel	
	carbidopa-levodopa	Sinemet	
	dronabinol	Marinol	2%
	ephedrine		
	fluphenazine hydrochloride	Permitil Hydrochloride	
	indomethacin	Indocin	
	lidocaine		
	meperidine	Demerol	
	naltrexone	Trexan	
	NSAIDs		
	perphenazine	Trilafon	
	perphenazine and amitriptyline	Etrafon, Triavil	
	phenylephrine		
	sympathomimetics		
	triazolam	Halcion	
Parkinson-like symptoms	asparaginase	Elspar	
	chlorothiazine and reserpine	Diupres	
	chlorprothixene	Taractan	common
	chlorthalidone and reserpine	Demi-Regroton	
	fluphenazine hydrochloride	Permitil Hydrochloride, Prolixin Hydrochloride	
	haloperidol	Haldol	
	hydrochlorothiazide and reserpine	Hydropres-25	
	hydroflumethiazide	Saluron	
	indomethacin	Indocin	
	mesoridazine	Serentil	

PSYCHIATRIC DRUG REACTIONS *(continued)*

SYMPTOM	GENERIC NAME	TRADE NAME	INCIDENCE
Parkinson-like symptoms *(continued)*	methychlothiazide and reserpine	Diutensen-R	
	methyldopa	Aldomet	
	methyldopa and chlorothiazide	Aldoclor	
	methyldopa and hydrochlorothiazide	Aldoril	
	metoclopramide	Octamide	
	metyrosine	Demser	
	perphenazine	Trilafon	
	perphenazine and amitriptyline	Etrafon, Triavil	
	pimozide	Orap	
	polythiazide	Renese	
	prochlorperazine	Compazine	
	rauwolfia serpentina	Raudixin	
	reserpine	Ser-Ap-Es, Serpasil	
	thiothixene	Navane	
	trichlormethiazide and reserpine	Metatensin	
	trifluoperazine	Stelazine	
	trimethobenzamide	Tigan	
Psychiatric disturbances	guanadrel	Hylorel	3.8%
	phenacemide	Phenurone	17%
Psychosis	amantadine	Symmetrel	
	bromocriptine	Parlodel	
	chlorprothixene	Taractan	
	cimetidine	Tagamet	
	clonazepam	Klonopin	
	cycloserine	Seromycin	
	dapsone	Avlosulfon	
	dextrothyroxine sodium	Choloxin	
	digoxin	Lanoxicaps, Lanoxin	1% to 4%
	divalproex sodium	Depakote	
	ethionamide	Trecator-SC	
	hydrochlorothiazide and reserpine	Hydropres-25	
	hydroxychloroquine	Plaquenil	
	Iohexol	Omnipaque	
	methadone (I.V.)		
	methyldopa	Aldomet	
	metrizamide	Amipaque	
	morphine sulfate	Duramorph	
	perphenazine	Trilafon	
	phendimetrazine	Plegine	
	phentermine	Adipex-P	
	prednisolone sodium phosphate	Hydeltrasol	
	procainamide	Pronestyl	
	sulfisoxazole and phenazopyridine	Azo Gantrisin	
	valproic acid	Depakene	
	vidarabine	Vira-A	

(continued)

PSYCHIATRIC DRUG REACTIONS *(continued)*

SYMPTOM	GENERIC NAME	TRADE NAME	INCIDENCE
Psychosis, activation	bromocriptine	Parlodel	
	desipramine	Pertofrane	
	fluphenazine hydrochloride	Prolixin Hydrochloride	
	perphenazine and amitriptyline	Etrafon, Triavil	
	prochlorperazine	Compazine	
Psychosis, exacerbation	desipramine	Norpramin	
	fluphenazine hydrochloride	Permetil Hydrochloride, Prolixin Hydrochloride	
	imipramine	Tofranil	
	nortriptyline	Pamelor	
	perphenazine and amitriptyline	Etrafon	
	protriptyline	Vivactil	
	thiethylperazine	Torecan	
	thioridazine	Mellaril	
	trimipramine	Surmontil	
Psychosis, toxic	isoniazid (INH)		
	methylphenidate	Ritalin	
	morphine sulfate	Duramorph	
Rage reactions	indomethacin	Indocin	
	sulindac	Clinoril	
Seizures	alprazolam	Xanax	2 to 3 days (after abrupt discontinuation)
	bromocriptine	Parlodel	
	chloroquine	Aralen	
	chlorpromazine	Thorazine	
	cyclosporine	Sandimmune	>3%
	desipramine	Pertofrane	
	esmolol	Brevibloc	
	fluphenazine	Permitil	
	lidocaine	Xylocaine	
	lithium	Cibalith-S, Eskalith, Lithane, Lithobid	
	methdilazine hydrochloride	Tacaryl	
	methocarbamol	Robaxin	
	metoclopramide	Reglan	
	metronidazole	Flagyl, Protostat	
	mezlocillin	Mezlin	
	paramethadione	Paradione	
	pemoline	Cylert	
	penicillin		
	perphenazine	Etrafon, Triavil	
	promethazine	Phenergan	
	ticarcillin/clavulanate	Timentin	
	tocainide	Tonocard	
	trimeprazine	Temaril	
	trimethadione	Tridione	

PSYCHIATRIC DRUG REACTIONS (continued)

SYMPTOM	GENERIC NAME	TRADE NAME	INCIDENCE
Sensorium, clouded	atenolol	Tenormin	
	CNS depressants		
	labetalol	Trandate	
	labetalol and hydrochlorothiazine	Normozide	
	mepivacaine	Carbocaine	
	nadolol and bendroflumethiazide	Corzide	
	propranolol	Inderal	
	propranolol and hydrochlorothiazide	Inderide	
	timolol	Blocadren, Timoptic	
Sleep disturbances	bromocriptine	Parlodel	
	diazepam	Valium	
	ethosuximide	Zarontin	
	guanabenz	Wytensin	3%
	guanadrel	Hylorel	2.1%
	imipramine	Tofranil	
	metoprolol	Lopressor	
	mexiletine	Mexitil	7.1%
	naltrexone	Trexan	>10%
	nifedipine	Adalat, Procardia	2%
Suicidal ideation	amitriptyline	Elavil	
	carbidopa-levodopa	Sinemet	
	chlorthalidone and reserpine	Demi-Regroton, Regroton	
	clonazepam	Klonopin	
	desipramine	Pertofrane	
	meprobamate	Meprospan, Miltown	
	perphenazine	Trilafon	
Tardive dyskinesia	chlorpromazine	Thorazine	
	chlorprothixine	Taractan	
	fluphenazine hydrochloride	Permitil Hydrochloride, Prolixin Hydrochloride	
	haloperidol	Haldol	
	loxapine hydrochloride	Loxitane C	
	mesoridazine	Serentil	
	metoclopramide	Octamide, Reglan	
	molindone	Moban	
	perphenazine	Trilafon	
	perphenazine and amitriptyline	Etrafon, Triavil	
	pimozide	Orap	
	prochlorperazine	Compazine	
	thioridazine	Mellaril	
	thiothixine	Navane	
	trifluoperazine	Stelazine	
Tourette's syndrome	dextroamphetamine	Dexedrine	
	methamphetamine	Desoxyn	
	pemoline	Cylert	

PSYCHOTROPIC DRUGS: TRADE NAMES AND MANUFACTURERS

In the chart below, psychotropic drugs are listed alphabetically by trade name and followed by generic name and manufacturer. The accompanying telephone number provides access to the manufacturer's information, for example, in the case of overdose or another clinical problem.

Adapin (doxepin)	Fisons Corporation Prescription Products (U.S.)	(716) 475-9000
Adipost (phendimetrazine)	B. F. Ascher & Company, Inc. (U.S.)	(913) 888-1880
Akineton (biperiden)	Knoll Pharmaceuticals (U.S.)	(800) 526-0221, (201) 428-8250
	Knoll Pharmaceuticals (Canada)	(416) 475-7070
Ak-Zol (acetazolamide)	Akorn, Inc. (U.S.)	(800) 535-7155
Alurate (aprobarbital)	Roche Laboratories (U.S.)	(800) 526-6367
Alzapam (lorazepam)	Major Pharmaceutical Inc. (U.S.)	(800) 521-5340
Amitril (amitriptyline)	Parke-Davis (U.S.)	(201) 540-3950, (201) 540-2117 (evenings and weekends)
Amytal (amobarbital)	Eli Lilly and Company (U.S.)	(317) 276-3714
	Eli Lilly Canada Inc.	(416) 694-3221
Anafranil (clomipramine)	Ciba Pharmaceutical Company (U.S.)	(201) 277-5000
	Geigy Pharmaceuticals (Canada)	(800) 387-8395
Anorex (phendimetrazine)	Dunhall Pharmaceuticals (U.S.)	(501) 787-5232
Anxanil (hydroxyzine)	Econo Med Pharmaceuticals, Inc. (U.S.)	(919) 226-1091
Aparkane (trihexyphenidyl)	ICN Pharmaceuticals, Inc. (Canada)	(800) 556-1937
Aphen (trihexyphenidyl)	Major Pharmaceutical Inc. (U.S.)	(800) 521-5340
Apo-Chlordiazepoxide (chlordiazepoxide)	Apotex Inc. (Canada)	(416) 749-9300, (800) 268-0599 (Canada except Ontario, Quebec)
Apo-Diazepam (diazepam)	Apotex Inc. (Canada)	(416) 749-9300, (800) 268-0599 (Canada except Ontario, Quebec)
Apo-Flurazepam (flurazepam)	Apotex Inc. (Canada)	(416) 749-9300, (800) 268-0599
Apo-Haloperidol (haloperidol)	Apotex Inc. (Canada)	(416) 749-9300, (800) 268-0599 (Canada except Ontario, Quebec)

PSYCHOTROPIC DRUGS: TRADE NAMES AND MANUFACTURERS *(continued)*

Apo-Imipramine (imipramine)	Apotex Inc. (Canada)	(416) 749-9300, (800) 268-0599 (Canada except Ontario, Quebec)
Apo-Lorazepam (lorazepam)	Apotex Inc. (Canada)	(416) 749-9300, (800) 268-0599 (Canada except Ontario, Quebec)
Apo-Meprobamate (meprobamate)	Apotex Inc. (Canada)	(416) 749-9300, (800) 268-0599 (Canada except Ontario, Quebec)
Apo-Oxazepam (oxazepam)	Apotex Inc. (Canada)	(416) 749-9300, (800) 268-0599 (Canada except Ontario, Quebec)
Apo-Perphenazine (perphenazine)	Apotex Inc. (Canada)	(416) 749-9300, (800) 268-0599 (Canada except Ontario, Quebec)
Apo-Thioridazine (thioridazine)	Apotex Inc. (Canada)	(416) 749-9300, (800) 268-0599 (Canada except Ontario, Quebec)
Apo-Trifluoperazine (trifluoperazine)	Apotex Inc. (Canada)	(416) 749-9300, (800) 268-0599 (Canada except Ontario, Quebec)
Apo-Trihex (trihexyphenidyl)	Apotex Inc. (Canada)	(416) 749-9300, (800) 268-0599 (Canada except Ontario, Quebec)
Aquachloral (chloral hydrate)	Webcon Pharmaceuticals (U.S.)	(817) 293-0450
Artane (trihexyphenidyl)	Lederle Laboratories (U.S.)	(914) 735-2815, (914) 732-5000 (evenings and weekends)
	Lederle-Cyanamid Canada Inc.	(416) 470-3600
Asendin (amoxapine)	Lederle Laboratories (U.S.)	(914) 732-5000
	Lederle-Cyanamid Canada Inc.	(416) 470-3600
Atarax (hydroxyzine)	Roerig Division (U.S.)	(212) 573-2187
Ativan (lorazepam)	Wyeth-Ayerst Laboratories (U.S.)	(215) 688-4400
	Wyeth Ltd. (Canada)	(416) 736-4056

(continued)

PSYCHOTROPIC DRUGS: TRADE NAMES AND MANUFACTURERS *(continued)*

Atozine (hydroxyzine)	Major Pharmaceutical Inc. (U.S.)	(800) 521-5340
Aventyl (nortriptyline)	Eli Lilly and Company (U.S.)	(317) 276-3714
	Eli Lilly Canada Inc.	(416) 694-3221
Bacarate (phendimetrazine)	Reid-Rowell (U.S.)	(404) 578-9000
Banflex (orphenadrine)	Forest Pharmaceuticals, Inc. (U.S.)	(314) 569-3610
Barbased (butabarbital)	Major Pharmaceutical Inc. (U.S.)	(800) 521-5340
Barbita (phenobarbital)	Vortech Pharmaceuticals (U.S.)	(313) 584-4088
Beldin (diphenhydramine)	Halsey Drug Company (U.S.)	(718) 467-7500
Benadryl (diphenhydramine)	Parke-Davis (U.S.)	(201) 540-3950, (201) 540-2117 (evenings and weekends)
Benylin (diphenhydramine)	Parke-Davis (Canada)	(416) 288-2200
Bontril (phendimetrazine)	Carnrick Laboratories, Inc. (U.S.)	(201) 267-2670
BuSpar (buspirone)	Mead Johnson Pharmaceuticals (U.S.)	(812) 429-5000
	Bristol Laboratories of Canada	(613) 596-5850
Butalan (butabarbital)	Lannett Company, Inc. (U.S.)	(215) 333-9000
Butatran (butabarbital)	Hauck Pharmaceuticals (U.S.)	(404) 475-4758
Buticaps (butabarbital)	Wallace Laboratories (U.S.)	(609) 655-6000, (609) 799-1167 (evenings and weekends)
Butisol (butabarbital)	Wallace Laboratories (U.S.)	(609) 655-6000, (609) 799-1167 (evenings and weekends)
	Frank W. Horner Inc. (Canada)	(514) 731-3931
Calan (verapamil)	G. D. Searle & Co. (U.S.)	(800) 323-4204 (outside Illinois) (312) 982-7000 (within Illinois)
Carbolith (lithium carbonate)	ICN Pharmaceuticals, Inc. (Canada)	(800) 556-1937

PSYCHOTROPIC DRUGS: TRADE NAMES AND MANUFACTURERS *(continued)*

Celontin **(methsuximide)**	Parke-Davis (U.S.)	(201) 540-3950, (201) 540-2117 (evenings and weekends)
	Parke-Davis (Canada)	(416) 288-2200
Centrax (prazepam)	Parke-Davis (U.S.)	(201) 540-3950, (201) 540-2117 (evenings and weekends)
Chlorpromanyl **(chlorpromazine)**	Technilab Inc. (Canada)	(514) 337-6030
Chlorpazine **(prochlorperazine)**	Major Pharmaceutical Inc. (U.S.)	(800) 521-5340
Cibalith-S (lithium citrate)	Ciba Pharmaceuticals Company (U.S.)	(201) 277-5000
Clozaril (clozapine)	Sandoz Pharmaceutical Corporation (U.S.)	(201) 503-7500
Cogentin **(benztropine)**	Merck Sharp & Dohme (U.S.)	(215) 661-5000
	Merck Sharp & Dohme Canada	(514) 695-7550
Compazine **(prochlorperazine)**	Smith, Kline & French Laboratories (U.S.)	(215) 751-4000
Compoz **(diphenhydramine)**	Jeffrey Martin (U.S.)	(201) 687-4000
Cylert (pemoline)	Abbott Laboratories (U.S.)	(800) 255-5162
	Abbott Laboratories, Limited (Canada)	(514) 340-7100
Dalmane (flurazepam)	Roche Laboratories (U.S.)	(800) 526-6367
	Hoffmann-La Roche Limited (Canada)	(416) 620-2800
Desoxyn **(methamphetamine)**	Abbott Laboratories (U.S.)	(800) 255-5162
Desyrel (trazodone)	Mead Johnson Pharmaceuticals (U.S.)	(812) 429-5000
	Bristol Laboratories of Canada	(613) 596-5850
Dexedrine **(dextroamphetamine)**	Smith, Kline & French Laboratories (U.S.)	(215) 751-4000
	Smith, Kline & French Canada Ltd.	(416) 821-2200
Diamox **(acetazolamide)**	Lederle Laboratories (U.S.)	(914) 732-5000
	Lederle-Cyanamide Canada Inc.	(416) 470-3600
Didrex **(benzphetamine)**	The Upjohn Company (U.S.)	(616) 329-8244, (616) 323-6615

(continued)

PSYCHOTROPIC DRUGS: TRADE NAMES AND MANUFACTURERS *(continued)*

Dilantin (phenytoin)	Parke-Davis (U.S.)	(201) 540-3950, (201) 540-2117 (evenings and weekends)
	Parke-Davis (Canada)	(416) 288-2200
Diphen (diphenhydramine)	Pharmaceutical Basics, Inc.	(708) 967-5600
Diphenadryl (diphenhydramine)	Schein Pharmaceutical, Inc. (U.S.)	(516) 625-9000
Diphenylan (phenytoin)	Lannett Company, Inc. (U.S.)	(215) 333-9000
Disipal (orphenadrine)	Riker/3M Pharmaceuticals (U.S.)	(612) 736-4930
	Riker/3M Canada Inc.	(519) 451-2500
Dopar (levodopa)	Norwich Eaton Pharmaceuticals, Inc. (U.S.)	(607) 335-2565
Doral (quazepam)	Baker Cummins Pharmaceuticals, Inc. (U.S.)	(305) 590-2200, (305) 590-2254
Doriglute (glutethimide)	Major Pharmaceutical Inc. (U.S.)	(800) 521-5340
Duralith (lithium carbonate)	McNeil Pharmaceutical (Canada) Limited	(416) 640-6900
Durapam (flurazepam)	Major Pharmaceutical Inc. (U.S.)	(800) 521-5340
E-Pam (diazepam)	ICN Pharmaceuticals, Inc. (Canada)	(800) 556-1937
E-Vista (hydroxyzine)	The Seatrace Company (U.S.)	(205) 442-5023
Elavil (amitriptyline)	Merck Sharp & Dohme (U.S.)	(215) 661-5000
	Merck Sharp & Dohme Canada	(514) 695-7550
Eldepryl (selegiline)	Somerset Pharmaceutical (U.S.)	(201) 586-2310
Emitrip (amitriptyline)	Major Pharmaceutical Inc. (U.S.)	(800) 521-5340
Endep (amitriptyline)	Roche Laboratories (U.S.)	(800) 526-6367
Enovil (amitriptyline)	Hauck Pharmaceuticals (U.S.)	(404) 475-4758
Epitol (carbamazepine)	Lemmon Company (U.S.)	(800) 545-8800
Equanil (meprobamate)	Wyeth-Ayerst Laboratories (U.S.)	(215) 688-4400
	Wyeth Canada Ltd.	(416) 736-4056
Eskalith (lithium carbonate)	Smith, Kline & French Laboratories (U.S.)	(215) 751-4000
Ferndex (dextroamphetamine sulfate)	Ferndale Laboratories (U.S.)	(800) 621-6003, (313) 548-0900

PSYCHOTROPIC DRUGS: TRADE NAMES AND MANUFACTURERS *(continued)*

Flexoject (orphenadrine)	Mayrand Pharmaceuticals, Inc. (U.S.)	(919) 292-5347
Flexon (orphenadrine)	Keene Pharmaceutical Inc. (U.S.)	(817) 645-8083
	Wesley Pharmacal Co., Inc. (U.S.)	(215) 953-1680
Gemonil (metharbital)	Abbott Laboratories (U.S.)	(800) 255-5162
Halcion (triazolam)	The Upjohn Company (U.S.)	(616) 329-8244, (616) 323-6615
	The Upjohn Company of Canada	(800) 268-7888
Haldol (haloperidol)	McNeil Pharmaceutical (U.S.)	(800) 542-5365
Hydramine (diphenhydramine)	Dixon-Shane, Inc. (U.S.)	(215) 673-7770
Hydril (diphenhydramine)	Blaine Company, Inc. (U.S.)	(606) 341-9437
Hydroxacen (hydroxyzine)	Central Pharmaceuticals, Inc. (U.S.)	(812) 522-3915
Hyzine (hydroxyzine)	Hyrex Pharmaceuticals (U.S.)	(901) 794-9050
Impril (imipramine)	ICN Pharmaceuticals, Inc. (Canada)	(800) 556-1937
Inapsine (droperidol)	Janssen Pharmaceutica Inc.	(800) 253-3682
Inderal (propranolol)	Wyeth-Ayerst Laboratories (U.S.)	(215) 688-4400
	Ayerst Laboratories (Canada)	(514) 744-6771
Insomnal (diphenhydramine)	Welcker-Lyster Ltd. (Canada)	(514) 381-5631
Isoptin (verapamil)	Knoll Pharmaceuticals (U.S.)	(800) 526-0221, (201) 428-8250
	Knoll Pharmaceuticals Canada	(416) 475-7070
Janimine (imipramine)	Abbott Laboratories (U.S.)	(800) 255-5162
Kemadrin (procyclidine)	Burroughs Wellcome Co. (U.S.)	(800) 443-6763
	Burroughs Wellcome Inc. (Canada)	(514) 694-8220
Klonopin (clonazepam)	Roche Laboratories (U.S.)	(800) 526-6367
Largactil (chlorpromazine)	Rhône-Poulenc Pharma Inc. (Canada)	(514) 384-8220
Larodopa (levodopa)	Roche Laboratories (U.S.)	(800) 526-6367
	Hoffmann-La Roche Limited (Canada)	(416) 620-2800
Levate (amitriptyline)	ICN Pharmaceuticals, Inc. (Canada)	(800) 556-1937

(continued)

PSYCHOTROPIC DRUGS: TRADE NAMES AND MANUFACTURERS *(continued)*

Libritabs (chlordiazepoxide)	Roche Laboratories (U.S.)	(800) 255-5162
Librium (chlordiazepoxide)	Roche Laboratories (U.S.)	(800) 255-5162
	Hoffmann-La Roche Limited (Canada)	(416) 620-2800
Lipoxide (chlordiazepoxide)	Major Pharmaceutical Inc. (U.S.)	(800) 521-5340
Lithane (lithium carbonate)	Miles Pharmaceuticals (U.S.)	(800) 468-0894, (203) 937-2000
	Pfizer Canada Inc.	(514) 695-0500
Lithizine (lithium carbonate)	Paul Maney Laboratories (Canada)	(800) 361-9754 (Quebec), (800) 361-6667
Lithobid (lithium carbonate)	Ciba Pharmaceutical Company (U.S.)	(201) 277-5000
Lithonate (lithium carbonate)	Reid-Rowell (U.S.)	(404) 578-9000
Lithotabs (lithim carbonate)	Reid-Rowell (U.S.)	(404) 578-9000
Loxapac (loxapine)	Lederle-Cyanamide Canada Inc	(416) 470-3600
Loxitane C (loxapine)	Lederle Laboratories (U.S.)	(914) 732-5000
Ludiomil (maprotiline)	Ciba Pharmaceutical Company (U.S.)	(201) 277-5000
	Ciba Pharmaceuticals (Canada)	(800) 387-8395
Luminal (phenobarbital)	Winthrop Pharmaceuticals (U.S.)	(212) 907-2000
Marflex (orphenadrine)	Vortech Pharmaceuticals (U.S.)	(313) 584-4088
Marplan (isocarboxazid)	Roche Laboratories (U.S.)	(800) 526-6367
Mazanor (mazindol)	Wyeth-Ayerst Laboratories (U.S.)	(215) 688-4400
Mazepine (carbamazepine)	ICN Pharmaceuticals, Inc. (Canada)	(800) 556-1937
Mebaral (mephobarbital)	Winthrop Pharmaceuticals (U.S.)	(212) 907-2000
	Winthrop Pharma (Canada)	(416) 773-1122, Ext. 112
Medilium (chlordiazepoxide)	Medic Laboratory Limited (Canada)	(514) 668-9750
Meditran (meprobamate)	Medic Laboratory Limited (Canada)	(514) 668-9750

PSYCHOTROPIC DRUGS: TRADE NAMES AND MANUFACTURERS *(continued)*

Drug	Manufacturer	Phone
Mellaril (thioridazine)	Sandoz Pharmaceuticals Corporation (U.S.)	(201) 503-7500
	Sandoz Canada Inc.	(800) 363-8883
Meprospan (meprobamate)	Wallace Laboratories (U.S.)	(609) 655-6000, (609) 799-1167 (evenings and weekends)
Mesantoin (mephenytoin)	Sandoz Pharmaceuticals Corporaton (U.S.)	(201) 503-7500
	Sandoz Canada Inc.	(800) 363-8883
Meval (diazepam)	Medic Laboratory Limited (Canada)	(514) 668-9750
Millazine (thioridazine)	Major Pharmaceutical Inc. (U.S.)	(800) 521-5340
Milontin (phensuximide)	Parke-Davis (U.S.)	(201) 540-3950, (201) 540-2117 (evenings and weekends)
	Parke-Davis (Canada)	(416) 288-2200
Miltown (meprobamate)	Frank W. Horner Inc. (Canada)	(514) 731-3931
Moban (molindone)	Du Pont Pharmaceuticals (U.S.)	(302) 992-4240, (302) 892-1980 (evenings and weekends)
Modecate Decanoate (fluphenazine)	Squibb Canada Inc.	(514) 331-7423
Moditen Enanthate (fluphenazine)	Squibb Canada Inc.	(514) 331-7423
Multipax (hydroxyzine)	Rorer Canada Inc.	(416) 792-1212
Myidone (primidone)	Major Pharmaceutical Inc. (U.S.)	(800) 521-5340
Myolin (orphenadrine)	Hauck Pharmaceuticals (U.S.)	(404) 475-4758
Mysoline (primidone)	Wyeth-Ayerst Laboratories (U.S.)	(215) 688-4400
	Ayerst Laboratories (Canada)	(514) 744-6771
Nardil (phenelzine)	Parke-Davis (U.S.)	(201) 540-3950, (201) 540-2117 (evenings and weekends)
	Parke-Davis (Canada)	(416) 288-2200
Navane (thiothixine)	Roerig Division (U.S.)	(212) 573-2187
	Pfizer Canada Inc.	(514) 695-0500
Neocyten (orphenadrine)	Central Pharmaceuticals, Inc. (U.S.)	(812) 522-3915

(continued)

PSYCHOTROPIC DRUGS: TRADE NAMES AND MANUFACTURERS *(continued)*

Nembutal (pentobarbital)	Abbott Laboratories	(800) 255-5162
Neuramate (meprobamate)	Halsey Drug Company (U.S.)	(718) 467-7500
Nidryl (diphenhydramine)	Geneva Generics, Inc. (U.S.)	(303) 466-2400
Nobesine (diethylproprion)	Rougier Inc. (Canada)	(514) 381-5631
Noctec (chloral hydrate)	E. R. Squibb & Sons, Inc. (U.S.)	(609) 243-6305, (609) 243-6306
	Squibb Canada Inc.	(514) 331-7423
Noludar (methyprylon)	Roche Laboratories (U.S.)	(800) 526-6367
	Hoffmann-La Roche Limited (Canada)	(416) 620-2800
Nordinyl (diphenhydramine)	Vortech Pharmaceuticals (U.S.)	(313) 584-4088
Norflex (orphenadrine)	Riker/3M Pharmaceuticals (U.S.)	(612) 736-4930
	Riker/3M Canada Inc.	(519) 451-2500
Norpramin (desipramine)	Marion Merrell Dow Inc. (U.S.)	(800) 552-3656, (513) 948-9111 (evenings and weekends)
	Merrell Dow Pharmaceuticals (Canada) Inc.	(416) 883-1915
Novochlorpromazine (chlorpromazine)	Novopharm Limited (Canada)	(800) 268-4127
Novochlorhydrate (chloral hydrate)	Novopharm Limited (Canada)	(800) 268-4127
Novoclopate (clorazepate)	Novopharm Limited (Canada)	(800) 268-4127
Novodipam (diazepam)	Novopharm Limited (Canada)	(800) 268-4127
Novoflurazine (trifluoperazine)	Novopharm Limited (Canada)	(800) 268-4127
Novoflupam (flurazepam)	Novopharm Limited (Canada)	(800) 268-4127
Novohexidyl (trihexyphenidyl)	Novopharm Limited (Canada)	(800) 268-4127
Novolorazem (lorazepam)	Novopharm Limited (Canada)	(800) 268-4127
Novomepro (meprobamate)	Novopharm Limited (Canada)	(800) 268-4127

PSYCHOTROPIC DRUGS: TRADE NAMES AND MANUFACTURERS *(continued)*

Novoperidol (haloperidol)	Novopharm Limited (Canada)	(800) 268-4127
Novopoxide (chlordiazepoxide)	Novopharm Limited (Canada)	(800) 268-4127
Novopramine (imipramine)	Novopharm Limited (Canada)	(800) 268-4127
Novoridazine (thioridazine)	Novopharm Limited (Canada)	(800) 268-4127
Novosecobarb (secobarbital)	Novopharm Limited (Canada)	(800) 268-4127
Novotriptyn (amitriptyline)	Novopharm Limited (Canada)	(800) 268-4127
Novoxapam (oxazepam)	Novopharm Limited (Canada)	(800) 268-4127
Nytol with DPH (dipyhenhydramine)	Block Drug Company, Inc. (U.S.)	(201) 434-3000
Obalan (phendimetrazine)	Lannett Company, Inc. (U.S.)	(215) 333-9000
Orap (pimozide)	Gate Pharmaceuticals (U.S.)	(800) 292-GATE
	McNeil Pharmaceutical (Canada) Limited	(416) 640-6900
Orflagen (orphenadrine)	Goldline Laboratories, Inc. (U.S.)	(305) 491-4002
Ormazine (chlorpromazine)	Hauck Pharmaceuticals (U.S.)	(404) 475-4758
Orphenate (orphenadrine)	Hyrex Pharmaceuticals (U.S.)	(901) 794-9050
Oxpam (oxazepam)	ICN Pharmaceuticals, Inc. (Canada)	(800) 556-1937
Oxydess II (dextroamphetamine)	Vortech Pharmaceuticals (U.S.)	(313) 584-4088
Peganone (ethotoin)	Abbott Laboratories (U.S.)	(800) 255-5162
Pamelor (nortriptyline)	Sandoz Pharmaceuticals Corporation (U.S.)	(201) 503-7500
Paradione (paramethadione)	Abbott Laboratories (U.S.)	(800) 255-5162
Parlodel (bromocriptine)	Sandoz Pharmaceuticals Corporation (U.S.)	(201) 503-7500
Parnate (tranylcypromine)	Smith, Kline & French Laboratories (U.S.)	(215) 751-4000
	Smith, Kline & French Canada Ltd.	(416) 821-2200

(continued)

PSYCHOTROPIC DRUGS: TRADE NAMES AND MANUFACTURERS *(continued)*

Paxipam (halazepam)	Schering Corporation (U.S.)	(800) 526-4099, (201) 298-4000 (evenings and weekends)
Permax (pergolide)	Eli Lilly and Company (U.S.)	(317) 276-3714
Permitil (fluphenazine)	Schering Corporation (U.S.)	(800) 526-4099
	Schering Canada Inc.	(514) 695-1320
Pertôfrane (desipramine)	Rhône-Poulenc Rorer Pharmaceuticals Inc. (U.S.)	(215) 540-5613, (215) 628-6000
	Geigy Pharmaceuticals (Canada)	(800) 387-8395
Phenazine (perphenazine)	Keene Pharmaceuticals Inc. (U.S.)	(817) 645-8083
Phenurone (phenacemide)	Abbott Laboratories (U.S.)	(800) 255-5162
Phenzine (phendimetrazine)	Hauck Pharmaceuticals (U.S.)	(404) 475-4758
Placidyl (ethchlorvynol)	Abbott Laboratories (U.S.)	(800) 255-5162
	Abbott Laboratories, Limited (Canada)	(514) 340-7100
PMS Thioridazine (thioridazine)	Pharmascience Inc. (Canada)	(514) 340-1114
Pondimin (fenfluramine)	A. H. Robins Company, Inc. (U.S.)	(215) 688-4400
Prelu-2 (phendimetrazine)	Boehringer Ingelheim Pharmaceuticals, Inc. (U.S.)	(203) 798-9988
Prolixin Decanoate, Prolixin Enanthate (fluphenazine)	Princeton Pharmaceutical Products (U.S.)	(609) 243-6000
Prolixin (fluphenazine)	Princeton Pharmaceutical Products (U.S.)	(609) 243-6000
Promaz (chlorpromazine)	Keene Pharmaceuticals Inc. (U.S.)	(817) 645-8083
Prozac (fluoxetine)	Dista Products Company (U.S.)	(317) 276-3714
	Eli Lilly Canada Inc.	(416) 694-3221
Prozine (promazine)	Hauck Pharmaceuticals (U.S.)	(404) 475-4758
Quiess (hydroxyzine)	Forest Pharmaceuticals, Inc. (U.S.)	(314) 569-3610
Reposans-10 (chlordiazepoxide)	Wesley Pharmacal Co., Inc. (U.S.)	(215) 953-1680
Restoril (temazepam)	Sandoz Pharmaceuticals Corporation (U.S.)	(201) 503-7500

PSYCHOTROPIC DRUGS: TRADE NAMES AND MANUFACTURERS *(continued)*

Drug	Manufacturer	Phone
Ritalin (methylphenidate)	Ciba Pharmaceuticals (U.S.)	(201) 277-5000
	Ciba Pharmaceuticals (Canada)	(800) 387-8395
Rivotril (clonazepam)	Hoffmann-La Roche Limited (Canada)	(416) 620-2800
Sarisol No.2 (butibarbital)	Halsey Drug Company (U.S.)	(718) 467-7500
Seconal (secobarbital)	Eli Lilly and Company (U.S.)	(317) 276-3714
	Eli Lilly Canada Inc.	(416) 694-3221
Serentil (mesoridazine)	Boehringer Ingelheim Pharmaceuticals, Inc. (U.S.)	(203) 798-9988
Serax (oxazepam)	Wyeth-Ayerst Laboratories	(215) 688-4400
	Wyeth Ltd. (Canada)	(416) 736-4056
Sinemet (carbidopa-levodopa)	Merck Sharp & Dohme (U.S.)	(215) 661-5000
	Merck Sharp & Dohme Canada	(514) 695-7550
Sinequan (doxepin)	Roerig Division (U.S.)	(212) 573-2187
	Pfizer Canada Inc.	(514) 695-0500
Sleep-Eze 3 (diphenhydramine)	Whitehall Laboratories Inc. (U.S.)	(800) 343-0856
Solazine (trifluoperazine)	Frank W. Horner, Inc. (Canada)	(514) 731-3931
Solfoton (phenobarbital)	Poythress Laboratories, Inc. (U.S.)	(804) 644-8591
Solium (chlordiazepoxide)	Frank W. Horner Inc. (Canada)	(514) 731-3931
Sominex (diphenhhdyramine)	Beecham Laboratories (U.S.)	(215) 751-4000
Somnol (flurazepam)	Frank W. Horner Inc. (Canada)	(514) 731-3931
Som-Pam (flurazepam)	ICN Pharmaceuticals, Inc. (Canada)	(800) 556-1937
Sonazine (chlorpromazine)	Geneva Generics, Inc. (U.S.)	(303) 466-2400
Sparine (promazine)	Wyeth-Ayerst Laboratories (U.S.)	(215) 688-4400
Sprx-1, Sprx-2, Sprx-3 (phendimetrazine)	Reid-Rowell (U.S.)	(404) 578-9000
Statobex (phendimetrazine)	Lemmon Company (U.S.)	(800) 545-8800
Stelazine (trifluoperazine)	Smith, Kline & French Laboratories (U.S.)	(215) 751-4000

(continued)

PSYCHOTROPIC DRUGS: TRADE NAMES AND MANUFACTURERS *(continued)*

Stemetil (prochlorperazine)	May & Baker Pharma (Canada)	(514) 384-8220
Suprazine (trifluoperazine)	Major Pharmaceutical Inc. (U.S.)	(800) 521-5340
Surmontil (trimipramine)	Wyeth-Ayerst Laboratories (U.S.)	(215) 688-4400
	Rhône-Poulenc Pharma Inc. (Canada)	(514) 384-8220
Symmetrel (amantadine)	Du Pont Pharmaceuticals (U.S.)	(302) 992-4240, (302) 892-1980 (evenings and weekends)
Taractan (chlorprothixene)	Roche Laboratories (U.S.)	(800) 526-6367
Tarasan (chlorprothixene)	Hoffmann-La Roche Limited (Canada)	(416) 620-2800
Tegretol (carbamazepine)	Geigy Pharmaceuticals (U.S.)	(201) 277-5000
	Geigy Pharmaceuticals (Canada)	(800) 387-8395
Tenuate (diethylpropion)	Marion Merrell Dow Inc. (U.S.)	(800) 552-3656, (513) 948-9111 (evenings and weekends)
Tepanil (diethylpropion)	Riker/3M Pharmaceuticals (U.S.)	(612) 736-4930
Terfluzine (trifluoperazine)	ICN Pharmaceuticals, Inc. (Canada)	(800) 556-1937
Thor-Pram (chlorpromazine)	Major Pharmaceutical Inc. (U.S.)	(800) 521-5340
Thorazine (chlorpromazine)	Smith, Kline & French Laboratories (U.S.)	(215) 751-4000
Tindal (acetophenazine)	Schering Corporation (U.S.)	(800) 526-4099
Tofranil (imipramine)	Geigy Pharmaceuticals (U.S.)	(201) 277-5000
	Geigy Pharmaceuticals (Canada)	(800) 387-8395
Tranmep (meprobamate)	Reid-Rowell (U.S.)	(404) 578-9000
Tranxene (clorazepate)	Abbott Laboratories (U.S.)	(800) 255-5162
	Abbott Laboratories, Limited (Canada)	(514) 340-7100
Triadepin (doxepin)	Fisons Corporation, Limited (Canada)	(416) 479-9200
Tridione (trimethadione)	Abbott Laboratories (U.S.)	(800) 255-5162

PSYCHOTROPIC DRUGS: TRADE NAMES AND MANUFACTURERS *(continued)*

Trihexy-2, Trihexy-5 (triphexyphenidyl)	Geneva Generics, Inc. (U.S.)	(303) 466-2400
Trilafon (perphenazine)	Schering Corporation (U.S.)	(800) 526-4099
	Schering Canada Inc.	(514) 695-1320
Trimtabs (phendimetrazine)	Mayrand Pharmaceuticals, Inc. (U.S.)	(919) 292-5347
Triptil (protriptyline)	Merck Sharp & Dohme Canada	(514) 695-7550
Tusstat (diphenhydramine)	Century Pharmaceuticals (U.S.)	(317) 849-4210
Twilite (diphenhydramine)	Pfeiffer Company (U.S.)	(717) 826-9000
Valium (diazepam)	Roche Laboratories (U.S.)	(800) 526-6367
	Hoffmann-La Roche Limited (Canada)	(416) 620-2800
Valrelease (diazepam)	Roche Laboratories (U.S.)	(800) 526-6367
Vistacon (hydroxyzine)	Hauck Pharmaceuticals (U.S.)	(404) 475-4758
Vistaject (hydroxyzine)	Mayrand Pharmaceuticals, Inc. (U.S.)	(919) 292-5347
Vistaquel (hydroxyzine)	Pasadena Research Labs (U.S.)	(714) 492-4030
Vistazine (hydroxyzine)	Keene Pharmaceuticals Inc. (U.S.)	(817) 645-8083
Vivactil (protriptyline)	Merck Sharp & Dohme (U.S.)	(215) 661-5000
Vivol (diazepam)	Frank W. Horner Inc. (Canada)	(514) 731-3931
Wehless-105 (phendimetrazine)	Hauck Pharmaceuticals (U.S.)	(404) 475-4758
Wellbutrin (buproprion)	Burroughs Wellcome Co. (U.S.)	(800) 443-6763
Xanax (alprazolam)	The Upjohn Company (U.S.)	(616) 329-8244, (616) 323-6615
	The Upjohn Company of Canada	(800) 268-7888
Zapex (oxazepam)	Laboratoire Riva Ltée (Canada)	(514) 389-6701, (514) 669-5398
Zarontin (ethosuximide)	Parke-Davis (U.S.)	(201) 540-3950, (201) 540-2117 (evenings and weekends)
	Parke-Davis (Canada)	(416) 288-2200

MANAGEMENT OF ACUTE SUBSTANCE ABUSE

SUBSTANCE	SIGNS AND SYMPTOMS	INTERVENTIONS
Alcohol (ethanol)		
• beer and wine • distilled spirits • other preparations, such as cough syrup or mouthwash	• Ataxia • Seizures • Coma • Hypothermia • Alcohol breath odor • Respiratory depression • Bradycardia • Hypotension • Nausea and vomiting	• Induce vomiting or perform gastric lavage if ingestion occurred within the past 4 hours. Give activated charcoal and a saline cathartic. • Start I.V. fluid replacement and administer dextrose, thiamine, B-complex vitamins, and Vitamin C, to prevent dehydration and hypoglycemia and to correct nutritional deficiencies. • The patient may need padded bed rails and cloth restraints for protection from injury. • Control seizures with an anticonvulsant such as diazepam (Valium). • Monitor for hallucinations and alcohol withdrawal syndrome. If these occur, treat with chlordiazepoxide (Librium), chloral hydrate, or paraldehyde. • Monitor for crackles or rhonchi, possibly indicating aspiration pneumonia. Treat with antibiotics, as appropriate. • Clearly monitor neurologic status and vital signs until the patient is stable. Consider dialysis if the patient's vital functions are severely depressed.
Amphetamines		
• amphetamine sulfate (Benzedrine) — bennies, greenies, cartwheels • dextroamphetamine sulfate (Dexedrine) — dexies, hearts, oranges • methamphetamine — speed, meth, crystal	• Dilated reactive pupils • Altered mental status (from confusion to paranoia) • Hallucinations • Tremor and seizure activity • Hyperactive deep tendon reflexes • Exhaustion • Coma • Dry mouth • Shallow respirations • Tachycardia • Hypertension • Hyperthermia • Diaphoresis	• If the drug was taken orally, induce vomiting or perform gastric lavage; give activated charcoal and a sodium or magnesium sulfate cathartic. • Acidify the patient's urine by adding ammonium chloride or ascorbic acid to I.V. solution to lower pH to 5. • Force diuresis with mannitol. • Use short-acting barbiturate, such as pentobarbital, to control stimulant-induced seizures. • Restrain the paranoid or hallucinating patient so that he won't injure himself and others. • Treat agitation or assaultive behavior with haloperidol (Haldol) I.M. • Treat hypertension with an alpha-adrenergic blocking agent, such as phentolamine (Regitine). • Monitor for cardiac arrhythmias. Treat tachyarrhythmias or ventricular arrhythmias with propranolol or lidocaine. • Treat hyperthermia with tepid sponge baths or a hypothermia blanket. • Provide a quiet environment to avoid overstimulation. • Monitor for signs and symptoms of withdrawal, such as abdominal tenderness, muscle aches, and prolonged periods of sleep. • Observe suicide precautions, especially if the patient shows signs of withdrawal.

MANAGEMENT OF ACUTE SUBSTANCE ABUSE *(continued)*

SUBSTANCE	SIGNS AND SYMPTOMS	INTERVENTIONS
Antipsychotics		
• haloperidol (Haldol) • phenothiazines such as chlorprom-azine (Thorazine) or thioridazine (Mellaril)	• Constricted pupils • Photosensitivity • Extrapyramidal (dys-kinesia, opisthotonos, muscle rigidity, ocular deviation) • Dry mouth • Decreased level of consciousness • Decreased deep tendon reflexes • Seizures • Hypothermia or hyperthermia • Dysphagia • Respiratory depres-sion • Hypotension • Tachycardia	• Perform gastric lavage if the patient ingested the drug within the past 6 hours. (Don't administer ipecac, because phenothiazines have an antiemetic effect.) Give activated charcoal and a cathartic. • Treat extrapyramidal adverse reactions with diphen-hydramine (Benadryl) or benztropine (Cogentin). • Give physostigmine salicylate (Antilirium) to reverse the drug's anticholinergic effects in severe cases. • Replace fluids I.V. to correct hypotension; monitor vital signs. • Monitor respiratory rate and provide supplemental oxygen to treat respiratory depression. • Control seizures with an anticonvulsant, such as di-azepam, or a short-acting barbiturate, such as pento-barbital sodium (Nembutal). • Keep the patient's room dark to avoid exacerbating his photosensitivity.
Anxiolytic sedative-hypnotics		
• benzodiazepines such as chlordiaze-poxide hydrochlo-ride (Librium) and diazepam (Valium)	• Confusion • Drowsiness • Stupor • Decreased reflexes • Seizures • Coma • Shallow respirations • Hypotension	• Induce vomiting or perform gastric lavage; give acti-vated charcoal and a cathartic. • Provide supplemental oxygen to correct hypoxia-induced seizures. • Administer fluids I.V. to correct hypotension; monitor the patient's vital signs frequently. • In severe toxicity, give physostigmine salicylate (Anti-lirium) to reverse respiratory and CNS depression.
Barbiturate sedative-hypnotics		
• amobarbital so-dium (Amytal Sodium) – blue an-gels, blue devils, blue birds • phenobarbital (Luminal) – phen-nies, purple hearts, goofballs • secobarbital sodium (Se-conal) – reds, red devils, seccy	• Poor pupil reaction to light • Nystagmus • Depressed level of consciousness (from confusion to coma) • Flaccid muscles and absent reflexes • Hyperthermia or hypothermia • Cyanosis • Respiratory depres-sion • Hypotension • Blisters or bullous lesions	• Induce vomiting or perform gastric lavage if the pa-tient ingested the drug within the past 4 hours; give ac-tivated charcoal and a saline cathartic. • Maintain blood pressure with I.V. fluid challenges and vasopressors. • After phenobarbital overdose, give sodium bicarbon-ate I.V. to alkalinize urine and speed the drug's elimina-tion. • Provide a hyperthermia or hypothermia blanket to help return the patient's temperature to normal. • Consider hemodialysis or hemoperfusion if toxicity is severe. • Closely monitor neurologic status and vital signs. • Monitor for respiratory distress or pulmonary edema and signs of withdrawal, such as hyperreflexia, general-ized tonic-clonic seizures, and hallucinations. • Provide symptomatic relief of withdrawal symptoms, as appropriate.

(continued)

MANAGEMENT OF ACUTE SUBSTANCE ABUSE *(continued)*

SUBSTANCE	SIGNS AND SYMPTOMS	INTERVENTIONS
Cocaine		
● cocaine hydrochloride ● crack ● "free-base"	● Dilated pupils ● Confusion ● Alternating euphoria and apprehension ● Hyperexcitability ● Visual, auditory, and olfactory hallucinations ● Spasms and seizures ● Coma ● Tachypnea ● Hyperpnea ● Pallor or cyanosis ● Respiratory arrest ● Tachycardia ● Hypertension or hypotension ● Fever ● Nausea and vomiting ● Abdominal pain ● Perforated nasal septum or oral sores	● If cocaine was ingested, induce vomiting or perform gastric lavage; give activated charcoal followed by a saline cathartic. ● Administer an antipyretic to reduce fever. ● Monitor blood pressure and heart rate and treat symptomatic tachycardia with propranolol. ● Control seizures with an anticonvulsant, such as diazepam (Valium). ● Scrape the inside of the patient's nose to remove residual amounts of inhaled cocaine. ● Monitor cardiac rate and rhythm – ventricular fibrillation and cardiac standstill can occur as a direct cardiotoxic result of cocaine. Defibrillate and initiate cardiopulmonary resuscitation, as indicated.
Glutethimide (Doriden)		
● blues ● CD ● cibas	● Small, reactive pupils ● Nystagmus ● Drowsiness ● Irritability ● Impaired thought processes (memory, judgment, attention span) ● Slurred speech ● Twitching, spasms, and seizures ● Hypothermia ● CNS depression (unresponsive to deep coma) ● Apnea ● Respiratory depression ● Hypotension ● Paralytic ileus ● Poor bladder control	● If the drug was taken orally, induce vomiting or perform gastric lavage; give activated charcoal and a cathartic. ● Maintain the patient's blood pressure with I.V. fluid challenges and vasopressors. ● Consider hemodialysis or hemoperfusion if the patient has hepatic or renal failure or prolonged coma. ● Control seizures with an anticonvulsant, such as diazepam (Valium). ● Closely monitor neurologic status. Coma may recur because of the drug's slow release from fat deposits. ● Monitor for signs of increased intracranial pressure, such as decreasing level of consciousness and widening pulse pressure. Give mannitol I.V. as indicated. ● Watch for signs of withdrawal, such as hyperreflexia, generalized tonic-clonic seizures, and hallucinations. ● Provide symptomatic relief of withdrawal symptoms.

MANAGEMENT OF ACUTE SUBSTANCE ABUSE *(continued)*

SUBSTANCE	SIGNS AND SYMPTOMS	INTERVENTIONS
Hallucinogens		
• lysergic acid diethylamide (LSD) — hawk, acid, sunshine • mescaline (peyote) — mese, cactus, big chief	• Dilated pupils • Intensified perceptions • Agitation and anxiety • Synesthesia • Impaired judgment • Hyperactive movement • Flashback experiences • Hallucinations • Depersonalization • Moderately increased blood pressure • Increased heart rate • Fever	• Impose safety precautions to protect the patient from injuring himself and others. • If the drug was taken orally, induce vomiting or perform gastric lavage; give activated charcoal and a cathartic. • Control seizures with diazepam (Valium) I.V.
Narcotics		
• codeine • heroin — smack, H, junk, snow • hydromorphone (Dilaudid) — D, lords • morphine — mort, monkey, M, Miss Emma	• Constricted pupils • Depressed level of consciousness (but the patient is usually responsive to persistent verbal or tactile stimuli) • Seizures • Hypothermia • Slow, deep respirations • Hypotension • Bradycardia • Skin changes (pruritus, urticaria, and flushed skin)	• Repeat naloxone (Narcan) administration until the drug's CNS depressant effects are reversed. • Replace fluids I.V. to increase circulatory volume. • Correct hypothermia as indicated. • Auscultate frequently for crackles, possibly indicating pulmonary edema. (Onset may be delayed.) • Provide oxygen via nasal cannula, mask, or mechanical ventilation to correct hypoxemia from hypoventilation. • Monitor cardiac rate and rhythm, being alert for atrial fibrillation. (This should resolve spontaneously when hypoxemia is corrected.) • Monitor for signs of withdrawal, such as piloerection (goose flesh), diaphoresis, and hyperactive bowel sounds.
Nonbarbiturate sedative-hypnotics		
• methaqualone (Quaaludes) — ludes, soapers, love drug	• Dilated pupils • Nystagmus • Disorientation • Slurred speech • Hypertonicity • Ataxia • Twitching and seizures • Coma • Dry mouth • Anorexia • Nausea, vomiting, or diarrhea	• Induce vomiting or perform gastric lavage if the patient ingested the drug within the past 2 to 4 hours. Give activated charcoal and a cathartic. • Maintain blood pressure with I.V. fluids and vasopressors. • Consider hemodialysis or hemoperfusion for severe toxicity. • Initially treat hypertonicity with diazepam (Valium). If hypertonicity doesn't improve, the patient may require treatment with curare and mechanical ventilation. • Control seizures with diazepam, phenytoin (Dilantin), or phenobarbital (Luminal).

(continued)

MANAGEMENT OF ACUTE SUBSTANCE ABUSE *(continued)*

SUBSTANCE	SIGNS AND SYMPTOMS	INTERVENTIONS

Nonbarbiturate sedative-hypnotics (continued)

| | | ● Monitor for crackles, rhonchi, or decreased breath sounds, possibly indicating aspiration pneumonia. Provide supplemental oxygen and antibiotics, as indicated.
● Monitor for signs of withdrawal, such as hyperreflexia, generalized tonic-clonic seizures, and hallucinations.
● Treat withdrawal signs and symptoms with pentobarbital or phenobarbital, as indicated. |

Phencyclidine (PCP)

| ● angel dust
● hog
● peace pill | ● Blank staring
● Nystagmus
● Amnesia
● Decreased awareness of surroundings
● Recurrent coma
● Violent behavior
● Hyperactivity
● Seizures
● Gait ataxia
● Muscle rigidity
● Drooling
● Hyperthermia
● Hypertensive crisis
● Cardiac arrest | ● If the drug was taken orally, induce vomiting or perform gastric lavage; instill and remove activated charcoal repeatedly.
● Force acidic diuresis by acidifying the patient's urine with ascorbic acid to increase excretion of the drug. Continue to acidify urine for 2 weeks, because toxic symptoms may recur when fat cells release their stores of PCP.
● Control agitation or psychotic behavior with diazepam (Valium) and haloperidol (Haldol).
● Control seizures with diazepam.
● Treat hypertension and tachycardia with propranolol or, if the patient's hypertension is severe, nitroprusside.
● Closely monitor urine output and serial renal function tests—rhabdomyolysis, myoglobinuria, and renal failure may occur in severe intoxication.
● If the patient develops renal failure, perform hemodialysis. |

Tricyclic antidepressants

| ● amitriptyline (Elavil)
● imipramine (Tofranil) | ● Dilated pupils
● Blurred vision
● Altered mental status (from agitation to hallucinations)
● Loss of deep tendon reflexes
● Seizures
● Coma
● Anticholinergic effects (dry mucous membranes, diminished secretions)
● Tachycardia
● Hypotension
● Nausea and vomiting
● Urine retention | ● Induce vomiting or perform gastric lavage if the patient ingested the drug within the past 24 hours. (Anticholinergic effects of these drugs decrease gastric emptying.) Give activated charcoal and a magnesium sulfate cathartic.
● Replace fluids I.V. to correct hypotension.
● Give hypertonic sodium bicarbonate I.V. to correct hypotension and arrhythmias; if bifascicular or complete heart block occurs, a temporary transvenous pacemaker may be required.
● Treat seizures with diazepam (Valium) or phenobarbital I.V.
● Some clinicians administer physostigmine salicylate (Antilirium) to reverse central anticholinergic effects. |

SCHEDULES OF CONTROLLED SUBSTANCES

The Drug Enforcement Administration (DEA) within the U.S. Department of Justice enforces the Controlled Substances Act of 1970, which regulates the manufacturing, distribution, and dispensing of drugs that have potential for abuse.

D.E.A. SCHEDULES

The DEA divides drugs under its jurisdiction into five schedules based on their potentials for abuse and physical and psychological dependence. Controlled substances are identified by schedule in the following list.

Schedule I (C-I)

Drugs in this category have high abuse potential and no accepted medical use.

heroin

marijuana

LSD

Schedule II (C-II)

Drugs in this category have high abuse potential associated with severe risk of dependence (opiates, amphetamines, barbiturates).

alfentanil

amobarbital

amobarbital sodium

amphetamine mixtures

amphetamine sulfate

cocaine

codeine phosphate

codeine sulfate

dextroamphetamine sulfate

fentanyl citrate

fentanyl citrate and droperidol

hydrocodone bitartrate

hydromorphone hydrochloride

levorphanol tartrate

meperidine hydrochloride

methadone hydrochloride

methamphetamine hydrochloride

methylphenidate hydrochloride

morphine hydrochloride

morphine sulfate

opium tincture

oxycodone hydrochloride

oxymorphone hydrochloride

pantopon (hydrochlorides of opium alkaloids)

pentobarbital

pentobarbital sodium

phenmetrazine hydrochloride

secobarbital

secobarbital sodium

sufentanil

Schedule III (C-III)

Drugs in this category have less abuse potential than schedule II drugs and a smaller risk of dependence (nonbarbiturate sedatives, nonamphetamine stimulants, limited amounts of certain opiates, and anabolic steroids).

aprobarbital

benzphetamine hydrochloride

butabarbital

butabarbital sodium

chlorphentermine hydrochloride

fluoxymesterone

glutethimide

methyltestosterone

methyprylon

nandrolone decanoate

nandrolone phenpropionate

oxymethalone

paregoric tincture

phendimetrazine

phendimetrazine tartrate

stanozolol

testolactone

testosterone

testosterone cypionate

testosterone enanthate

testosterone propionate

thiamylal sodium

thiopental sodium

(continued)

SCHEDULES OF CONTROLLED SUBSTANCES *(continued)*

Schedule IV (C-IV)

Drugs in this category have less abuse potential than schedule III drugs and a limited risk of dependence (some sedative-hypnotics, anxiolytics, nonopiate analgesics, and CNS stimulants).

alprazolam	oxazepam
chloral hydrate	paraldehyde
chlordiazepoxide	pemoline
clonazepam	pentazocine
clorazepate	phenobarbital
clorazepate dipotassium	phenobarbital sodium
diazepam	phentermine hydrochloride
diethylpropion hydrochloride	prazepam
estazolam	propoxyphene hydrochloride
ethchlorvynol	propoxyphene hydrochloride and acetaminophen
fenfluramine hydrochloride	propoxyphene hydrochloride and aspirin
flurazepam hydrochloride	propoxyphene napsylate
halazepam	propoxyphene napsylate and acetaminophen
lorazepam	propoxyphene napsylate and aspirin
mazindol	quazepam
mephobarbital	temazepam
meprobamate	triazolam
methohexital sodium	

Schedule V (C-V)

Drugs in this category have limited abuse potential: primarily small amounts of opiates (codeine) used as antitussives or antidiarrheals. Under federal law, limited quantities of certain C-V drugs may be purchased without a prescription directly from a pharmacist. The purchaser must be at least age 18 and must furnish suitable identification. All such transactions must be recorded by the dispensing pharmacist.

Index

Page numbers in boldface refer to major entries.

prochlorperazine edisylate, **124**
prochlorperazine maleate, **124**
procyclidine hydrochloride, **90,** 261t
Prolixin Decanoate, 107
Prolixin Enanthate, 107
Prolixin Hydrochloride, 107
Promaz, 100
promazine hydrochloride, **128,** 265-266t
propranolol hydrochloride, **160**
ProSom, 193
protriptyline hydrochloride, **58,** 259t
Prozac, 46
Prozine-50, 128
psychiatric disturbances, as drug reaction, 279t
psychosis
    activation, 280t
    as drug reaction, 279t
    exacerbation, 280t
    toxic, 280t

Q

quazepam, **206,** 268t
Quiess, 152

R

rage reactions, as drug reaction, 280t
Razepam, 210
Regibon, 168
Restoril, 210
Ritalin, 174
Ritalin-SR, 174
Rivotril, 8
Ro-Diet, 168

S

Sanorex, 171
Sarisol No. 2, 189
secobarbital sodium, **207,** 269t
Seconal, 207
Sedabamate, 155
sedative-hypnotics, 183-213
    adverse reactions to, 184
    clinical considerations for, 184-185
    comparison of, 184t
    mechanism of action of, 183
    pharmacokinetics of, 183-184
    pharmacologic effects of, 183
seizures
    classification of, 2-3t
    as drug reaction, 280t
selegiline hydrochloride, **92**
sensorium, clouded, as drug reaction, 281t
Serax, 156
Serentil, 115
Sinemet, 86
Sinequan, 44
SK-Bamate, 155
sleep disturbances, as drug reaction, 281t

Solazine, 136
Solfoton, 204
Som-Pam, 197
Sonazine, 100
Spancap No. 1, 166
Sparine, 128
Sprx-1, 178
Sprx-2, 178
Sprx-3, 178
Statobex, 178
Stelazine, 136
Stemetil, 124
succinimides, pharmacologic effects of, 1
suicidal ideation, as drug reaction, 281t
Suprazine, 136
Surmontil, 64
Symmetrel, 76

T

Taractan, 103
Tarasan, 103
tardive dyskinesia, as drug reaction, 281t
Tegretol, 6
Temaz, 210
temazepam, **210,** 269t
Tenuate, 168
Tepanil, 168
Terfluzine, 136
thioridazine, **130**
thioridazine hydrochloride, **130,** 266t
thiothixene, **133,** 266t
thiothixene hydrochloride, **133**
Thorazine, 100
Thor-Prom, 100
Tindal, 97
Tofranil, 48
Tofranil-PM, 48
tonic-clonic seizures, 3t
tonic seizures, 3t
Tranmep, 155
Tranxene-SD, 10
Tranxene-SD Half Strength, 10
Tranxene T-Tab, 10
tranylcypromine sulfate, **60,** 259t
trazodone hydrochloride, **62,** 259t
Triadapin, 44
Trialodine, 62
triazolam, **212,** 269t
tricyclic antidepressants, 234-235
    managing acute abuse of, 301t
Tridione, 28
trifluoperazine hydrochloride, **136,** 266t
Trihexane, 93
Trihexidyl, 93
Trihexy-2, 93
Trihexy-5, 93
trihexyphenidyl hydrochloride, **93,** 261t
Trilafon, 120
trimethadione, **28,** 254-255t
trimipramine maleate, **64,** 260t
Trimtabs, 178
Triptil, 58

t refers to a table